Zygmunt L. OSTROWSKI

HEALTH AND NUTRITIONAL STATUS

OF THE NILOTIC POPULATION IN THE SOUTHERN SUDAN

L'Harmattan

Published by Ahfad University for Women, Omdurman, Sudan

5-7, rue de l'Ecole-Polytechnique, 75005 Paris

http://www.harmattan.fr

ISBN : 978-2-343-12837-5
EAN : 9782343128375

I would like acknowledge to:

Dr Marie-Christine Josse, for her full participation in this study, for her scientific advices and the logistic help during the seven years in the Sudan.

Dr Gaffar Ibn Auf Suliman for his scientific advices and administrative help.

Professor Yousif Badri for his special support with his Ahfad University College.

Professor Pierre Aymard for his biological analyses and advices.

French medical doctors Alexis Armengaud, Bruno Semichon, and Arcade Davion.

A.D.E. local team, especially to Elisabeth, Martha, Joseph, Luciano and James as well as to the Nilotic population for their cooperation.

French Company CCI-GTM for their logistic support during the study and all donators (IBM, Air France, Peugeot, Zodiac, Kemo Mat, Coulter counter, etc.).

Dr Katerine Kreisel, Dr Jerzy J. Ostrovsky and Madame Valery Robertson, for the English revising of the text.

A.D.E. RESEARCH CENTER
Hôpital Armand Trousseau, 21, Ave. Dr A. Netter, 75012 Paris, France

The A.D.E. study was carried out with the participation of an international team of scientists :

- Ministry of Health of the Republic of the Sudan, Khartoum
- WHO in Cairo and Khartoum as well as FAO in Rome and Khartoum.
- World Health Organisation, Dept. Nutrition, Geneva (Dr Keller)
- Ahfad University College for Women, Omdurman (Prof. Yousif Badri)
- Emergency Children's Hospital, Khartoum (Dr G. Ibn Auf Suliman)
- Faculty of Medicine, Biochemistry Dept, Khartoum (Prof. R.Bayoumi)
- West African Health Community, Lagos (Dr N.A. De Heer)
- Nutrition Unit, Control Disease Institute, Atlanta (Prof. A. Roche)
- Laboratoire de Biochimie, Hôpital Trousseau, Paris (Prof. P. Aymard, Dr M. Pressac, Dr D. Feldmann and A. Jardel)
- Service de Parasitologie, Hôpital Pitié-Salpêtrière, Paris (Prof. Gentilini and Dr Datry)
- Laboratoire de Physiologie, Faculté de Pharmacie, Chatenay Malabry, (Dr G. Morgant)
- Centre du Secteur d'Hémobiologie-Transfusion, Hôpital Saint-Louis, Paris, (Dr J. Reviron)
- Département de Nutrition, Hôpital Bichat, Paris (Prof. M. Apfelbaum and Dr M.C. Bertier)
- London School of Hygiene and Tropical Medicine (Dr D.I. Turnham)
- Institute of Child Health, London (Prof. Tanner and Dr Cameroun)
- Courtault Institute of Biochemistry, Middlesex Hospital, London, (Dr D. Bender)
- Department of Child Health, Cardiff (Prof. J.A. Dodge)
- European Institute E.I.A.S.M., Bruxelles (Prof. O. Faure)
- Faculté de Wetenschappen, Université de Bruxelles (Dr Hauspie)
- Institut für Soziale Pädiatrie, Uniwersität München (Dr Koehler)
- Dep. of Human Anthropology, Polish Academy of Science, Warsaw (Prof. N. Wolanski)

The study was approved by the A.D.E. Scientific Committee, the Minister of Health of the Republic of Sudan and the directors of Health Departments in Juba and Malakal as well as the National Research Council.

A.D.E. organized and supervised by Dr Zygmunt L. Ostrowski and Dr Marie-Christine Josse, a team of collaborators: Miss E. Ojaba (field leader), Dr A. Armengaud, Dr B. Semichon, Dr G. Habib, Dr A. Davion, Dr A. Bouagina, Dr Nicole Heidrecheid, Mr H. van Rooij, Dr Ch. Helenon and Mr E. Cazaux Devy.

CONTENTS

PREFACE

In 1978 **Dr Zygmunt L. Ostrowski** visited Ahfad University College and met with the late professor Yousif Badri.

In that meeting **Dr Ostrowski** presented his idea of conducting a study of child nutrition in the Jonglei Canal area with **Dr Marie-Christine Josse**.

It was expected that after the digging of the Jongli Canal there will be vast ecological changes which will influence the life of the population. Hence the study aimed at documenting the existing way of life in particular to food and nutrition.

Ahfad University College graduated at that time several young women from South Sudan. One of them Ms. Elizabeth Ojaba was selected to be the Sudanese counters part.

Although this book is published three decades after the completion of the research yet its significance remains today valid as it provides the only information about the nutritional and socio cultural habits of that region.

We hope that this book will provide researchers with information they can hardly find any where else.

Gasim Badri
Omdurman January 2014

HEALTH, NUTRITIONAL AND SOCIO CULTUTAL STATUS OF THE NILOTIC POPULATION IN THE SOUTHERN SUDAN

ABSTRACT

This book presents the results of a large study realised between 1979 and 1984, in the Upper Nile State, on a significant sample of a southern Sudanese population belonging to three Nilotic tribes (Dinka, Nuer and Shilluk). In 1979, these populations still lived in a very traditional way and were subject to rapid changes due to the construction of the 365 km long Jonglei canal. The study was interrupted by the civil war, in February 1984.

This book is divided into four distinct parts:
The population and the environment are described in the first part.
The objectives of the studies and their methodology are presented in the second part.
The results of a cross-sectional study (300 children, men and women) and of a longitudinal study of 400 pregnant women and their newborn child until the age of three years are presented in the third part. The anthropometrical, clinical, biological and nutritional data are included.
The traditional way of life, beliefs as well as the socio-cultural aspects (customs, social activities, magic, dreams, death, relationship and freedom, libido or sexual desires, diseases, and collective activities) are described in the fourth part. Genealogical trees of two families, one a Dinka and another Shilluk (from the 13th century), are presented in Annexe.
This book can serves as a guide for medical doctors, public health workers, epidemiologists, NGO-s… and for comparatives studies in Africa.

Key words: Health, morbidity, mortality, anthropometry, biology, nutrition, psycho-sociology, customs, culture, genealogy, methodology, survey, South-Sudan.

RESUME

LA SANTE, LA NUTRITION ET L'ETAT SOCIO CULTUREL D'UNE POPULATION NILOTIQUE DU SUD SOUDAN

Cet ouvrage présente les résultats d'une vaste étude réalisée entre 1979 et 1984, dans l'Etat du Haut-Nil, auprès d'un échantillon représentatif de la population nilotique sud-soudanaise appartenant à trois tribus (Dinka, Nuer et Shilluk). En 1979, cette population vivait encore de façon très traditionnelle, mais le percement d'un canal de 365 km de long allait modifier leur mode de vie. L'étude était interrompue par la guerre civile, en février 1984.

Le livre est divisé en plusieurs parties distinctes :
Dans une première partie sont décrites la population et l'environnement.
Dans une seconde partie sont présentés les objectifs des études et leur méthodologie.
Dans une troisième partie sont présentés les résultats d'une étude transversale (300 enfants, hommes et femmes) et d'une étude prospective réalisée sur 400 femmes enceintes et leurs nouveau-nés. Les données recueillies concernent la santé, l'anthropométrie, la biologie et la nutrition.
Dans une quatrième partie sont décrits la vie traditionnelle, les croyances ainsi que l'aspect socio-culturel (coutumes, activités sociales, magie, rêves, relations et liberté, libido ou désirs sexuels, maladies, et activités collectives).
En annexe, les arbres généalogique de deux familles, l'une Dinka, l'autre Shilluk (jusqu'au 13ème siècle), sont montrés.
Ce livre peut servir de référence pour des médecins, des responsables de Santé publique, des épidémiologistes, des ONG… et pour des études comparatives en Afrique.

Mots clés : Santé, morbidité, mortalité, anthropométrie, biologie, nutrition, psycho-sociologie, coutumes, culture, généalogie, méthodologie, enquête, Sud-Soudan.

هذا الكتاب

هذا الكتاب هو خلاصة دراسات عريضه تم تحقيقها بين الأعوام 1979 – 1984 في ولاية أعالي النيل بجنوب السودان علي عينه من السكان الذين ينحدرون من أصل ثلاث قبائل نيليه (الدينكا – النوير – الشلك). وقد عاشت تلك العينات من السكان في العام 1979 بطرق تقليديه لكنها تعرضت لمتغيرات متلاحقه نتيجه لعمليات إنشاء قناة جونقلي التي يبلغ طولها 360 كيلومترا. غير ان الدراسة قد توقفت بسبب الحرب الأهليه التي اشتعلت في فبراير من العام 1984.

وينقسم هذا الكتاب الي أربعه أجزاء: الجزء الأول يحتوي علي وصف تفصيلي للسكان والبيئه. وحوي الجزء الثاني أهداف الدراسه وطرقها. الجزء الثالث يحتوي علي دراسة استعراضيه لعينه تتكون من 300 شخصا من الأطفال والرجال والنساء، ودراسه طوليه لـ 400 من النساء الحوامل وأطفالهم بعد الولادة حتي العام الثالث. ويضم هذا الجزء ايضا بيانات تتعلق بالنواحي القياسيه للجنس البشري ، والطبيه والبيولوجيه وانواع الغذاء لمواطن جنوب السودان.

الجزء الرابع يحتوي علي وصف تفصيلي لطرق الحياة التقليديه، والمعتقدات، والجوانب الثقافيه الاجتماعيه (من عادات وأنشطه اجتماعيه ومعتقدات السحر والسحرة، والأحلام والموت والعلاقات والحريه، والشهوة والرغبات الجنسيه، والأمراض والأنشطه الجماعيه).
وحوي هذا الجزء ايضا وصفا جينيا " لشجرتي عائلتين من قبيلتي الدينكا والشلك في القرن الثالث عشر الميلادي.

يعتبر هذا الكتاب مرشدا" للأطباء، وعمال الصحه العامه، والمتخصصين في علم الأوبئه والمنظمات غير الحكوميه، ومن أجل الدراسات المقارنه في افريقيا بشكل عام.

كلمات مفتاحيه:
الصحه، إنتشار الأمراض ، الوفيات ، الأنثروبومتريه (قياس الجسم البشري) ، علم الأحياء ، التغذيه ، علم النفس الاجتماعي ، العادات والتقاليد ، الثقافه ، علم الأنساب والسلالات ، طرق الدراسه ، المسح ، جنوب السودان.

PART I

GENERALITIES

1. INTRODUCTION
by Z. L. Ostrowski

The World Health Assembly (1980) resolved as one of its most important issues to assure the best possible development of the individual by the year 2000. This objective could be achieved through optimal psychomotor development during early childhood. But still, thirty years later this goal has not been reached, especially in Africa.

Malnutrition in children was, and is still, a major public health problem in many developing countries. About 230 million (43%) of children younger than 5 years in developing countries are reported by Fawzi (1) and Onis (2) to be stunted, whereas ~50 million (9%) were wasted. The trend for stunting is very disturbing. For the Sub-Saharan African less progress has been made in reducing the prevalence of child malnutrition over the past 30 years. Of course, in 1997, the Third Report of the World Nutrition Situation (3) mentioned that there is some improvement with important differences amongst African countries (35,2% to 52%). IN 1985, Sudan was classified by the World Health Organization as a country where xerophthalmia and vitamin A deficiency were public health problems (4).

Few studies in early childhood are available and none in very remote areas, especially in the South Sudan. Rowland (5) studied the impact of infection on growth of children in West Africa, Shears (6) studied the Ethiopian refugees in Sudan, and Coulter (7) studied clinical malnutrition in northern Sudan. The few studies in Africa are mostly in urban areas. As to Pagezy (8), in tropical regions, the survey of babies and infants is, for practical reasons of organization and cost, easier to perform in urban than in rural areas. A longitudinal study of 120 children has been performed by Cornu (9) in Yaounde, but only 63 children remained for statistical analyses with two examinations at 8 and 23 months.

In the late 1970s some of the Nilotic tribes in Southern Sudan, like many others in Africa, still lived in a very traditional way (Photos 1 to 4).

Since growth and nutritional status reflect the general health status of the population, it was important to conduct a study of health and nutrition in children and particularly in the rural areas where rapid development and change took place. At the same time, primary health care needed to be provided because many people living in the remote areas of Sudan still lacked access to any form of health services. The lack of schools left these populations, and especially children, without education. They were not prepared to meet the rapid change of society, the passage from the traditional way of life of the past to the advanced technology of the late 20th century.

In 1977, in the framework of the national project to develop Southern Sudan (the construction by French company GTM of the 365 km long Jonglei Canal between Nile-Sobat Mouth and Bor, exploration of petrol by Chevron and Total) a rapid socio-economic and environmental change was expected. It was urgent to describe the health and nutritional status of this population as well as to collect data concerning their psycho-social status, before any changes occurred. The choice of a study in the Jonglei Canal Area was dictated by the fact that basic data should be obtained before the canal was finished (a 4-5 year time frame).

A general protocol for a research project was signed with the Ministry of Health in 1979. A health and nutritional longitudinal study on pregnant women and their offspring until three years of age was planned between 1979-1984 in the Jonglei Canal Area to determine the main health and nutrition problems and to provide information for the establishment of an adequate health and nutritional policy. As part of this survey, a cross-sectional study on children and adults was carried out in three ethnic areas (Shilluk, Dinka and Nuer) near the future Jonglei canal under construction. A psycho-social study was carrying out to better understand the tradition and habits of this population.

The first study started in 1979 and was supposed to end in 1984. A second study was planed 10-20 years later. Because of the civil war which interrupted (February 1984) the first study, the second comparative study could not start because of the continuous fighting in the study area.

The results of this A.D.E. study were published only recently because of the 21 year long civil war in Sudan. This delay in publication does not, however, diminish the value of the scientific study. Some other studies have also been published with a delay. Broeck's semi-longitudinal study in Zaire (12) was published 8 years after our studies. Also the longitudinal study of pregnant women carried out in 1975 by Rush (13) was published 13 years later, in 1988.

In the mean time, some studies on children in rural African areas have been published but they concern small observations, like Robert's study (10) of a Dinka village, or are limited to one subject, like Herrera's study on vitamin A in north Sudan (11), based on data from Fawzi's study (1).

2. POPULATION AND ENVIRONMENT
by Z.L. Ostrowski and M.-Ch. Josse

At the time of this study, Sudan was the largest country in Africa (map 1a) with about 27 million habitants; about 7 million were living in Southern Sudan. More than half of them were under 15 years of age.

The World Development Report (1985) indicated that the fertility rate in Sudan was 6.3. The perinatal mortality was 78, the life expectancy at birth increased from 46 to 57 years (between 1960 and 1990) and decreased again to 51 years (in 1991). The child mortality rate decreased from 203 to 152 (between 1969 and 1975), in 1990 it was 104. Concerning nutrition and health behaviour, the same reference indicated that 32% of children were affected by stunting (*) (ages 24-59 months) and 13% by wasting (**) (ages 12-23 months), that 84% of children (ages 0-3 months) were fully breastfed (1985-1990). A study on anaemia in pregnant women (1970-1980) indicated 36% below the norm for haemoglobin.

The adult illiteracy rate in 1990 was 88% for females and 73% for males: between 1970-1990 less than 38% to 49% were enrolled in primary education and only 7% to 20% in secondary education (***). No data was available for the southern Sudanese population because no scientific studies have been carried out in Southern Sudan.

2.1. DESCRIPTION OF STUDY AREA

The area selected for this study in the Upper Nile region, south from Malakal (see map 1b and map 2) is the Jonglei Canal Area. It is an area of about 20.000 km². It lies within the zone of the grassland savannah climate. It experiences rainfall peaks averaging 600 to 900 mm. The whole region was subject to a greater or lesser degree of flooding during the rainy seasons due to the flatness of the land, impermeability of the soils and the comparatively heavy rainfall with few, generally insufficient, drainage channels.

The estimated population in the Jonglei Canal Area, about 240.000, decreased with time. Already in 1977 a considerable number of the potential economically active males migrated away from their birth place (29,6% in the 20-29 years old group), as described by Payne (10). Part of the population was living a semi nomadic life. This population belongs to Nilotic tribes: Dinka, Nuer and

(*) *Stunting signifies slowing in skeletal growth (17).*
(**) *Wasting indicates a deficit in tissue and fat mass compared with the amount expected in a child of the same height or length; it can develop very very rapidly*
(***) *Published for the World Bank by Oxford University Press, 1993.*

Shilluk (map 3). These three tribes share similarities of culture, lifestyle, physical characteristics and a basic language (although their languages are less mutually intelligible). Both the Dinka and the Nuer are divided into a number of sections and practice a mixed economy in which cattle plays a predominant social and economic role.

Most people live in compounds consisting of 1-3 huts (*tukul*) and a luak. The compounds are scattered throughout the area. There are no villages in the sense of a large number of homesteads, but groupings of few huts which have been used to number each household (map 4) (photo 25). A household was defined as a group of people habitually eating and sleeping together on the same compounds and one demographic survey form was used for each household (*).

The Shilluk (photos 5 and 6) are the third largest Nilotic ethnic group of Southern Sudan (about 500.000), after the Dinka and Nuer. The Shilluk live on the west bank of the Nile between Lake No in the south and Kosti in the north. A great number of the Shilluk live along the Nile, from Tonga to Kodok and along the Sobat River from Malakal to Gojak. Some Shilluk settlements are also on the east bank of the Nile, up to Anakdier. The Shilluk capital is Fashoda. The community is formed as a cluster of hamlets headed by members of a dominant lineage. Their country is flat lying plains. The Shilluk are less dependent on animal husbandry than on crop husbandry and fishing. The Shilluk are mostly sedentary, engaging in subsistence agriculture (sorghum, maize, simsim, beans), but they also have some livestock (cattle, goats and sheep). They also fish as they have easy access to the Nile and its numerous tributaries. The Shilluk language is related to other Luo languages, as well as to Nuer and Dinka languages. The Shilluk are a more compact group and have a relatively organized political system with a king known as "Reth" at the top.
For the Shilluk the king has the following titles: "the first born of God", "child of God", etc. (**).

(*) *At the beginning of the construction of the 365 km long Jonglei Canal from the Nile-Sobat Mouth (35 km south from Malakal), the future canal area was less inhabited. In 1982, along the first 150 km of the canal only a few villages were registered. On the west side of the canal, 41 km away was the small village of Arickwer and 80 km away was Achwil Bong. A great agglomeration of huts known as Yei is situated east of the canal (116,8 km - 135,7 km away) with a greater concentration around 125-126 km, and partly situated west of the canal between km 128,8 and 135,7. At 140 km was a small village Ogar with a great water hole, created by CCI at this place. Only two hospitals were available for the whole Jonglei Canal area: 35 km north from the Nile-Sobat mouth in Malakal, and about 400 km south in Bor. A.D.E. created few dispensaries at km 41, 70 and 125 on the east side of the canal.*
(**) *Mbiti J.S., African religious and Philosophy, New York, 1990, pages 91-94.*

The Dinka, a semi-nomadic population (photo 7), live further south than the Shilluk. At the northern extremity of the Dinka region (Duk Fadiat/Duk Fawil) the people build their *tukuls* and *luaks* on the southern part of the sandy highland areas of the Duk ridge. They have access to very large areas of intermediate grazing lands known as *aying* and, in the west, to very large *toiches* (*a swampy area for grazing*).

The Nuer also a nomadic population (photo 8) live mostly to the south-east of the Shilluk, but also to the west (see map 5). This tribe has a similar lifestyle to the Dinka.

2.2. HEALTH

Healthcare in the whole Jonglei area was very poor. Only two hospitals existed in the towns of Malakal and Bor. The hospitals were very badly equipped with no laboratory or X-ray facilities and without medicines. The hospital in Bor was worst: next to useless.

Between these two hospitals, over a distance of approximately 400 km, no medical care from a doctor was available. Only three dispensaries with paramedical staff existed in Ayoud, Duk Fawil and Kongor, and a few dressing stations without medical personnel in the study area. For the most part healthcare was provided by witch doctors using only herbal medicine and magic (photo 17)!

In 1981, A.D.E. established a Nutritional Centre and in 1983 some dispensaries near the Sobat-Nile mouth (see map 2).

2.3. CATTLE

The livestock population was still important. In the southern Dinka area of Jonglei Province alone, at that time (1976) an aerial survey suggested that there were approximately 228.000 cattle, 33.500 sheep and 101.000 goats (18). Due to the primordial role played by cattle in the life of this population it is important to describe the health status of the domestic animals.

The Dinka manage a Nilotic type of cattle similar to those owned by the Nuer and the Shilluk. There was very considerable variation between those owned by Shilluk and those owned by Dinka living south of Duk Fadiat, as well as between the types of cattle owned by different families.

Dinka cattle are bred and raised primarily to produce milk, which was the staple diet of the people. Average milk production of Dinka cows under indigenous management was probably of the order of 1,000 ml per day. The percentages of fat, total solids and ash in the milk were 8.2, 17.8 and 1.4 percent respectively (in the early rain season the percentage of fat decreased to 4.2%). In addition the majority of the cows would suckle and raise a calf (18).

The Dinka rear their cattle in the *toc*, which, as mentioned by John Wuol Makec (19), is vital to the life of Dinka for a variety of reasons. *Toc* is a very suitable area for their cattle to graze as it consists of large, rich pastures. Besides these pastures there is always plenty of water throughout the year for the cattle. Secondly, the fishing areas are in *toc*. Thirdly, the *toc* attracts a variety of wild game because of the rich pastures and water. It therefore constitutes a good hunting area. In the *toc* area the whole land was subject to communal usage, with very few exceptions.

Cattle meat is eaten when cattle have died, are sacrificed or are specifically killed for food (consumption of meat was relative high). Cattle hides are used for a variety of purposes. These cattle are very hardy and are presumably tolerant to some extent to a variety of diseases and internal and external parasites (18).

Sheep provide meat and are used for minor ritual sacrifice. These sheep are extremely tolerant of disease and parasites (18).

Goats are usually milked, the milk being drunk by women and children. Occasionally a child will be seen directly suckling a lactating goat. They are obviously tolerant of diseases and parasites (18).

Poultry have been introduced into the Dinka livestock economy. Chicken eggs as well as the eggs of wild birds (including guinea fowl, goose and ostrich) are consumed.

Because of close cohabitation with animals, some major diseases are a threat for both children and adults:

- Anthrax is a bacterial disease affecting cattle, sheep, goats and humans. Diseased carcases are a prime source of infection.
- Tuberculosis is a bacterial disease affecting cattle and humans.
- Leptospirosis, another bacterial disease of cattle, sheep and goats, is also dangerous for humans (transmitted in urine).
- Rift Valley fever is a viral infection usually affecting cattle and sheep, but also humans (transmitted mainly by mosquitoes).
- Tick-borne disease: Amblyomma variegatum (cattle, sheep, goats, pigs, dogs and wild game) and Haemophysalis eachi leachi (dogs, wild carnivores) transmits Q-fever (Coxiella burnetii) in humans.
- Trypanosomiasis, a proteoal disease, transmitted by tsetse flies is rare in this

area.

- Brucelliosis is a bacterial disease of cattle which causes miscarriages.
- Contagious bovine pleurisy-pneumonia is an endemic disease only in cattle.

The cycle of the human tape worm (Tania saginata and Cysticerus bovis) in cattle exists in the Jonglei Area as human faeces are scattered throughout the grazing areas surrounding the settlements. Eisa (18) reported an incidence of 75% in the Pibor Area District).

Fascioliasis is the dominant fluke infecting the liver of cattle, sheep and goats in the Jonglei Area (16.6 - 30%).

Schistosomiasis is an internal parasitic disease of cattle, sheep and goats caused by schistosomia whose alternate hosts are aquatic snails. 11.8% were infected in Malakal area (18).

The presence of sleeping sickness in southern Sudan threatens millions of people. According to Kigotho (20) the problem is due to the high density of tsetse flies.

Because no veterinary services existed in this area, a great number of cattle died and many of the above mentioned diseases affected the population.

MAP 1 a
THE SUDAN

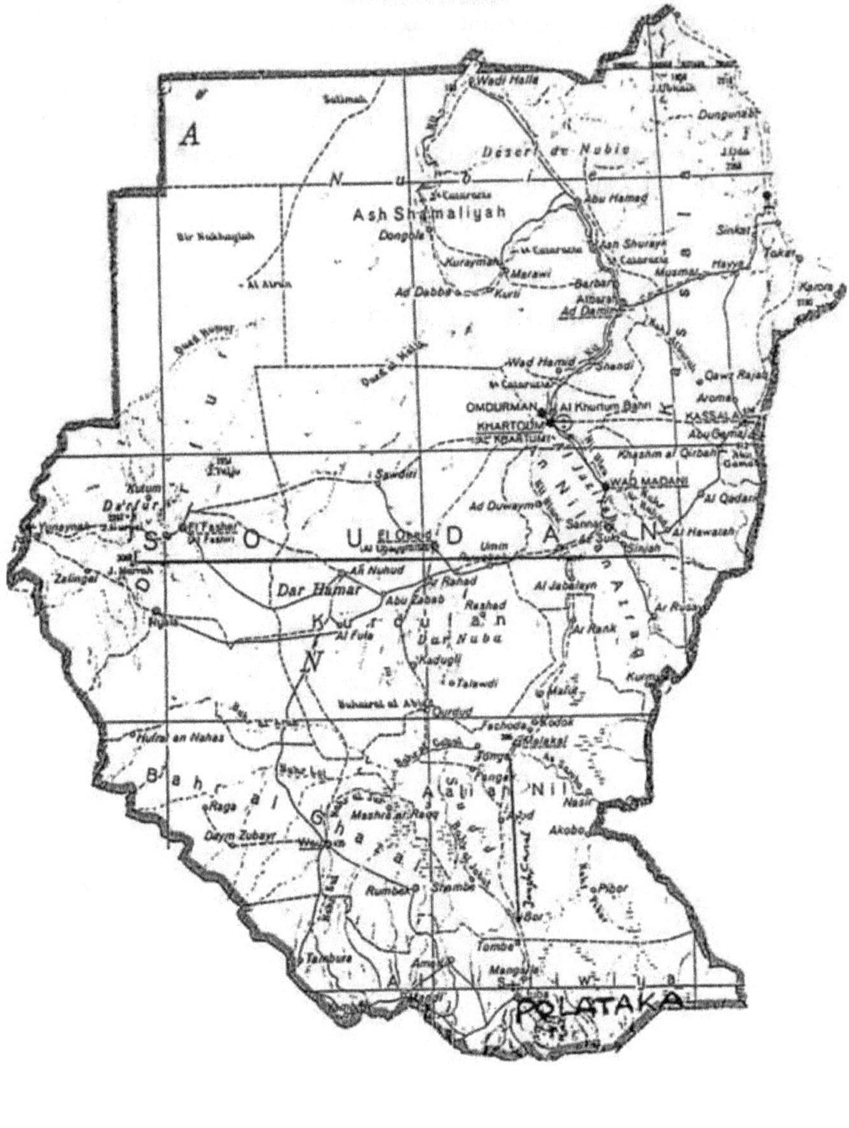

MAP 1b

UPPER NILE REGION OF THE SOUTH SUDAN

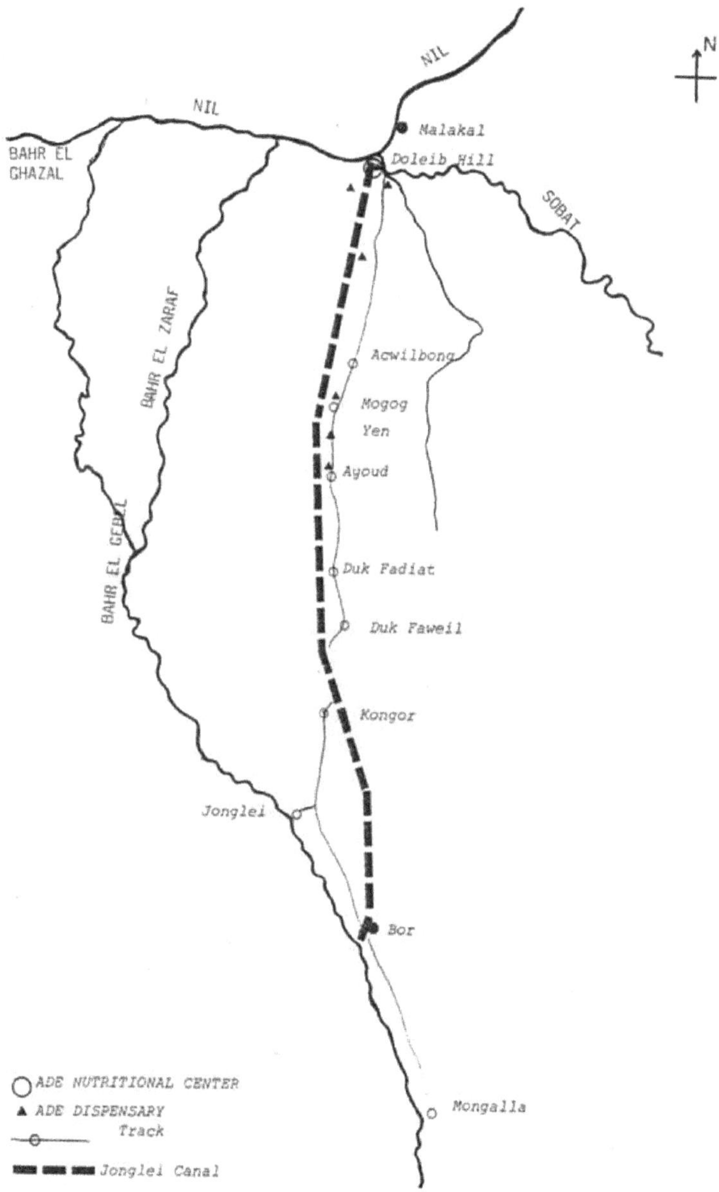

MAP 2

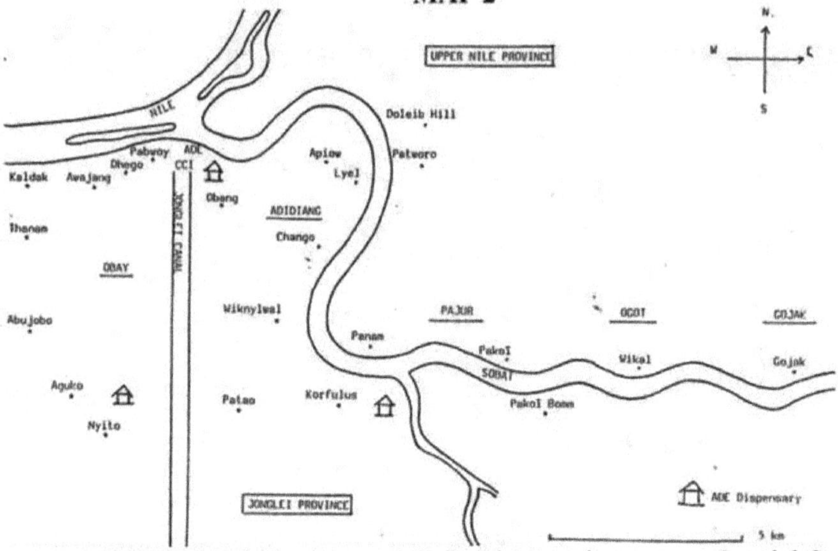

O A.D.E. Research Center **x** A.D.E. Dispensaries ==== Jonglei Canal

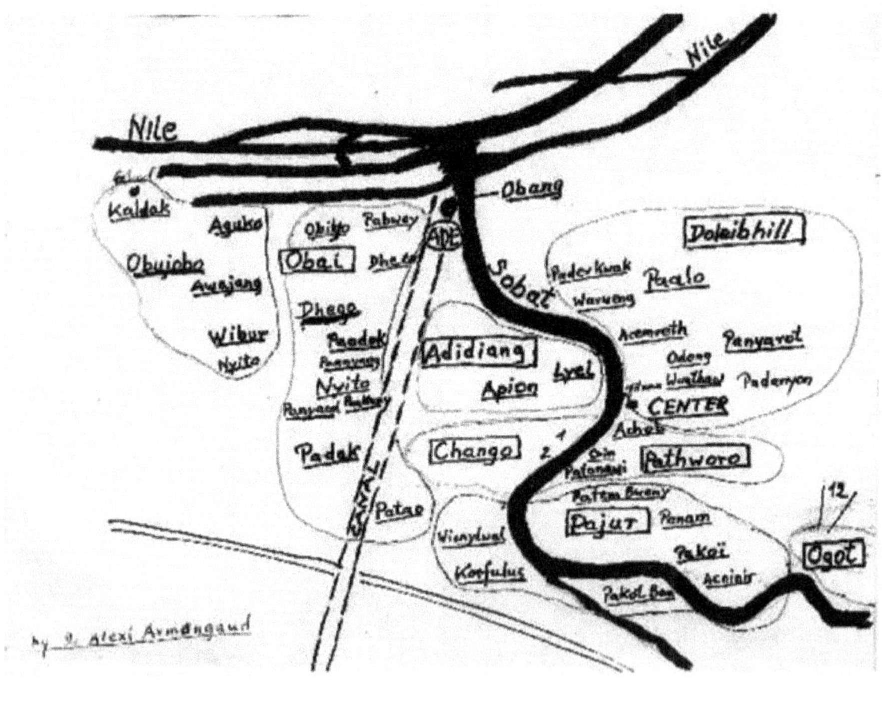

MAP 3
Nilotic tribes: Dinka, Nuer and Shilluk

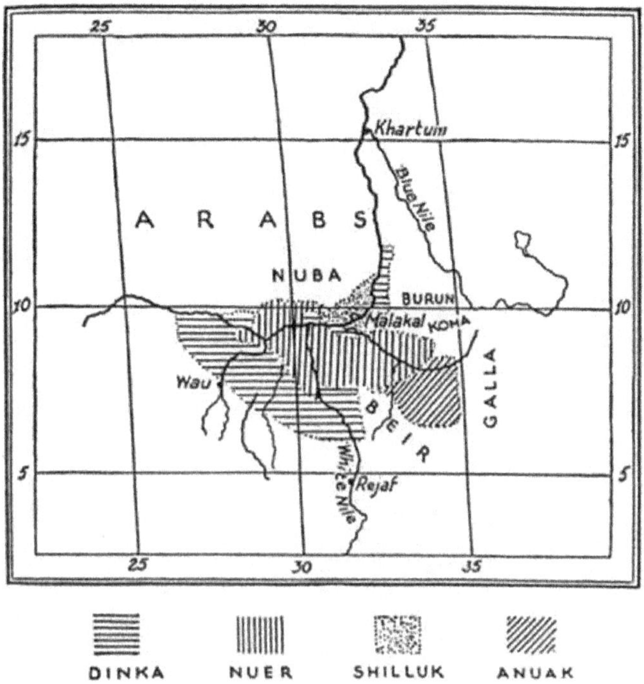

MAP 4
THE VILLAGE

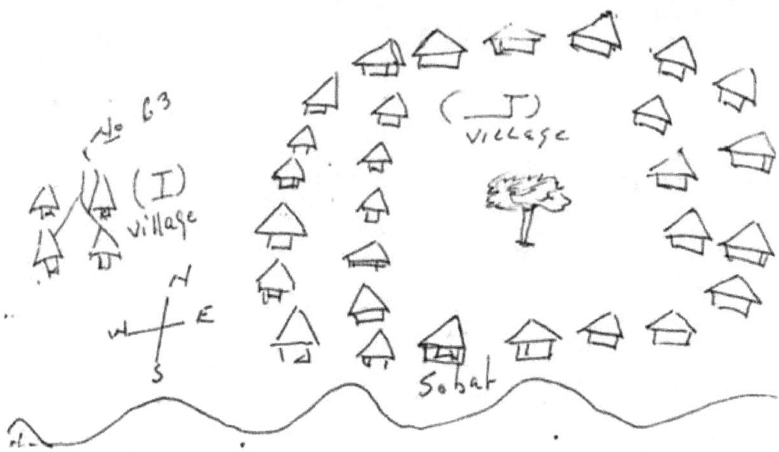

MAP 5
YAI, a village in the Nuer area

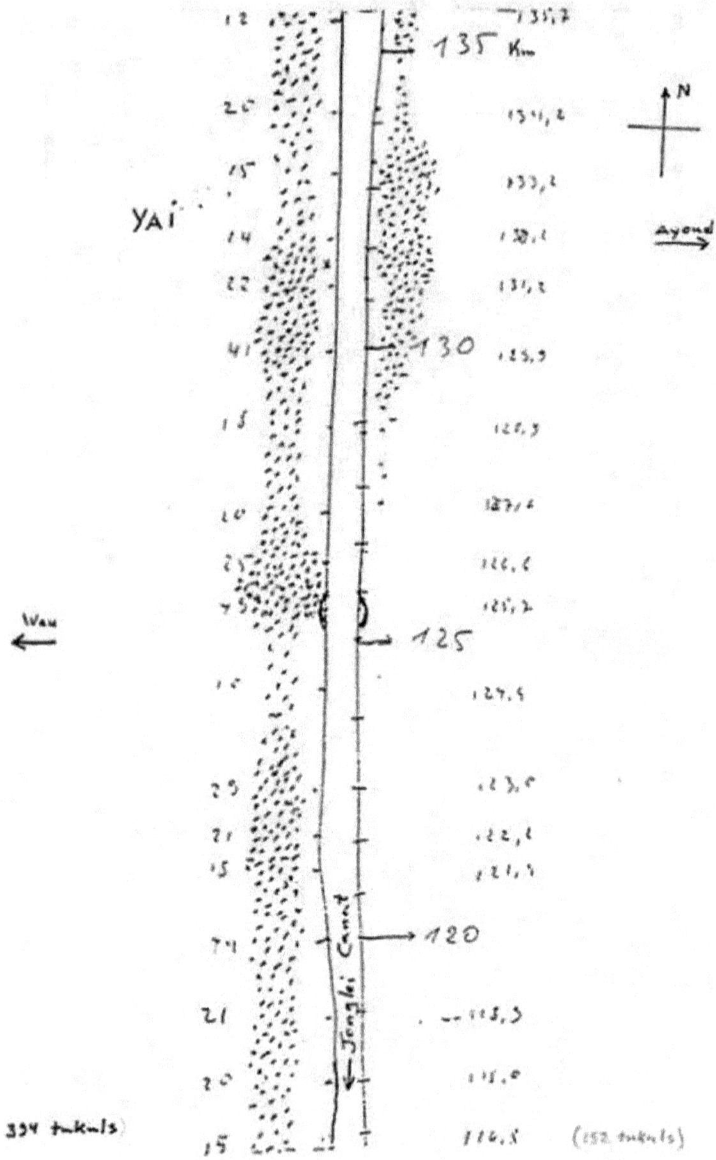

PART II

METHODOLOGICAL ASPECTS

1. OBJECTIVES
by Z.L. Ostrowski and M.-Ch. Josse

The general aim of this longitudinal epidemiological survey was to provide the Sudanese Government with quantitative information which could allow the competent authorities (Ministry of Health, Jonglei Executive Organ) to identify the main health problems in the most vulnerable group of the population (pregnant women and children) of Southern Sudan and to determine the health infrastructure for disease control activities.

The primary objectives of this study were to determine the nutritional and clinical status of a minimum of 300 pregnant women and their offspring in Southern Sudan. At the same time, a cross-sectional study of the whole population (men, women and children) and a socio-psychological study of 89 families in the study area were carried out. A previous pilot study carried out by Ostrowski and coll. (21) was the basis for this research project.

The objectives were as follows:

a) - To obtain a qualitative and a quantitative assessment of the health and nutritional status of the most vulnerable group of the population;
   - that the collected anthropometrical data might help establish a regional growth chart as a guide for children and pregnant women,
   - that accurate data on morbidity and mortality during pregnancy and early childhood could be used as base line information for the prevalence of endemic diseases (malaria, diarrhoea, infectious diseases, anaemia...) and assessment of major public health problems,
   - that the biological values might help in diagnosis and detection of pathology.

b) - To study the relationship between nutritional status during pregnancy, outcome of pregnancy and growth during early childhood.

c) - To determine infectious, social behaviour and altitudes and different environmental risk factors which might influence observed disease patterns and growth.

d) - To provide the necessary information for the development of preventive measures and for the establishment of a nutritional policy.

e) - To establish a health system survey to identify major public health problems which might result from considerable environmental changes due to the construction of the Jonglei Canal.

In the course of the project, other objectives were added:

a) - Establishment of primary health care units, construction of dispensaries, training of paramedical staff and education on village level (home gardening)

b) - Establishment of a Research Centre to study the impact of changes which might occur in this population.

The collected data of this survey could be used, as in Ostrowski and Josse European's study (22), as a baseline of information against which to assess, after a period of several years, the necessity of reinforcing and increasing public health measures and preventive medicine activities (environmental sanitation, vector control, immunization programs, epidemiological surveillance, etc.).

It was clear that the survey could not attempt to identify all health problems in the Jonglei Canal Area.

2. PRELIMINARY STUDY

by Z.L. Ostrowski

To undertake such a longitudinal study on Growth and Developpement in a remote area of Africa it was necessary to visit the study area to better understand the population, the environmental and the logistic possibilities

A pilote study was carry out by Ostrowski and Heidrecheid (*), of a sample of children and adults of the three tribes : Shillouk, Dinka and Nuer, between 1977-1978. It showed that the population lived in a very precarious way and that it was important to provide the Sudanese government with quantitative information for an adequate health policy for the Southern population. The results of this pilote study were the base for the methodology of the longitudinal study.

(*) Ostrowski Z.L. and Heidrecheid N., Some aspects of nutritional status in the South of the Sudan, J.Trop. Pediatrics, 1982, 28:153-158.

3. METHODS FOR DATA COLLECTION, DATA PROCESSING and DATA ANALYSIS (PROSPECTIVE STUDY)

By M.-Ch. Josse

To carry out a prospective study on pregnant women and their children in a very remote area like the Sobat region, where field conditions are notoriously difficult, it was essential to establish a specific methodology for data collection, data processing and data analysis. In this chapter, we describe two stages:

- The conception of a written tool - "questionnaire" - used for data collection,
- The creation of a "software" for data storage and computer treatment.

3.1. RECALL ON THE STUDY'S SCHEDULE

Three linked samples could be treated separately in this prospective study:

- Pregnant women ==> STUDY " PW "
- Their children ==> STUDY " CH "
- Lactating women ==> STUDY " LW "

Each woman was visited every month (a maximum of 6 times), and their children every three months. Lactating women were a sub-sample drawn from the pregnant women's sample: they were visited 6, 18 and 36 months after giving birth.

3.2. CONCEPTION OF THE PRE-FORMED QUESTIONNAIRE

All data was collected through pre-determined structured questionnaires for an efficient use of data and to aid with further statistical analysis. To meet this goal, we built a set of three questionnaires corresponding to each study ("PW", "CH", "LW"). Each questionnaire was composed of five files:

1) ***General*** (to fill out during the first visit, for each of the three studies):
   - For the "PW" study: data concerning the socio-demographic characteristics of the parents (age, occupation, highest level of education); data concerning the parity, marital status, outcome of previous pregnancies; items for anthropometrics: measurements of the father were recorded.

   - For the "CH" study: the outcome of the delivery, the characteristics of perinatal period and the health status of the newborn child.

   - For the LW" study: the health status of the mother after delivery.

2) ***Anthropometrical*** (to fill out at each visit for the three studies);
3) ***Clinical*** (to fill out at each visit for the three studies);
4) ***Biological*** (to fill out at specific visits);
5) ***Nutritional*** (to fill out at specific visits). Dietary intakes for one day were collected by a semi-quantitative 24 hour recall method. The women were asked to describe what they had eaten the previous day. The amount they had eaten was estimated by a Sudanese nutritionist. A nutritional survey involving weighing was done on a sub-sample. The nutritional questionnaire was based on the survey Ostrowski-Josse (22) with opened-closed questions about general foods habits.

From one study to another, the same structure was maintained for all the files: a hybrid questionnaire with numerical and alpha-numeric questions, rating and ranking questions, open-ended and closed-ended questions (figures 2, 3, 4, and 5 in Annex 1). It was necessary to design the paper "questionnaire" with data collection and data analysis in mind.

Several surveys were taken into consideration as the basis for the conception of this questionnaire: the Jerusalem perinatal study; the London School of Hygiene and Tropical medicine's survey on growth; the INSERM's survey on growth and nutrition, etc. (References 4, 5, 6, 8, 10, 12 and 15 in the bibliography, Annex 1).

Remarks on the first five items

To further facilitate the handling of data between these three related studies (multi-file exploitation), special attention was given to the identification of the study, the type of examination, and the subject. At the top of each questionnaire and of each file, five items are found:

1. "**STUDY N°**" (1= pregnant woman, 2= her children, 3= lactating woman);
2. "**TYPE OF EXAMINATION**" (1= general, 2= anthropometric, 3= clinical, 4=biological, 5=nutritional);
3. "**EXAMINATION N°**" (range of examination);
4. "**DATE OF SURVEY**" (dd/mm/yy);
5. "**INVESTIGATOR**" (as a number).

Identification of statistical units (ID)

We developed a participant specific identification number (ID). This ID was used to link a PW (or a lactating woman) and her children. Each pregnant woman was identified by a code of 3 digits between 001-400 (item n°6 from the general questionnaire). Each child was identified by the same code added by one 4th digit (1=simple birth, 2=stillbirth, 3= first twin, 4= second twin).

This codification (4 digits numbers) added to codes (village, household, etc.) permits a unique identification of every study, and subject, and establishes a relationship between the mother - pregnant or lactating - and her child.

3.3. DATA STORAGE

To store (then to manipulate) all the different data, we developed a data-entry program, a software package called "PWCHLW", in the A.D.E. Centre in Paris (23). This software was built and run on a mini-computer (IBM 5110) in Basic language (*). It was developed and tested over eight months.

3.3.1. <u>Design goal for the "PWCHLW" software system:</u>

a) To record the data from the three types of survey of the prospective and cross-sectional study in a data bank,
b) To be easy to use - by providing one easy interface between user and machine. The questionnaires were reproduced as faithfully on the screen; data were entered interactively through a series of display screens. The user is guided in a logical manner through the data entry process.
c) To reduce data entry errors via immediate data validation.
d) To realize multi-file exploitation.
e) To treat the data via classical statistical methods, multivariate methods, then to edit some results.

3.3.2. <u>Program files, data files for data source storage (data entry)</u>

3.3.2.1. General organisation of the "PWCHLW" package

The "PWCHLW" package contained three types of files:

a) *Program files.* These files made it possible to present on the screen of the IBM 5110 computer the structure of the five questionnaires (general, anthropometric, clinical, biological and nutritional) from the three surveys for data entry purposes. They permitted the user to pass from one survey to another at any time.

b) Fifteen *data files* which stored the *raw data* from the three surveys in their respective data files "PW.DATA", "CH.DATA" and "LW.DATA", each of them divided into 5 data files, e.g. for the survey PW: "GEN.PW.DATA", "ANT.PW.DATA","CLIN.PW.DATA","BIO.PW.DATA,"NUT.PW.DATA"

c) Some *table files* generated automatically (VILLAGES.LIST; SCHEDULE. PW, SCHEDULE.CH…) as data entry progressed.

* We appreciated the Basic language and its operating commands like RUN, CHAIN… essential for the operation and development of programs.

3.3.3. Constitution of the data files

3.3.3.1. Methods of Data Collection

The program files of "PWCHLW" package resided on the IBM 5110 computer as executable files. By entering the command "PROC 55", the program file named "SELEC.DEPART" would be executed and started. The first screen to appear (image 1, figure 6) permitted the user to choose any value from a list:

1 = Longitudinal (prospective) study
2 = Cross-sectional study
3 = WHO-code (creation, modification, suppression)
4 = WHO-code (impression)
5 = Food-code (creation, modification, impression)
6 = Food-code (impression)
7 = List of pregnant women 8 = List of children
9 = List of villages 0 = End of job

Selecting the options menu item displayed submenus.

Remarks on some options

...Option 3 "*WHO-code (creation, modification, suppression)*" ran a program named "WHO.CODE", and saved data (WHO-code in four digits and name of the corresponding disease of the international classification in 14 characters maximum) in a data file named "WHO.DATA" which could be printed (figure 8, Annex 1) if the user selected option 4 "*WHO-code, (impression)*". The same principle applies to options 5 and 6 in relation to food codes.

...Options 7 and 8 - *"List of pregnant women'* and *"list of children"* - ran the programs files "SCHEDULE.PRINT.PW" and "SCHEDULE. PRINT.CH". A table could be printed to find where the user had got to in their data entry (example: schedule of pregnant women's survey, see figure 9, Annex 1).

... As is typical in interactive programs, the "End of job" option was included in all the « PWCHLW » screens. This option caused the screen to be closed.

Examples:

The on-line data entry was performed by operator menus. The program files "PWCHLW" worked by displaying screens (submenus) to which the user responded, making the system easy to use with minimal training.

a) In a first example (figure 6, pp. 224-225) we showed the different screens displayed and the progression in conversational mode when the operator wanted to access the clinical questionnaire of the "survey PW".

When the questionnaire was found, options (1 to 6) appeared on the screen:

- 1=Input *(allows operator to enter the record),*
- 2=impression *(allows operator to edit the record),*
- 3=Modification *(allows operator to modify existing data),*
- 4=annulation *(allows operator to delete a record),*
- 5=impression of list PW *(allows operator to edit some record*),
- 6=End of Job *(allows operator to exit)*

b) In another example (figure 10, Annex 1) we showed how the questionnaire was reproduced on the computer screen. The program file displayed successively on the visualisation screen:

The *variable name*, some *blanks cases* (the number of blanks always corresponded to the field length; the blanks were blinking to make computer data entry easier); the right side of the screen contained some *information (coding methods) to assist the operator.*

The validation of data, data checking... an important step in the data input.

The periods between examinations have been automatically adapted to the exact day of the examinations so that a longitudinal follow up could be easy determined.
The program files allowed immediate validation of data: if a technical mistake appeared - for example instead of 87 cm of body length, 78 cm was recorded - the program did not accept this number if referring to data from the previous exam information. An error display appeared, the input data stopped and allowed immediately to correct collected data.
"PWLW software" did some data checking in order to reduce the chance for errors, but the checking was not exhaustive. Further, no amount of checking could detect data-entry errors in which a reasonable but incorrect value was entered by mistake. It was still possible **to verify that the raw data were accurate by a visual inspection.** So, the output files always could be examined to make sure that data had been defined as intended. To help with this, the command "impression" allowed operators to edit some records

3.4. DATA MANIPULATION AND INTERROGATION

The software automatically created three *raw* data files, namely *"PW.DATA"*, *"CH.DATA"* and *"LW.DATA"*, organised as **sequential files in a fixed data format** where each variable was arranged within the data files in columns and rows, as in a table. Each row represented a subject record (PW, CH or LW) identified by its ID, and each column was a list of related values. Within each record, a given variable always appeared in the same column(s), in a fixed position.

3.4.1. Data recoding, data transformation, creation of new variables

After data were checked for entry errors and before the primary statistical analysis was performed, much *raw data* often required recoding for preparation of the primary analysis for two general reasons: a) the raw data were awkward to work with and/or b) the data did not meet the assumptions of the preferred statistical methods. The data were checked for reliability and validity (frequency distributions study).

From the raw data files, we generated **new variables** using an expression that could combine constants, variables, functions, arithmetic and logical operators (example: Quetelet's indices). **Some variables could be recoded** in preparation for applying statistical tests through a variety of techniques: collapse a categorical variable into fewer categories (for example to regroup a numeric variable such as "woman's age in years" into categories: 15-19 years = 1, 20-24 years =2, 25-29 years =3, 30-34 years =4…), break a categorical variable up into several sub-variables with fewer categories or combine several categorical variables into fewer variables with more categories. Continuous data could be recoded into another continuous variable through either linear or nonlinear transformation (an important transformation used in our study was the Z-score).

3.4.2. Interrogation and statistics

To extract information from data collected, some statistical analyses have been performed in A.D.E. Research Centre in Paris, at University Kremlin-Bicêtre in Paris, and at WHO in Geneva. Some statistical analyses have been done using software packages: SPSS/PC+ package, BMDP, SAS package, Graph-in-the-Box programmes and Epi-Info-CDC-Atlanta (25).

A mix of statistical methods was used. Classical statistical methods were implemented: the simplest (mean/variance, median/quartile, chi-2, matched-pair case control studies, histograms, cross-tabulations, analysis of variance (t-test), Mann-Whittney U test) as well as some advanced statistical methods (multivariate regression analysis, factorial analysis of correspondence, principal components methods, discriminant analysis).

4. SAMPLE PROCEDURE

In the study area, demography and sanitary statistical data were absent: basic information on the magnitude of the measurements (e.g. expected prevalence of anaemia, malnutrition, diarrhoea, etc.) was not available. In consequence, it was impossible to determine the sample size with mathematical formulas. A judgement in the selection of the sample to be used was necessary. Ostrowski and Josse (22) studies in Europe served as a baseline; additionally, several epidemiologists from WHO and the London School of Hygiene and Tropical Medicine suggested a sampling procedure to ensure the maximum representative character of the sample.

The sample of pregnant women needed to be large enough from a statistical point of view to provide data on 100 boys and 100 girls at three years of age. Because of unknown morbidity-mortality rates and levels of migration, a survey covering approximately 400 pregnant women could give adequate information.

In view of the homogenous social structure and living conditions of the population in the Jonglei Canal area, the first 400 pregnant women (between 3rd to 9th month of pregnancy) met in the first villages and compounds along the Nile and Sobat banks, as well as on the canal road, in the vicinity of the A.D.E. Research Centre were included in this study. However, an area of the first 10 km from the A.D.E. camp was excluded because of the vicinity to the CCI camp (see map 2). It was impossible to conduct the village's selection in a strict statistical, systematic manner.

Between April 1981 and January 1984, a cohort study was conducted in the selected rural community. The study subjects were recruited over a period of 36 months. Because of the movement of the population and local fighting it was sometimes difficult to find all missing pregnant women and children. In case they didn't return to their village, the follow up was suspended. The climate conditions were another obstacle to follow up all the subjects of the sample.

PART III

HEALTH AND NUTRITION

1. SAMPLE DESCRIPTION
By Z.L. Ostrowski and M.-Ch. Josse

The cross-sectional study was carried out near the Jonglei Canal, between Malakal and Kongor in the dry season of 1982 (see map 1b). The study was carried out over 7 consecutive days in the villages between Doleib Hill and Obai (Shilluk area), 3 days in Ayod (Nuer area) and 1 to 2 days in villages between Obai and Ayod (Dinka area). The entire population present in these villages at the time of the survey were included in this study. We considered each examined child as a new observation, like Fawzi (27) in his study on Sudanese children.

Due to seasonal migration of the Nuer youth with cattle at the time of the survey, the Nuer sample constitutes mostly adults. In the Dinka villages only 33 people were present due to local fighting between the Dinka and Shilluk at the time of the survey.

A total of 286 people (106 children and 180 adults) attended the survey (139 Shilluk, 114 Nuer and 33 Dinka) (tables 1.1a and 1.1b).

1.1. FAMILY SIZE

The family size was difficult to determine with accuracy because of polygamy, mostly in the Nuer tribe. Women indicated always a higher family size than men: men indicated only children from their actual wife or wives, women indicated all persons living in their families (Tables 1.2 and 1.3). However the mean family size was about four people (between 1 and 10 people). Among the three ethnicities, Shilluk had higher family size and polygamy was common (table 1.4).

1.2. MORBIDITY AND MORTALITY

The number of children living in each family was seriously reduced due to high rates of miscarriage, stillbirth and infant mortality. The number of miscarriages per woman was higher in the Nuer than in the other ethnic groups (3 to 4 per woman!) (Table 1.5). Also, the stillbirth rate was very high in the Nuer. Two Nuer women had 5 stillbirths and one even 6 stillbirths! (Table 1.6).

The mortality rate in the study area is shown in table 1.7. In 46 % of the population more than 3 children died per family. Amongst the Nuer the mortality was highest: 33% lost more than 5 children. The information concerning the age at death of the children could be obtained only from the last child. Table 1.8 shows that around 50% died in the first year.

The number of living children was much reduced, but was always important. In the study sample, the mean number of living children was more than two per family, rarely reaching 5 per family (table 1.9).

1.3. SOCIO-ECONOMICAL STATUS

The socio-economical status of the whole studied population was as follows: women had no occupation and no education (except for 3 Shilluk); 84% of men had no education; only a few Shilluk had some higher education (table 1.10).

Among the studied male population, the majority of Dinka (70%) and Shilluk men (67%) cultivated spontaneously (mainly sorghum) around their huts, while only 3% of Nuer men cultivated (table 1.11). An average family had 1 to 3 huts and sometimes a luak (big hut for cows), depending on their family size and on the number of wives. Shilluk and Dinka mostly had more than two huts per family (table 1.12) as well as a luak (table 1.13).

1.4. DISCUSSION

The way of life observed in the population under study was similar to their ancestors. A high morbidity and mortality rate, especially in early childhood, was equilibrated by high birth rate.

Roth (28) reported high levels of childhood mortality in Southern Sudan. Also Ibrahim (29) observed in his study in a rural area in Sudan the high risk of an unfavourable outcome in multiple pregnancies, which was more than nine times that of singletons. The high level of stillbirths was also observed by Taha (30) who related it to malaria during pregnancy. In Tanzania, Kitange (31) described crude mortalities ranged from 6.1/1000/year for women in Hai to 15.9/1000 per year for men in Morogororo rural area. Age specific mortalities were up to 43 times higher than rates in England. Seaman (32) reported also a high death rate (38%-57%).

According to Bergsjo (33), traditional medicine with a home birth was the only solution available, as in the majority of the African rural population.

Polygamy is normal in Africa. In our study, because of their young age, only 11% of men had more than one wife. The average family size was between 1 and 10 persons. Taylor (34) and Maynard (35) mentioned that polygamy and large family size characterized the African population. They mentioned also that there was no, or very little, education (84%) and that the majority of the people live in a very simple way. Ali (36) reported that the simple way of living exists also in the Shendi area of Sudan. The main occupation was cattle rearing, hunting, fishing and sometimes agriculture.

Table 1.1a Number of cases for the three cross-sectional studies for each studied item.

Ethnicity	Category	Age	General	Clinical	Anthropom	Nutritional	Haematology	Biological
	Children	0- 5 years	33	33	31	27	20	2
SHILLUK	Children	6-14	38	38	38	35	28	19
	Women	years	30	29	30	29	23	20
	Men		38	38	38	38	35	32
	Children	0- 5 years	8	8	7	7	5	-
DINKA	Children	6-14	7	7	6	6	7	-
	Women	years	8	8	8	8	5	4
	Men		10	10	10	10	7	7
	Children	0- 5 years	9	9	8	8	2	-
NUER	Children	6-14	11	11	10	11	6	9
	Women	years	61	61	58	58	28	35
	Men		33	33	31	33	21	17
TOTAL			286	285	275	271	186	145
%			*100%*	*100%*	*96%*	*95%*	*65%*	*51%*

41

TABLE 1.1b : NUMBER OF CASES BY ETHNICITY, SEX AND AGE

AGE GROUPS	SHILLUK			NUER			DINKA			TOTAL		
	♂	♀	Σ	♂	♀	Σ	♂	♀	Σ	♂	♀	Σ
0 - 5 years	20	13	33	6	3	9	4	4	8	30	20	50
6 – 14 years	25	13	38	8	3	11	5	2	7	38	18	56
ADULTS	38	30	68	33	61	94	10	8	18	81	99	180
TOTAL	83	56	139	47	67	114	19	14	33	149	137	286
%	*60%*	*40%*		*41%*	*59%*		*58%*	*42%*		*52%*	*48%*	

TABLE 1.2 : FAMILY SIZE INDICATED BY 105 WOMEN

SIZE NUMBER	SHILLUK			NUER			DINKA			TOTAL		
	n	%	Cum%	n	%	Cum%	n	%	Cum%	n	%	Cum%
1	0	-	-	1	1,64	1,64	0	-	-	1	0.95	0,95
2	1	2,78	2,78	9	14,75	16,39	1	12,5	12,5	11	10,48	11,43
3	5	13,89	16,67	12	19,66	36,05	2	25,0	37,5	19	18,09	29,52
4	6	16,66	33,33	20	32,78	68,83	1	12,5	50,0	27	25,71	55,23
5	10	27,78	61,11	10	16,40	85,23	3	37,5	87,5	23	21,91	77,14
6	10	27,78	88,89	4	6,56	91,79	1	12,5	100	15	14,29	91,43
7	2	5,55	94,44	2	3,28	95,07	0	-	-	4	3,81	95,24
8	1	2,78	97,22	0	-		0	-	-	1	0,95	96,19
9	0	-		0	-		0	-	-	0	-	
10>	1	2,78	100	0	-		0	-	100	1	0,95	97,14
Unknown	0			3	4,92	100	0			3	2,86	100

TABLE 1.3. FAMILY SIZE INDICATED BY MEN

SIZE N°	SHILLUK n	%	Cum%	NUER n	%	Cum%	DINKA n	%	Cum%	TOTAL n	%	Cum%
0	1	3	3	2	7	7	0	-	-	3	4	4
1	1	3	6	1	3	10	0	-	-	2	3	7
2	3	8	14	4	14	24	1	8	8	8	5	12
3	1	3	17	2	7	31	2	17	25	5	7	19
4	4	11	28	3	10	41	3	26	51	10	13	32
5	12	33	61	8	26	67	0	-	-	20	27	59
6	7	19	80	1	3	70	2	17	68	10	13	72
7	4	11	91	0	-	-	1	8	76	5	7	79
8	0	-	-	1	3	73	0	-	-	1	1	80
9	1	3	94	0	-	-	0	-	-	1	1	81
10>	1	3	97	5	17	90	1	8	84	7	11	92
?	1	3	100	3	10	100	2	16	100	6	8	100

TABLE 1.4. NUMBER of WIFES INDICATED BY MEN

NUMBER WIVES	SHILLUK n	%	NUER n	%	DINKA n	%	TOTAL n	%
No wives	8	21,05	4	12,12	1	10%	13	16,05
1 wife	26	69,43	18	55,55	7	70%	51	62,97
2 wives	2	5,26	3	9,09	2	20%	7	8,64
3 wives	-	-	1	3,03	-	-	1	1,23
Unknown	2	5,26	7	21,21	- -	-	9	11,11

TABLE 1.5. NUMBER OF ABORTIONS PER WOMAN

NUMBER OF ABORTIONS xi	SHILLUK ni	nixi	NUER ni	nixi	DINKA ni	nixi	TOTAL ni	nixi
0	31	0	37	0	6	0	74	0
1	4	4	10	10	-	-	14	14
2	1	2	7	14	2	4	10	20
3	0	0	6	18	-	-	6	18
4	0	0	1	4	-	-	1	4
TOTAL	36	6	61	46	8	4	105	56

TABLE 1.6. NUMBER OF STILLBORNS (SB) PER PREGNANT WOMAN (PW)

NUMBER OF STILLBORN Per woman xi	SHILLUK PW ni	SB nixi	NUER PW ni	SB nixi	DINKA PW ni	SB nixi	TOTAL PW ni	%
0	35	0	45	0	8	0	88	83,80
1	1	1	6	6			7	6,67
2			3	6			3	2,86
3			3	9			3	2,86
4			1	4			1	0,95
5			2	10			2	1,91
6			1	6			1	0,95
TOTAL	36	1	61	41	8	0	105	100%

TABLE 1.7. NUMBER OF DEAD CHILDREN PER FAMILY

NUMBER OF Dead children	SHILLUK		NUER		DINKA		TOTAL	
	n	Σ	n	Σ	n	Σ	n	Σ
1	5	5	8	8			13	13
2	3	6	5	10	1	2	9	18
3	4	12	8	24	1	3	13	39
4	5	20	8	32	1	4	14	56
5	1	5	3	15			4	20
6			5	30			5	30
7			2	14			2	14
8			2	16	1	8	3	24
9>			2	20			2	20
TOTAL	18	48	43	169	4	17	65	234

TABLE 1.8. AGE OF DEATH OF THE LAST CHILD PER WOMAN

AGE of death In years	SHILLUK			NUER			DINKA			TOTAL		
	n	%	Cum%	n	%	Cum%	n	%	Cum%	n	%	Cum%
<1	7	38,9	38,9	2	4,6	4,6	1	25	25	10	15,1	15,1
1	1	5,5	44,4	11	25,0	29,6				12	18,2	33,3
2				6	13,6	43,2	1	25	50	7	10,7	44,0
3	5	27,8	72,2	4	9,1	52,3				9	13,6	57,6
4				1	2,2	54,5				1	1,5	59,1
5	5	27,8	100	2	4,6	59,1	2	50	100	9	13,6	72,7
Unknow				18	40,9	100				18	27,3	100
TOTAL	18			44			4			66		

TABLE 1.9. NUMBER OF CHILDREN ALIVE PER FAMILY

NUMBER of ALIVE xi	SHILLUK				NUER			
	ni	∑ nixi	%	Cum%	ni	∑ nixi	%	Cum%
0	8				11			
1	6	6	21,4	21,4	14	14	28,0	28,0
2	4	8	14,3	35,7	22	44	44,0	72,0
3	11	33	39,3	75,0	12	36	24,0	96,0
4	6	24	21,4	96,4	2	8	4,0	100
5	1	5	3,6	100				
TOTAL	28	76	100%		50	102	100%	

NUMBER of ALIVE xi	DINKA				TOTAL			
	ni	∑ nixi	%	Cum%	ni	∑ nixi	%	Cum%
0	1				20			
1	1	1	14,3	14,3	21	21	24,7	24,7
2	3	6	42,9	57,2	29	58	34,1	58,5
3	2	6	28,6	85,8	25	75	29,4	88,2
4	1	4	14,2	100	9	36	10,6	98,8
5					1	5	1,2	100
TOTAL	7	17	100%		85	195	100%	

TABLE 1.10. EDUCATION LEVEL (amongst men)

EDUCATION	SHILLUK		NUER		DINKA		TOTAL	
	n	%	n	%	n	%	n	%
None	25	69	30	97	10	100	65	84
Elementary	2	6					2	3
Primary	5	14	1	3			6	8
Secondary	2	6					2	3
Higher	2	5					2	2
Unknown								
TOTAL	36		31		10		77	

TABLE 1.11. OCCUPATION (amongst men)

OCCUPATION	SHILLUK		NUER		DINKA		TOTAL	
	n	%	n	%	n	%	n	%
None	5	14	21				26	34
Cultivator	24	67	1	8	7	70	32	41
Fisher	2	5					2	3
Teacher	1	3					1	1
Nurse	0		1	3			1	1
Chief	1	3	5	16			6	8
Other	3	8	3	10	3	30	9	12
TOTAL	36		31		10	17	77	

TABLE 1.12. NUMBER OF HUTS PER FAMILY BASED ON INDICATIONS OBTAINED FROM 77 MEN

NUMBER of huts	SHILLUK			NUER			DINKA			TOTAL		
	n	%	Cum%	n	%	Cum%	n	%	Cum%	n	%	Cum%
0	1	3	3	2	7	7				3	4	4
1	8	22	25	14	52	59	3	30	30	25	34	38
2	17	47	72	7	26	85	5	50	80	29	40	78
3	8	22	94	4	15	100	1	10	90	13	18	96
3>	2	6	100				1	10	100	3	4	100
Unknown				4						4		
TOTAL	36			31			10			77		

TABLE 1.13. LUAKS PER FAMILY BASED ON INDICATION OBTAINED FROM MEN (> 18 YEARS)

LUAKS	SHILLUK		NUER		DINKA		TOTAL	
	n	%	n	%	n	%	n	%
Yes	23	64%	3	30%	21	68%	47	61%
No	13	36%	7	70%	9	29%	29	38%
Unknown					1	3%	1	1%
TOTAL	36	100%	10	100%	31	100%	77	100%

2. ANTHROPOMETRY
by Z. L. Ostrowski, M.-Ch. Josse, E. Ojaba

Among the anthropometrical measurements which can be used in nutritional studies, eight have been selected in our study: height, weight, and two skin fold thicknesses (tricipital and sub-scapular), arm length, mid-arm, calf and head circumferences. Two indexes were calculated: Z-score of weight to height by age and the Quetelet Index.

All measurements have been done by the same person using the same scales: for weight, a mechanical scale (obtained from WHO) to the nearest 0.1 kg; for height, a wooden meter or metal rolling meter (to the nearest 0.1 cm), for arm-length and arm-circumferences a metal rolling meter (to the nearest 0.1 cm), for skin fold thickness a Harpenden Calliper. The last three measurements have been done on the left side of the body. All measurements have been done following the standardised proceeding descripts by Jelliffe (38) and Ostrowski (39). Until 24 months, stature were measured with the infant recumbent, older children were measured in the standing position.

2.1. CROSS-SECTIONNAL STUDY

Due to the small sample of the studied population in the Dinka and Nuer villages (see chapter 1), these results concern mostly the Shilluk children and the Nuer and Shilluk adults (male and female).

The results of all measurements are shown in table 2.1 and 2.2 (mean "*m*", variance "*s*" and number "n"). The signification of differences between Shilluk and Nuer adults are shown in table 2.3.

2.1.1. AGE GROUPS

The 75 Shilluk children (boys and girls) were classified in 4 mean «age groups»: less than 2 yrs, 3-5 yrs, 6-9 yrs and 10-14 yrs but, because of uncertainty about the ages obtained, the data may not be exactly situated on the age scale.

The 64 Shilluk adults (men and women) were compared with the 92 Nuer adults. The mean age was not significantly different between the adult groups.

2.1.2. STATURE

The height by age curve was compared with WHO standard references (40). The height for age curve of the Shilluk children and adults does not obviously differ with the WHO standard (figure 2.1).

The height by age curve, for Nuer children and adults, is higher than WHO standard. The mean height of Nuer men are in the 80th centile of the standard references. The mean height of Nuer men is 182 cm and those of Shilluk men are 175 cm. The mean difference in height between the Nuer and Shilluk men is 7 cm ($p < 0.005$). The mean height of Nuer women is 169 cm and these of Shilluk women are 166 cm. The mean height of the 389 pregnant women from the longitudinal sample is 167,4 cm (table 2.6). The difference in height between the Nuer and Shilluk women is not significant (table 2.3).

2.1.3. WEIGHT

The weight for age curve of the Shilluk children is below WHO standard references (figure 2.2). The mean weight of Shilluk women is about 50 kg and that of men 56 kg without significant differences between the Shilluk and Nuer ethnicities (table 2.3). Compared with WHO references (<18 years), the mean weight of men (Shilluk and Nuer) is below the 10th centile and of women below the 20th centile.

2.1.4. Z-SCORE WEIGHT TO HEIGHT BY AGE

The Z-score, calculated using the CDC Atlanta anthropometry software package (25, 41), shows that Shilluk children are below zero (table 2.1) which is due to great weight difference between these children and the American. The histogram (figure 2.3) shows that only 13 % have a positive Z-score. The 50th centile of this sample is -1.7 S.D. of reference; the 10th centile is -2.6 S.D. (!) Figure 2.4 shows the evolution of the standard deviations (SD) of height, weight and Z-score in the first 30 months of life in the sample of *children from the longitudinal study.*

2.1.5. QUETELET INDEX

The Quetelet Index (weight/height^2), used very often in nutritional studies, decrease from 16,35kg/m^2 in infants to 13,27kg/m^2 in children 6-9 years old with a tendency to increase with age (table 2.1). In adults the Quetelet Index varies slightly between the two ethnicities: 17,16kg/m^2 for Nuer women and 18,88kg/m^2 for Shilluk women (table 2.2). It varies less than the Z-score.

2.1.6. ARM LENGTH

The arms and legs of the Nilotic population are longer than those of the Europeans. The mean adult arm length is 79 cm for women and 84 cm for men. The Nuer has longer arms than the Shilluk ($p < 0.01$) (table 2.3). But, because of higher stature, the arm length to height is the same (0,47) (table 2.1).

The correlation coefficient between the arm length and the stature in Shilluk is 0.9872 ($p < 0.001$) which shows a linear relation. However the proportion «arm length to stature» increases significantly with age ($r = 0.64$; $p < 0.001$) in children. In adults there is no visible difference between ethnicities and sex (table 2.3).

2.1.7. SKINFOLD THICKNESS

The thickness of the tricipital and sub-scapular skin folds in children was measured following the technique described by Ostrowski (39). The thickness of the two skin folds in children decreases with age. The tricipital skin fold decrease from 6,7 mm in infants to 4,2 mm in children 6-9 years old; the sub-scapular skin fold decrease from 5.3 mm to 3.7 mm respectively. At puberty both skin folds increase slightly (table 2.1). In adults the sub-scapular skin fold is between 5,6 and 6,8 mm. The tricipital skin fold varies more between men (4,0 - 4,5 mm) and women (6,4 - 6,8 mm) (Tables 2.2).

Compared for example, to French population, the mean of both skin fold thicknesses in children and adults is situated below 10th centile (39) compared to American population the difference is extremely high! (*)

2.1.8. MID-ARM AND CALF CIRCUMFERENCE

In children, the mid-arm and calf circumference increase with age, mostly between 6 and 14 years (table 2.1). In adults they are similar for both men and women in the two ethnicities (table 2.2). The muscle circumference is also equal in both ethnicities (21 cm).

2.1.9. HEAD CIRCUMFERENCE

The head circumference in Shilluk children increase from 43,07 cm, at age less than 2 year to 51,33 cm at age 10-14 years (table 2.1). In adults it is between 53,05 and 55,69 cm (table 2.2.). The head circumference in adult women, based on the sample of the 386 Shilluk pregnant women is 53,9 cm (table 2.6). The Nuer men have a slightly larger head circumference (55,69cm) than the Shilluk men (54,4cm) ($p<0.01$) (table 2.3).

2.1.10. STATISTICAL ANALYSIS

Some statistical analysis has been carried out between Z-score and Quetelet Index with some clinical and nutritional data. No correlation was found between clinical data and Z-score. For nutritional data one way analysis of variances with Z-score and Quetelet Index shows that in children less than 5 years old, more milk consumption is related to higher Z-score ($p<0.05$) and higher Quetelet Index ($p<0.005$). In children 5 to 9 years old there is no significant correlation. In adults there is only a significant correlation between Z-score and beer consumption ($p<0.05$). For milk and fish there is no significant correlation. An attempt was made by Cazaux Devy and Helenon (**) to get a longitudinal approach using the Jenss and Bayley (47) mathematical model for studying the growth of the child.

* *It is unwise to use American population as reference for studies in the third world, more than 1/3 of the American population is overweight or even obese.*

** *A.D.E. Research Centre, Paris*

TABLE 2.1. ANTHROPOMETRICAL VALUES FOR SHILLUK CHILDREN

AGE GROUPS		<2 years	3 – 5 years	6 – 9 years	10 – 14 years
AGE	m	**0,9**	**3,6**	**7,0**	**11,9**
(years)	S	0,4	0,9	0,9	1,5
	N	12	21	22	20
HEIGHT	m	**69,33**	**94,93**	**125,17**	**149,77**
(cm)	S	6,12	9,65	9,37	12,32
	N	12	19	22	20
WEIGHT	m	**7,90**	**12,52**	**20,88**	**31,93**
(kg)	S	1,58	2,22	3,42	7,46
	N	12	19	22	20
	M	**-0,67**	**-1,48**	**-1,76**	**-1,82**
Z-SCORE	S	1,13	1,03	0,84	0,82
	N	12	19	22	19
	M	**16,35**	**13,89**	**13,27**	**14,05**
QUETELET	S	1,92	1,52	0,92	1,35
	N	12	19	22	20
ARM LENGTH	m	**20,49**	**39,78**	**54,41**	**68,56**
(cm)	S	2,55	4,98	5,06	6,92
	N	12	19	22	20
ARM LENGHT	m	**0,43**	**0,42**	**0,43**	**0,46**
/ HEIGHT	S	0,01	0,01	0,02	0,01
	N	12	19	22	20
SUBSCAPULAR	m	**5,29**	**3,88**	**3,74**	**4,39**
(mm)	S	2,12	0,76	0,87	0,83
	N	10	16	22	15
TRICIPITAL	m	**6,66**	**6,63**	**4,21**	**4,65**
(mm)	S	2,15	1,28	0,68	1,53
	N	10	16	22	15
ARM CIRCUM	m	**13,14**	**13,52**	**15,24**	**17,80**
(cm)	S	1,84	1,00	1,03	2,01
	N	12	19	21	20
MUSCLE CIRC.	m	**11,14**	**11,44**	**13,86**	**16,39**
(cm)	S	1,71	0,98	1,00	1,74
	N	12	16	18	15
CALF CIRCUM	m	**15,31**	**17,51**	**20,88**	**23,59**
(cm)	S	1,63	1,33	1,45	2,52
	N	12	19	22	20
HAED CIRCUM	m	**43,07**	**47,21**	**50,00**	**51,33**
(cm)	S	1,92	1,85	1,94	1,69
	N	12	18	22	2O

TABLE 2.2. ANTHROPOMETRICAL VALUES FOR ADULTS (SHILLUK and NUER)

ETHNICITY		SH WOMEN	SH MEN	NU WOMEN	NU MEN
AGE	m	**33,6**	**38,9**	**40,1**	**42,0**
(years)	S	13,3	12,1	10,9	13,5
	N	28	36	59	33
HEIGHT	m	**165,93**	**175,33**	**168,61**	**181,79**
(cm)	S	5,59	7,82	7,82	7,15
	N	28	36	56	31
WEIGHT	m	**50,18**	**55,79**	**48,85**	**56,76**
(kg)	S	7,71	9,29	6,29	6,73
	N	28	36	56	31
	M	**-1,38**	**-1,24**	**-1,99**	**-2,19**
Z-SCORE	S	0,88	0,81	0,93	0,90
	N	28	35	56	31
	M	**18,88**	**18,06**	**17,16**	**17,16**
QUETELET	S	2,29	2,16	1,88	1,65
	N	28	36	56	31
ARM LENGTH	m	**77,27**	**82,32**	**79,85**	**85,53**
(cm)	S	3,68	3,56	4,42	4,07
	N	28	36	536	31
ARM LENGHT	m	**0,47**	**0,47**	**0,47**	**0,47**
/ HEIGHT	S	0,02	0,01	0,02	0,01
	N	28	36	56	31
SUBSCAPULAR	m	**6,76**	**5,73**	**5,96**	**5,59**
(mm)	S	1,50	1,07	1,73	0,61
	N	23	30	38	13
TRICIPITAL	m	**6,83**	**4,49**	**6,36**	**3,95**
(mm)	S	1,70	0,78	2,15	0,58
	N	23	30	38	13
ARM CIRCUM	m	**23,57**	**23,21**	**22,58**	**22,97**
(cm)	S	2,70	2,24	1,97	3,43
	N	27	36	56	31
MUSCLE CIRC.	m	**20,89**	**21,47**	**20,52**	**21,17**
(cm)	S	2,66	2,07	1,80	2,95
	N	22	30	38	13
CALF CIRCUM	m	**28,20**	**29,70**	**27,86**	**30,73**
(cm)	S	2,17	2,79	2,09	2,81
	N	28	36	56	31
HAED CIRCUM	m	**53,05**	**54,40**	**53,35**	**55,69**
(cm)	S	2,06	1,76	1,64	1,77
	N	28	36	56	31

TABLE 2.3. DIFFERENCES BETWEEN SHILLUK AND NUER (men and women) FOR ANTHROPOMETRICAL VALUES (Significances by Wilcoxon rank sum test)

	SIGNIFICANCES	
MEASUREMENTS	**MEN**	**WOMEN**
HEIGHT	* * *	NS
WEIGHT	NS	NS
Z – SCORE	* * *	* *
QUETELET	NS	*
ARM LENGTH	* * *	*
ARM LENGTH/ HEIGHT	NS	NS
SUBSCAPULAR	NS	*
TRICIPITAL	*	NS
ARM CIRCUMFERENCE	NS	NS
MUSCLE CIRCUMFERENCE	NS	NS
CALF CIRCUMFERENCE	NS	NS
HAED CIRCUMFERENCE	* *	NS

* $p < 0.05$; * * $p < 0.01$; * * * $p < 0.005$

FIGURE 2.1. HEIGHT WITH AGE FOR SHILLUK MALE (M) AND FEMALE (F); (WHO Reference for male ___ for female ---)

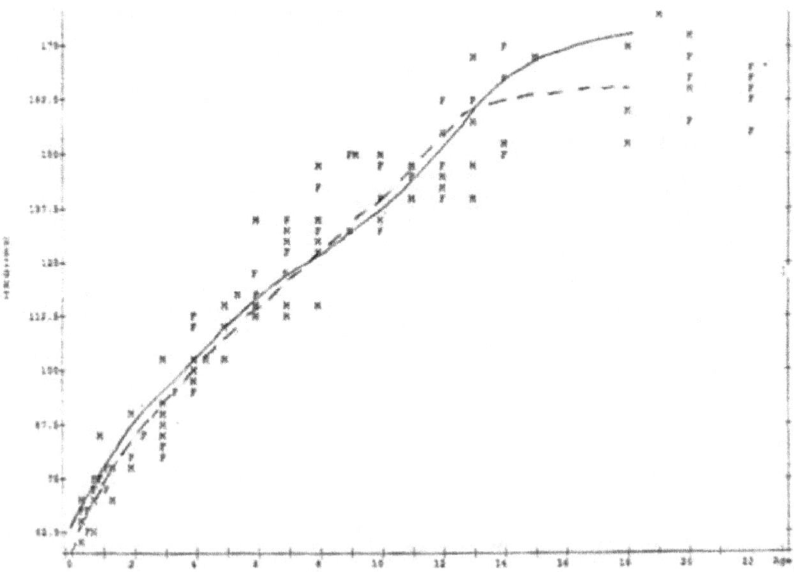

FIGURE 2.2. WEIGHT WITH AGE FOR SHILLUK MALE (M) AND FEMALE (F); (WHO Reference for male ___ for female ---)

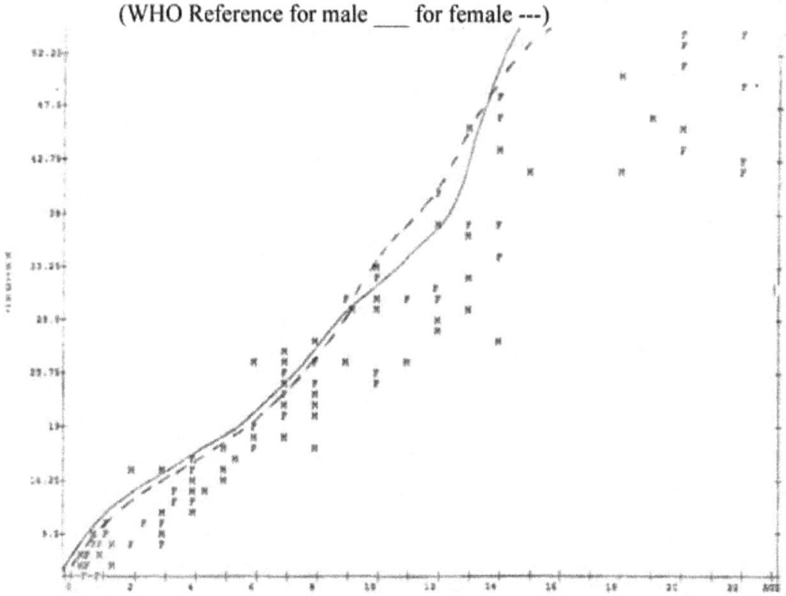

Figure 2.3. Z-SCORE weight for height for Shilluk children until 9 years (CDC Atlanta reference).

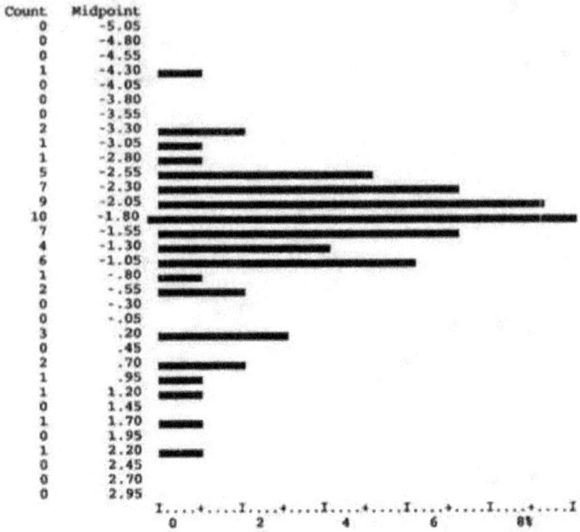

Percentile	Value	Percentile	Value	Percentile	Value	Percentile	Value
5.00	-3.132	10.00	-2.568	25.00	-2.240	50.00	-1.710
75.00	-1.140	80.00	-0.938	85.00	-0.405	90.00	0.480
95.00	1.193	99.00	.000	(Valid cases: 65	Missing cases : 198)		

FIGURE 2.4. Evolution of the standard deviations of height (SDH), weight (SDW) and Z-score (SDZ) in the first 30 months

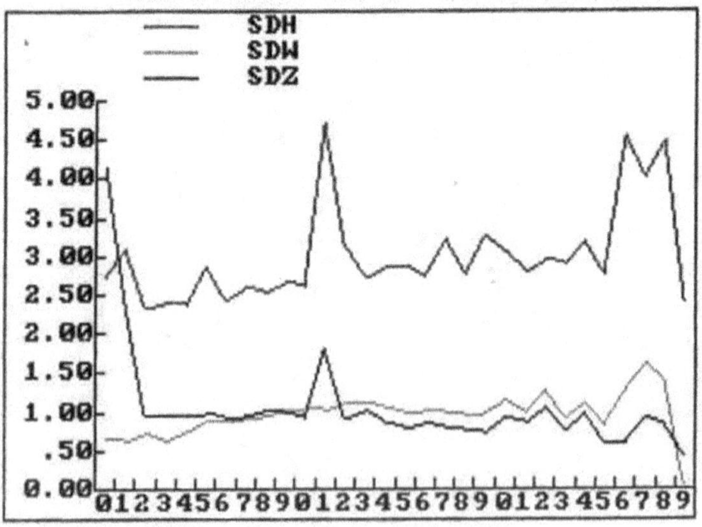

2.2. LONGITUDINAL STUDY

2.2.1. ANTHROPOMETRIC DATA DURING PREGNANCY

The period of pregnancy is a very special one. At this period some anthropometrical data can reflect the growth of the foetus and the health status of the pregnant woman. The weight gain is influenced by the changes of different organs. According to Hytten (42), the foetus represents one third of the total gain during pregnancy (4,4 kg); with placenta and amniotic liquid it presents more than 50% (6,7 kg). The other part of weight gain is due to the changes of mother's organs (7,6 kg) (table 2.4).

Some measurements of 359 pregnant women are shown in table 2.5. between the 3rd months and the middle of the 2nd and 3rd trimester. The mean age of the 394 pregnant women sample was 25,8 years (SD 5.6) and the mean parity 3,6 (SD 2.2). About 24% were primipara. In 105 non pregnant women the mean parity was 8.4.

The mean **height** was 167,4 cm (range 153-185 cm) (table 2.6). The evolution of **weight** gain between the 3rd and 9th month of pregnancy increased about 8 kg (figure 2.5). The differences (mean with percentiles) at each month are shown in table 2.7. If the weight is similar to kenyan pregnant women (Jansen – 43), the gain was more important in the last trimester in our sample (3,1 kg) than in Kenya (2 kg). Lawrence (44) found in his study of 50 rural Gambian pregnant women that the weight gain during first 35 weeks averaged 6,3 kg.

The mean **upper arm circumference** remained below 90 percent of the standard for non-pregnant women (Frisancho - 45). The brachial perimeter as well as the skinfold thickness (tricipital and sub scapular) decreased very slightly from the 5th month to the end of pregnancy (about 0,5 and 0,2 mm respectively) (table 2.8 and 2.9). In Kenyan women the skinfolds do not decrease.

The brachial perimeter and the **skinfold thickness** allowed calculating the brachial, muscular and adipose surface, which can better reflect the changes in repartition and use of body fat which decrease in the third trimester.

Similarly the **brachial, muscular and adipose surface** increased less than 1 cm^2 until the 5th month before starting to decrease (2,3cm^2-0,8cm^2-0,5cm^2) until the end of pregnancy (table 2.10). Other measurements are stable during the pregnancy except, of course, the abdominal perimeter which increase 13 cm (9-17cm) between the 3rd and 9th month of pregnancy (table 2.11).

After delivery, a sub-sample of 22 **lactating women** was examined. A group of 105 «non-pregnant non lactating women» (NP-NLW) were included in this study for comparison. For the non-pregnant and non-lactating women sample, the mean weight was 49 kg and the mean height 167 cm. The mean weight for height Z-score was - 1.6 SD, the mean skinfolds (tricipital and sub-scapular) was only about 6 mm and the arm circumference was about 23 cm.

TABLE 2.4 WEIGHT GAIN IN KG DURING PREGNANCY (45)

	TRIMESTER (*)		
	1st	2nd	3rd
FOETUS			
- Foetus		1.0	3.4
- Placenta		0.3	0.6
- Amiotic liquid		0.4	1.0
Total (1)		1.7	5.0
MOTHERS ORGANS			
- Uterus	0.3	0.8	1.0
- Brest	0.1	1.0	3.4
- Blood volume	0.3	1.0	3.4
- Intestinal liquid			1.7
Total (2)	0.7	2.4	4.5
Total (1+2)	0.7	4.1	9.5
General weight gain		14.3	

(*) At the end of each trimester

FIGURE 2.5. Evolution of weight gain during pregnancy

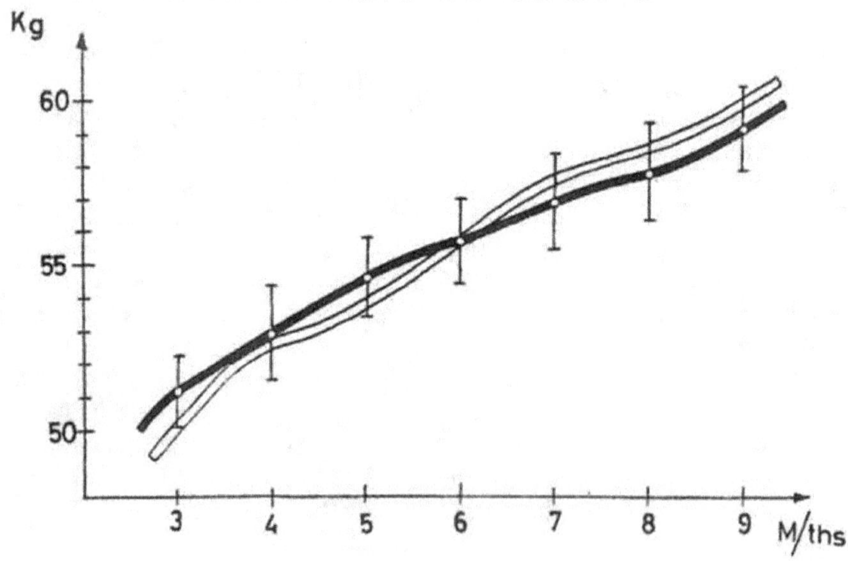

TABLE 2.5. CERTAIN MEASUREMENTS AT DIFFERENT MONTHS OF PREGNANCY
(Value and standart deviation)

TRIMESTER **Month of pregnancy**	**1 st** **3.0**	**2 nd** **5.2**	**3 rd** **7.8**
WEIGHT (kg)	51.2 5.2 (n=33) *52.5 7.0*	54.5 5.7 (n=264) *54.7 7.3*	57.6 6.2 (n=352) *56.7 7.0*
SUBSCAPULAR (mm)	8.2 2.6 (n=32) *12.2 4.6*	9.0 3.2 (n=261) *12.7 4.8*	8.4 2.9 (n=341) *12.9 5.6*
TRICIPITAL (mm)	**7.7** 2.8 (n=33) *14.2 5.4*	7.8 2.8 (n=269) *14.6 5.0*	7.3 2.5 (n=360) *14.6 8.5*
BRACHIAL PERIMETRE (cm)	24.2 2.0 (n=35) *24.8 3.1*	24.3 2.2 (n=270) 25.0 *3.4*	24.0 1.9 (n=364) *24.5 2.13*
BRACHIAL SURFACE (cm^2)	47.1 7.3 (n=35) *49.0*	47.5 8.7 (n=270) *49.8*	46.2 7.6 (n=364) *47.8*
MUSCULAR SURFACE (cm^2)	38.1 5.7 (n=33) *33.4 9.6*	38.3 6.3 (n=269) *34.0 12.1*	37.7 5.7 (n=360) 32.2 *5.6*
ADIPOSE SURFACE (cm^2)	8.9 3.8 (n=33) *49.0 3.1*	9.2 3.8 (n=269) 16.8 *7.4*	8.5 3.3 (n=360) 15.9 *6.9*
TIBIAL PERIMETER (cm)	29.6 2.2 (n=34)	30.0 2.1 (n=270)	29.9 2.1 (n=362)
CALF PERIMETER (cm)	47.1 4.5 (n=34)	47.5 3.9 (n=270)	47.3 4.1 (n=361)
THORAX PERIMETER (cm)	79.5 3.3 (n=34)	80.4 3.5 (n=270)	80.6 3.8 (n=361)
ABDOMINAL PERIMETER (cm)	70.1 4 .7 (n=33)	76.3 5.0 (n=269)	83.1 5.1 (n=364)

Data in italic concern Kenyan pregnant women (Jansen – 43)

TABLE 2.6. CERTAIN MEASUREMENTS FOR PREGNANT WOMEN

MEASUREMENTS in cm	n	mean	S.D.	Minimum	Maximum
HEIGHT	389	167.4	5.7	152.8	185.2
HAED CIRCUMFERENCE	386	53.9	1.5	49.8	58.8
ARM LENGTH	390	79.4	3.6	71.2	91.8

TABLE 2.7. WEIGHT (IN KG) AT DIFFERENT MONTHS OF PREGNANCY

MONTHS	n	mean	S.D.	Minimum	Maximum	**Percentils**		
						5°	**50°**	**95°**
3	33	51.2	5.2	39.3	60.9	42.6	50.8	60.8
4	55	52.6	6.0	37.8	66.2	42.2	52.3	63.4
5	91	54.5	5.4	43.8	68.5	46.8	54.7	64.3
6	118	55.4	5.7	42.7	69.5	46.8	54.7	66.2
2nd trimester	**264**	**54.5**	**5.7**	**37.8**	**69.5**	**46.1**	**54.2**	**65.4**
7	135	56.9	6.2	43.8	71.4	47.0	56.4	67.5
8	164	57.7	6.2	43.0	71.9	47.6	58.0	68.9
9	53	59.2	5.7	45.1	72.7	47.9	58.7	70.3
3rd trimester	**352**	**57.6**	**6.2**	**43.0**	**71.9**	**47.6**	**58.0**	**68.9**

As comparing with data from Kenyan pregnant women (Jansen – 43), the weight at the second trimester was similar (54.7 +- 7.3 kg) and at the third trimester it was slightly higher (56.7 +- 7.0 kg).

TABLE 2.8. BRACHIAL PERIMETER (IN CM) AT DIFFERENT MONTHS OF PREGNANCY

MONTHS	n	mean	S.D.	Minimum	Maximum	Percentils 5°	50°	95°
3	35	24.2	2.0	20.4	28.9	21.3	24.5	28.3
4	57	24.5	2.2	20.2	31.5	21.8	24.2	28.3
5	92	24.5	2.4	20.5	33.5	21.2	24.3	28.3
6	121	24.2	1.9	20.0	30.0	21.3	23.9	28.1
2nd trimester	**270**	**24.3**	**2.2**	**20.0**	**35.5**	**21.9**	**24.2**	**28.1**
7	139	24.2	2.0	20.1	31.6	21.2	24.2	27.3
8	169	24.0	2.1	19.7	31.3	20.6	23.9	27.5
9	56	23.9	1.5	20.0	27.5	21.3	23.6	26.5
3rd trimester	**364**	**24.0**	**1.9**	**19.7**	**31.6**	**21.0**	**23.9**	**27.3**

TABLE 2.9. SKINFOLD THICKNESS in *mm (REPARTITION IN PERCENTILS)*

	p 5	p 10	p 25	p 50	p 75	p 90	p 95
TRICIPITAL							
3rd month	3.8	4.3	5.9	7.1	8.9	10.6	15.8
2nd trimester	4.4	4.9	5.8	7.3	9.2	12.0	13.7
3rd trimester	4.0	4.5	5.5	6.8	8.8	10.8	12.2
SUB-SCAPULAR							
3rd month	4.8	5.6	6.8	7.8	8.8	12.0	15.1
2nd trimester	4.8	5.5	6.8	8.0	10.5	13.8	15.6
3rd trimester	4.7	5.2	6.4	7.8	9.8	12.0	13.7

TABLE 2.10. BRACHIAL, MUSCULAR AND ADIPOSE SURFACE in cm²
(mean and SD) AT DIFFERENT MONTHS OF PREGNANCY

Month of pregnancy		3	4	5	6	7	8	9
	n	34	57	92	121	139	169	56
Brachial surface	mean	47.1	48.1	48.0	46.8	46.7	46.0	45.7
	S.D.	7.9	8.7	9.9	7.7	7.7	7.9	6.1
	n	34	56	92	121	137	167	56
Muscular surface	mean	38.0	38.4	38.5	38.1	37.9	37.6	37.7
	S.D.	5.6	5.3	7.3	5.8	6.1	5.8	4.2
	n	33	56	92	121	137	167	56
Adipose surface	mean	8.9	9.6	9.5	8.8	8.8	8.4	8.0
	S.D.	3.8	4.2	3.9	3.5	3.4	3.3	3.0

The **muscular surface** (MS) was calculated using measurements of arm circumference (AC) and the tricipital skinfold (TS), based on the following formula :

$MS = n\, r^2$ or $r = AC/2n - TS/2$ or $MS = n^2\,(AC/n - TS)$

The **adipose surface** (AS) was calculated by difference of brachial surface (BS) and muscular surface (MS) : $AS = BS - MS$

TABLE 2.11. OMBILICAL CIRCUMFERENCE (IN CM) AT DIFFERENT MONTHS

MONTHS	n	mean	S.D.	Minimum	Maximum	Percentils 5°	50°	95°
3	33	70.1	4.7	61.0	81.0	63.0	70.0	79.6
4	57	72.7	4.7	62.0	85.0	64.0	73.0	80.0
5	91	76.1	4.6	66.0	88.0	68.0	75.0	85.0
6	121	78.2	4.6	63.0	91.0	71.0	78.0	86.9
2nd trimester	**269**	**76.3**	**5.0**	**62.0**	**91.0**	**68.0**	**76.0**	**85.0**
7	138	81.3	5.0	72.0	98.0	73.9	81.0	89.0
8	169	83.4	4.9	70.0	98.0	75.0	83.0	92.0
9	57	86.3	4.7	78.0	98.0	79.0	86.0	95.3
3rd trimester	**354**	**83.1**	**5.1**	**70.0**	**98.0**	**74.0**	**83.0**	**92.0**

2.2.2. ANTHROPOMETRIC DATA OF INFANTS

For all of the 247 children, 1497 measurements of weight and height were analysed in a transversal way and compared to the HCHS reference recommended in the WHO growth chart for international use in maternal and child health care (1978).

The weight of the infants was inferior to NCHS norms (46), but the height was superior. For boys, after age 14 months, the 97° percentile of weight became inferior to the median of the reference HCHS standards (figure 2.6). The same phenomena were observed for girls, after age 7 months (figure 2.7). The weight for height was -1.3 SD.

The attempt to get a model was carried out on a sub-sample of 67 children, based on the Berkey program (48). The predicted mean growth curve is different than those of American children: the growth speed was faster, followed by a more important bend (figure 2.8).

For analysing the growth of children in the first period of life in remote areas, some aspects have to be taken into consideration:

- difficulties to carry out anthropometrical, clinical and nutritional examinations at regular intervals («target times»),
- difficulties of determination maturity, due to some missing values of birth date, birth weight and height,
- problems of *choice* and application of existing models. We tried two models: Kouchi and Jenss-Bayley. It seems that the Jenss-Bayley model, modified to this particular study, may be the best fitting model to the irregularity of data and time intervals of examinations. However this model could be applied only to 67 children for the following reasons: 1°- the necessity to have a minimum of 5 measurements in the first 15 months of life, 2°- the first measurement has to be performed before the age of 4 months and the last may not be considered if done before the 12 months, 3°- 21 children owning the above characteristics had an «unsatisfying adjustment».

The weight and height curve during the first 30 months of life is shown in figure 2.9. Figure 2.10 shows the weight to height Z-score, the height to age Z-score and the weight to height Z-score. We observed a rapid decrease in the three curves between the 3rd and 9th month. When compared the height curve and the arm length curve (figure 2.11) it appears that the arm length doubles between the first three years. The curves of the tricipital and sub scapular skin fold thicknesses are shown in figure 2.12. It is obvious, that at age 0-30 months, less fat tissue is present. The tricipital skin fold is slightly increased in the third year of life. The mean head circumference (figure 2.13) increases rapidly with age, from 40 to 50 cm at the end of three years.

FIGURE 2.6. Weight growth curve of Sudanese boys and NCHS reference.

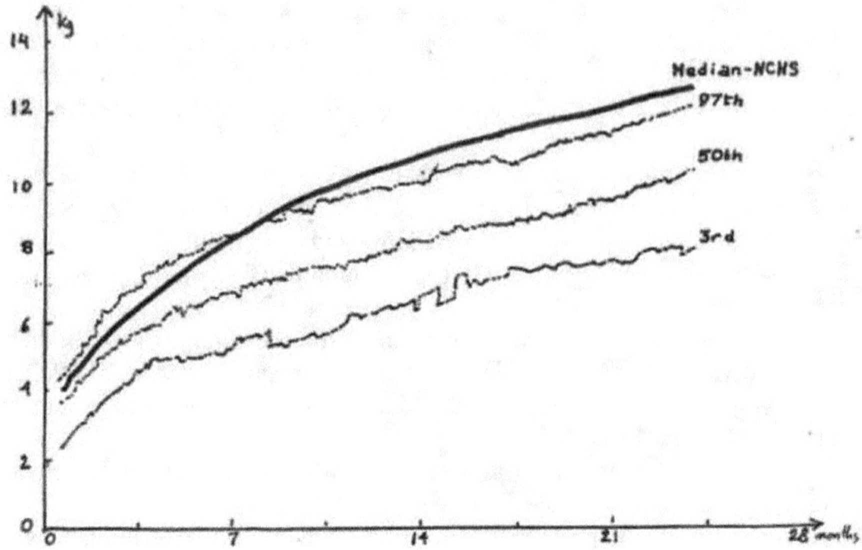

FIGURE 2.7. Weight growth curve of Sudanese girls and NCHS reference.

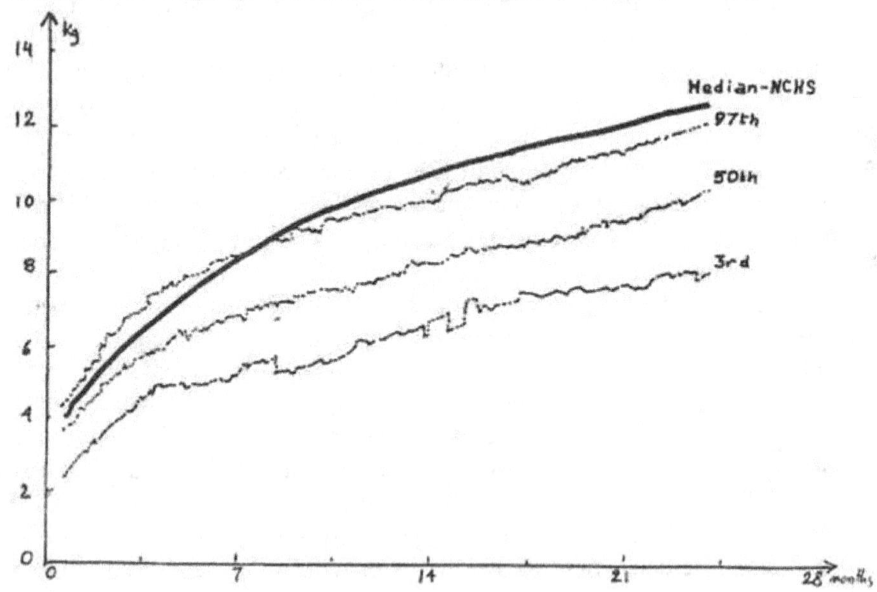

FIGURE 2.8. Predict mean growth curve of Sudanese children (A.D.E.) and other authors (Berkey, Manwani and Deming).

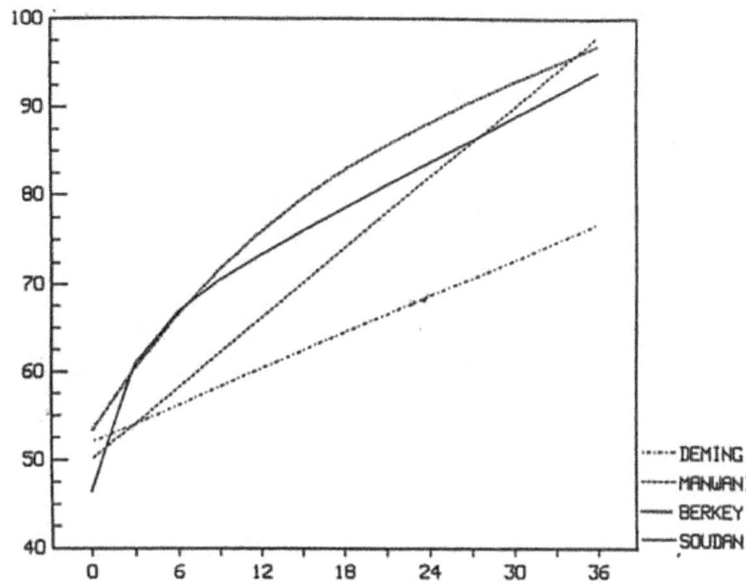

FIGURE 2.9. Weight and height curve during the first 30 months of life

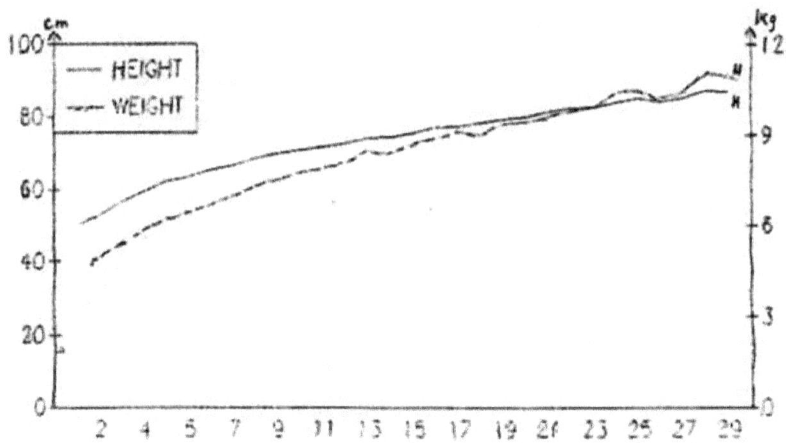

FIGURE 2.10. Weight to height Z-score, Height to Age Z-score and Weigh to Height Z-score in the first 30 months of life

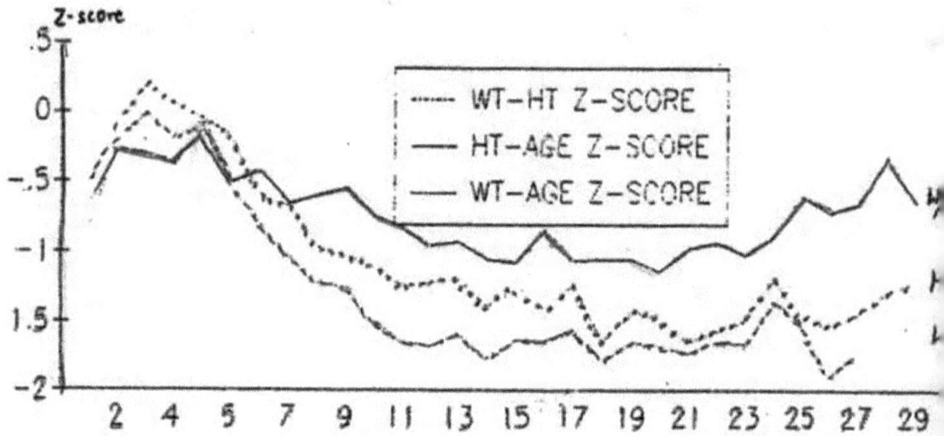

FIGURE 2.11. The height curve and the arm length curve in the first 30 months

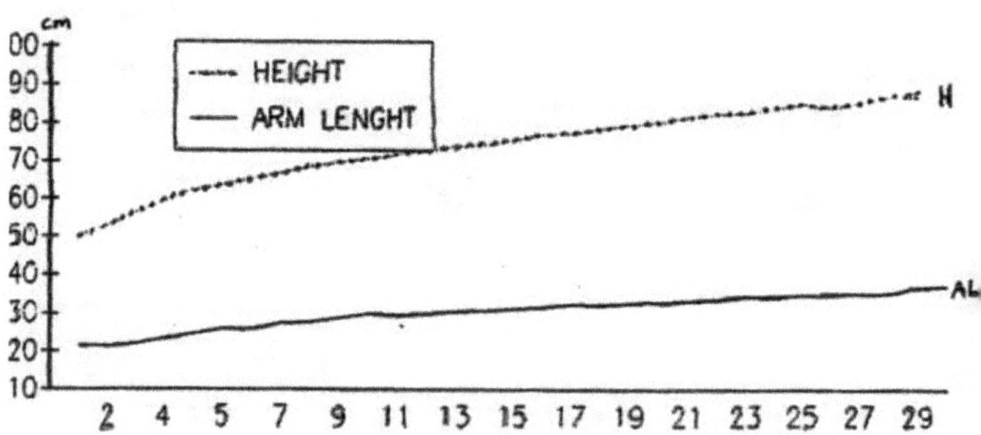

FIGURE 2.12.Tricipital and subscapular skin fold thickness in the first 30 months

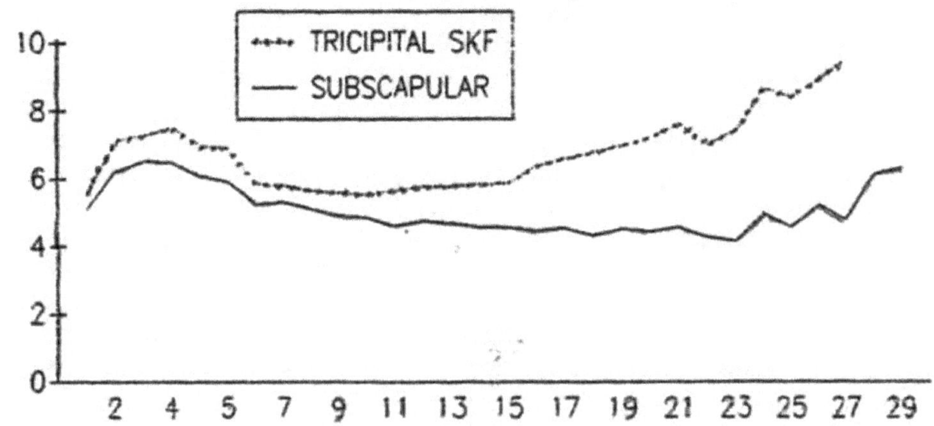

FIGURE 2.13. Mean head circumference in the first 30 months of life

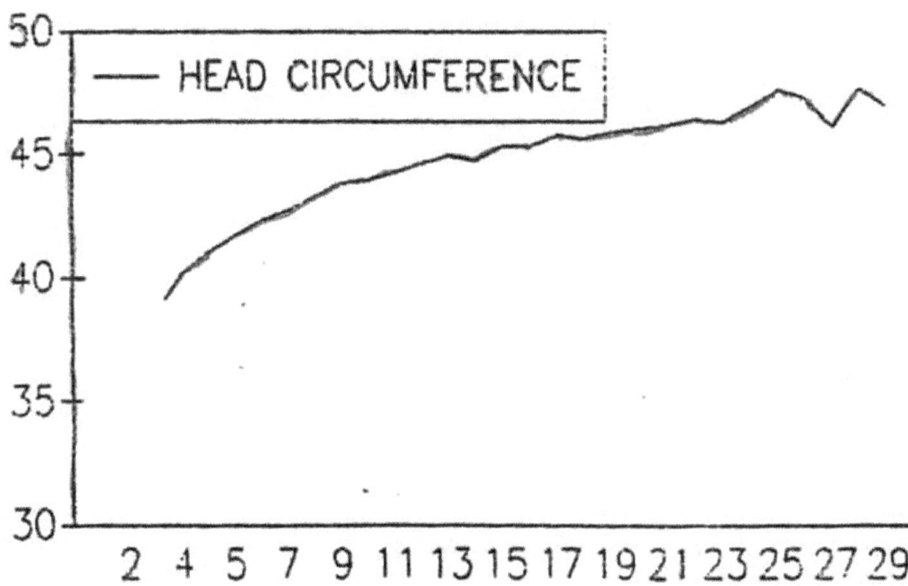

2.3. DISCUSSION

This is one of the largest complex studies on the health and nutritional status in a representative sample of a population of children, men and women, including pregnant and lactating women in the sub-saharian Africa.

In the group of 75 Shilluk children (less than 14 years old) and 156 adults (from the cross-sectional study), the anthropometrical measurements show that the Nilotic are tall and very slim. Their weight to height Z-score, based on CDC Atlanta reference show that with age (until 9 years) it decreases (- 1,80 S.D.). Wolff (49) found also a decrease in Z-score after age 4 years in children from a rural area in Peru. According to Dibley (37) Z-score is an important anthropometric indicator

The Quetelet Index shows the similar decrease in children from 16 to 13 kg/m². In adults it reached again 16 to 18 kg/m². This increase can be explained more by muscle development than by fat. The skin fold thickness was only ~5 mm. Brown (50) found similar skin fold thickness in children studied in a poor rural area in Bangladesh.

Chali (51) obtained data similar to ours, in a study of the same population (Dinka, Nuer and Shilluk) displaced by the civil war to a camp in Itang in Ethiopia. The mean height and weight of men were 175.9 +/-9cm and 59.7 +/-8kg and those of women were 169.0 +/-7cm and 54.0 +/- 8kg. The author observed also that the mean height of Dinka men (176.4 +/-9cm) and Nuer men (175.7 +/-9cm) were significantly higher than that of Shilluk men (172.6 +/-6.1cm). However in this large sample (2.233) the population was shorter and heavier than ours. Their height was shorter probably because of a mixture of different sub-groups and heavier because of better food in the Itang camp.

The mid upper arm circumference (MUAC) of the southern Sudaneses under A.D.E. study was in the range of normal for the Nilotic population. It is also similar to data obtained by Wolff (49) in his study of a poor population in Peru. It is one of sensitive indices in nutritional studies. Also Briend (52) choose MUAC as an indicator of the nutritional status. According to him, children with a MUAC of less than 11cm are obviously malnourished and growth charts are not needed to identify them. Many studies have already suggested that mid-upper arm is better than other anthropometric indices for screening and identification of children at high risk of death. Briend (52) mentioned that children with MUAC of less than 110 mm are obviously malnourished and growth charts are not needed to identify them. For Chen (53) mid upper arm circumference is better than other anthropometric indices for screening and identification of younger children at high risk of death.

Herrera (11) in his north-Sudanese study classified as stunted children who fell below -2 Z-score in height-for-age and as wasted those who fell below -2 Z-score in weight-for-height, calculated by reference to the National Centre for Health Statistics (NCHS) standard (46).

As to Broek (12), children below the customary cut-off point of -2 Z-score for weight-for-height may be at higher risk of death. For Fawzi (1) the risk of death was increased only for children less than -3 Z-score. This statement cannot be applied universally and especially to African population. In our case, the very tall Nilotic Nuer in the South-Sudan have a Z-score lower than -2 Z-score. Only for children less than 2 Z-score the normal range is around -0,7 Z-score. It is therefore unwise to use as reference the CDC data as reference (*) and to classify malnutrition even wasted or stunted in the African communities. The example of negative Z-score is contradictory with the low frequency of severe malnutrition in this population. Fawzi (27) considered as abnormal all values <-2 Z-Scores of the National Venter for Health Statistics. Also Brown (50) and Dibley (37) underlined that the children's patterns of growth differed from those of the NCHS references and can't be used directly for the local population.

Also other studies in the third world shows, that using NCHS references, the weight of children 0 - 60 months is «pathological» lower (Brown – 50).

For Stoltzfus (54) the prevalence of height-for-age Z-score <-2 rose from 14% in 7 years old Zanzibar children to 83% in 13 years old. Prevalence of weight-for-age Z-score <-2 in children <10 years was 10% or less. The variability in growth increments was explained by anaemia (for weight gain) and schistosomiasis (for height gain). The author suggests that appropriate prevention might prevent stunting in late childhood.

The hypothesis of Beaton (55) that the state of being stunted or «small» may be associated with a decreased capacity for physical work later in life, increased risk of morbidity and adverse effects of mental development is wrong because «tall» (as well as «small») adapted to their environment and way of life are healthy physically and mentally. We didn't find confirmation of Beaton's hypothesis.

Of course, if we change the environment rapidly and the way of life to an extremely different one, the Africans may not be able to follow this rapid change. It would be of interest to study the health and mental status, for example, of obese Americans exposed rapidly to an African environment.

(*) The references data are based on a population, where more than 30% are overweight or obese.

3. HEALTH STATUS

by Z. L. Ostrowski, M.-Ch. Josse, G. I. Suliman, G. Habib, A. Armengaud, B. Semichon, A. Davion

Clinical exams were carried out by a medical doctor and blood and urine samples were analysed at place by a medical laboratory assistant.

The morbidity was determined by a medical doctor based on a clinical examination and laboratory examination. Symptoms and diagnosis were registered using WHO codes (56). Diarrhoea, was registered if more than three loose or watery lotions per day for more than one day period have been observed.

Among the 295 adults and children under study, the most frequent symptoms in adults were fever, abdominal pain and headache, followed by cough and chest pain (table 3.1). The different abnormal clinical signs detected in each age group of children are presented in table 3.2. The most frequent detected signs were pallor, conjunctivitis, and splenomegalia. In children under 5 years mostly nasal discharges (33%) and conjunctivitis (26%) were observed. In elderly children more splenomegalia (27%) were detected.

The most important groups were infectious and parasitic diseases. Malaria which is endemic in this region was a major health problem (table 3.3), especially in children under five years (51%); it was confirmed by a positive blood film in some cases. Anemia or pallor was very frequent. 45% of children under five years of age had a level of haemoglobin below 11g/dl (blood sample analysed with Coulter Counter). Gastro-enteritis, intestinal amebiasis and intestinal gardiasis were grouped as intestinal infectious diseases which were mostly in early childhood (28% in the first five years).

During pregnancy, among past illnesses and symptoms, malaria and abdominal pain have been mentioned as the most frequent in the 3rd month. Backache and fever were more often in the third trimester (table 3.4). Final diagnosis by a medical doctor confirmed that most of the pregnant women suffered from malaria during pregnancy (table 3.5).

Table 3.1. The most frequent symptoms

SYMPTOMS	n	% (*)
Fever	88	29.8
Abdominal pain	50	16.9
Headache	39	13.2
Nausea and vomiting	23	7.8
Cough	23	7.8
Chest pain	20	6.8
No data	52	17.7

(*) The dominator is the total number of the population examined

TABLE 3.2. The abnormal signs and their frequency (*) in different age groups

SIGNS	Children 0-5 years		Children 6-14 years		Adults >14 years		Total	
	n	%	n	%	n	%	n	%
Conjunctivitis	22	26,2	14	12,2	64	23,5	100	23,8
Eye infections	2	2,4	3	4,7	53	19,4	58	13,8
Pallor	19	22,6	18	28,6	75	27,5	112	26,7
Nasal discharge	28	33,3	2	3,2	3	1,1	33	7,9
Kolimychia	-	-	1	1,6	-	-	1	0,2
Clubbing	1	1,2	2	3,2	8	2,9	11	2,6
Hepatomegalia	3	3,8	6	9,5	26	9,5	35	8,3
Splenomegalia	9	10,7	17	27,0	44	16,1	70	16,7

(*) The dominator is the total number of the population examined

TABLE 3.3. The most important diseases and their frequency in different age groups

DIAGNOSIS	Children 0-5 years n	%	Children 6-14 years n	%	Adults >14 years n	%	Total n	%
Malaria (acute attack)	33	50,8	29	55,8	68	42,8	130	46,7
Anaemia *	10	15,4	7	13,5	31	19,5	48	17,2
Intestinal infec-tious diseases	14	21,5	5	9,6	19	12,0	38	13,6
Malaria based On blood film **	6	9,2	7	13,4	26	16,3	39	14,0
Other parasitic diseases	2	3,1	4	7,7	15	9,4	21	7,5

(*) Laboratory diagnosis using Coulter counter S-5
(**) Positive blood films for malaria (thin and thick blood films)

TABLE 3.4. PAST ILLNESS AND SYMPTOMS DURING PREGNANCY (in percentage)

GESTIONAL AGE in months	3 n=34 %	4 n=57 %	5 n=92 %	6 n=121 %	7 n=140 %	8 n=169 %	9 n=58 %
Malaria	55.9	40.4	42.4	28.1	35.7	32.0	31.0
TTI & GTI		3.5	2.2	2.5	2.9	0.6	3.4
Jaundice				1.7	1.4	0.6	1.7
Fever	8.8	7.0	8.7	9.9	10.0	13.0	10.3
Vomiting		1.8	5.4	0.8	5.7	1.8	1.7
Abdominal pain	29.4	22.8	21.7	24.0	19.3	23.1	13.8
Diarrhoea	2.9		2.2	0.8	2.9	0.6	
Other digestive	5.3	3.3	5.0	3.6	6.5	5.2	
Caught	8.8	5.3	9.8	9.9	5.7	7.7	8.6
Palpitation		5.3	1.1	5.8	4.3	4.1	8.6
Chest pain		1.8	1.1	1.7	2.9	3.6	5.2
Headache	8.8	17.5	25.0	27.3	25.0	18.9	8.6
Backache	8.8	12.3	13.0	18.2	9.3	18.3	10.3
Joint pain	5.9	15.8	7.6	13.2	6.4	13.0	1.7
Body pain	2.9	5.3	7.6	7.4	9.3	5.9	5.2
Weakness		1.8	4.4	1.7	2.1	5.3	1.7
Genital bleeding		5.3	1.1				1.7
Skin symptoms			1.1	1.7	1.4	0.6	
Other	8.8	17.5	17.4	20.7	21.4	18.9	10.3

TABLE 3.5. FINAL DIAGNOSIS FOR PREGNANT WOMEN expressed in percentage

GESTIONAL AGE in months	3 n=34 %	4 n=57 %	5 n=92 %	6 n=121 %	7 n=140 %	8 n=169 %	9 n=58 %
Malaria	5.9	10.5	7.6	10.7	12.9	7.7	12.1
Anaemia	5.9	5.3	5.4	5.8	5.0	5.3	6.9
UTI	5.9	3.5	8.7	2.5	3.6	4.1	5.2
Other	5.9	1.5	9.8	9.1	8.6	18.9	1.7

3.1. MALARIA

Malaria was a major health problem in the studied area, especially in children under five. The diagnosis was based mainly on clinical examinations. In children malaria was often presented as gastro-intestinal symptoms. It was wise to start the treatment once the clinical diagnosis was achieved and not to wait for laboratory confirmation as negative blood film does not exclude the diagnosis. No resistance to chloriquine was detected in this area. Cerebral forms were rare in this population. According to our results, this area can be classified as meso-endemic. The splenic rate in children aged 2-10 years was found to be 28,6%.

Past history for malaria was given by 45% of pregnant women. Splenomegalia was found in 21% of cases with clinical malaria. Meanwhile the frequency of hepatomegalia was 5% and that of pallor was 36,2%. Thin and thick blood films were examined: 26% were positive for malaria. According to the laboratory results the most common plasmodium in this area was falciparum. (*Plasmodium Falciparum seems to be responsible for cerebral malaria. In this study, cerebral malaria was stated as rare and Plasmodium Falciparum showed not occur frequently. Probably the population has a good resistance to Plasmodium Falciparum. It would be preferable to carry out a second study*).

During the pilot study in 1981, Datry (57) found that 85% of the population had serological evidence of malaria parasites in their blood. However in the series of 60 blood films, all were negative for plasmodia. The explanation for these findings may be due to seasonal factors. When blood samples are obtained in the dry season, as many of the second batches were, then it was quite normal to find no parasites. However the amount of blood on the slides was not thick enough, for Datry, to exclude with complete confidence the possibility that parasites were not present.

Few years later (1993) in a control group of children from the same area, but displaced to Polataka at the southern borders of the Sudan due to a military conflict, parasites have been found in the blood samples. In a series of 132 blood films, analysed by Douay and Adam (*), 66 were negative for plasmodia. On the 66 positive blood films, 64 (97%) contain plasmodium falciparum and 2 (3%) plasmodium vivax (table 3.6). Between the 64 falciparum, 28% were gametocytes and 72% trophozoïtes (in 5 blood films gametocytes and trophozoïtes were present). An association of plasmodium falciparum and plasmodium vivax or plasmodium malaria was found in 5 blood films.

* *Douay and Adam, Hôpital Trousseau, Department of Hematology, Paris*

Table 3.6. PARASITOLOGICAL FINDINGS IN 66 POSITIVE BLOOD FILMS

PLASMODIUM	DIFFERENT FORMS	ASSOCIATIONS
PLASMODIUM FALCIPARUM 6 cases (97%)	46 Trophozoites (72%) (ring forms) 13 Gametocytes (20%) 5 Gametocytes + Trophozoites (8%)	Single : 59 cases Associations : 5 cases + pl. vivax : 3 cases + pl. malariae: 2 cases
PLASMODIUM VIVAX 2 cases (3%)	Trophozoites (ring forms) + Schizonts	

(*) Prof. Douay and Dr Adam, Department of Haematology, Hôpital Trousseau, PARIS

3.2. ANAEMIA

Anaemia was diagnosed on haemoglobin values (Hb%), using Coulter Counter S-5 which also gave other haematological values (white blood cells, red blood cells, haematocrite and mean cell volume). The diagnosis was established with reference to WHO Standards (1968) for age, sex or pregnancy status.

The general prevalence was 28% (table 3.7). The prevalence of anaemia was highest in children under 5 years (54,5% for 0-3yrs and 36,4% for 3-5yrs). This could be explained by a prolonged breastfeeding (more than 2 years) and a late introduction of solid foods, besides cow's milk. The main food during diversification was cow's milk, poor in iron. In this age group the mean cell volume (MCV) showed microcytosis. In children, above 5 years old, anaemia was less prevalent, mostly due to different factors (parasitic diseases, malaria, repeated infections and malnutrition...).

It was found that acute attack of clinical malaria does not affect the haemoglobin values (table 3.8). Nail signs of iron deficiency were not frequent in this population. Between ethnicities some difference was evident. The prevalence of anaemia was the same but iron deficiency was more prevalent in Nuer, especially in women.

In pregnant women, the haemoglobin levels were taken as an index of their nutritional status and the subjects were divided into four groups based on their haemoglobin status: 1° group < 8.5 g/dl (very low); 2° group : 8.5 - 10 g/dl (low); 3° group 10 - 11 g/dl (moderate); 4° group >11g/dl (normal). For the pregnant women sample, 2% were in the very low group, 10% in the low group, 22% in the moderate group and 66% in the normal group.

TABLE 3.7. Frequency of anaemia (as laboratory diagnosis) by age and sexes

Age and sexes group	sample size	n	%
6 - 35 months	11	6	54.5
3 - 5 years	11	4	36.4
6 - 13 years	34	7	20.6
Males 13> years	55	18	16.4
Females 13> years	51	12	23.5
Pregnant women	9	1	11.1
Total	171	48	28.0

TABLE 3.8. Mean haemoglobin levels (g/l) not affected by acute attack of malaria

Age and sexes group	**No Malaria**			**Malaria**			Signif.
	n	mean	SD	n	mean	SD	
0 - 5 years	5	11,3	1,13	17	10,9	1,18	N.S.
6 - 14 years	17	12,7	1,30	17	12,9	1,52	N.S.
Females 14> years	26	12,9	2,26	26	13,2	1,17	N.S.
Males 14> years	30	13,7	2,05	26	14,7	1,80	N.S.

** WHO reference : Children 6 months - 6 years = 11 g/dlHb*
Children 6 years - 14 years = 12 g/dlHb
Men = 13 g/dlHb
Women = 12 g/dlHb
Pregnant women = 11 g/dlHb

3.3. PARASITIC DISEASES

The most frequent parasitic diseases in this area, other than malaria, were intestinal amoebiasis and gardiasis. Table 3.9 shows the frequency of the different parasitic disease. No shistosomiasis was detected by laboratory analysis or it was difficult to confirm (in stool).

3.4. EYE INFECTIONS

The incidence of eye infections in children between 2 months and 5 years was 4%. Meanwhile in adults the higher incidence (28%) may be attributed to repeated severe infections.

TABLE 3.9. Frequency of different parasitic diseases

PARASITIC DISEASES	n	%
Malaria (acute attack)	130	62.2
Intestinal amoebiasis	25	12.0
Chronic visceral malaria	18	8.6
Intestinal gardiasis	13	6.2
Ascariasis	4	1.9
Urinary schistosomiasis *	2	1.0
Unspecified intestinal helmenthiasis	1	0.5
Other unspecified parasitic diseases	16	7.7
Total	209	100

(*) Not confirmed biologically (no urine)

3.5. CONJUNCTIVITIS AND NASOPHARYNGITIS

Conjunctivitis is a very common health problem in this population; most of the cases were mucopurulent conjunctivitis. Nasopharyngitis in children under 5 was very frequent (56%). The role of flies and lack of hygiene (personal and general) was the main cause. In children, very often purulent nasal discharge was followed by conjunctivitis. A simple prevention could be achieved by hygiene and control of house flies.

3.6. OTHER DISSEASES AND SYMPTOMS

Between a great number of rare diseases and symptoms the most impressive are :

- scarifications,(photo 9) often transformed into kyloides (photo 10), sometimes so important that there was a great restriction of body movement,
- goiter, especially between young women, with two to three great lobs (photo 11),
- hyperkeratose of skin mostly of knees in elderly population (photo 12),
- spteno- hepatomegaly, with dilated blood vessels on enlarged abdomen (photo 13),
- cachexia, mostly in elderly women population (photo 14),
- hunchbacked (photo 15),
- fractures (photo 16).

3.7. DISCUSSION

The health status of the Sudanese Nilotic population was not bad compared with other African populations. Malaria, anaemia and parasitic infections are the main diseases in this population. Eye infections, conjunctivitis and nasopharyngitis have been the most important symptoms. Cough, fever or accidents were largely observed and had no major impact of the health status.

According to DeMayer (58) 43% of all women and 34% of all men are anaemic in developing regions. Fawzi (1) using data from Herrera's study (11) of the northern Sudanese population mentioned that the main symptoms observed or collected by questioning the families and neighbours in case of death, were diarrhoea, cough, breathless, fever, rash, convulsions or accident. The relation between weight-for-height and mortality was more pronounced among children who were 2-4 years of age than among those younger or older. Following Haggaz and coll. (59) "*maternal anaemia was the main risk factor for LBW (odds ratio: 5.1, 95% Cl 1.7-15.2; P=0.003)*".

Broek (12) in his study among children 0-5 years old in Zaïre observed that the commonest causes of death were malaria and anaemia, when death directly attributed to marasmus or kwashiorkor were excluded.

According to Snow (60), malaria remains the most important health problem in Africa and a major public health challenge in sub-Saharian Africa. For Premji (61), plasmodium falciparum malaria was commonly associated with anaemia in children living in holo-endemic malaria areas.

In Sudan, following Abdalla and coll. (62), "*malaria incidence was estimated to be about 9 million episodes in 2002 and the number of deaths due to malaria was about 44.000. Children under five years of age had the highest burden*". Also for Giha and coll (63) "*severe malaria was recognized in all age groups, but 44.5% of patients were aged 2 to 4 years*". For Adam and coll. (64) in Eastern Sudan, "*not only primigravidae but all parities were infected with falciparum malaria and different manifestations of severity were detected*".

Snow (65) associated kwashiorkor, measles, trauma, convulsions and neonatal tetanus with childhood death, in rural east Africa. For Seaman (32) poor nutrition contributed to the risk of clinical infections.

Taha (66) reported that malaria was significantly associated with low birth weight and that stillbirth was significantly increased among women who reported malaria attacks in the first and second trimesters of pregnancy (30). The knowledge concerning malaria in the population is poor. In Elzubier's study (67) between students in eastern Sudan there were deficiencies regarding knowledge of the seriousness of malaria in primigravidas and children. Malaria attacks were always observed. Even after treatment malaria attacks persisted. Greenwood (68) showed in a study in Gambia that stopping chemoprophylaxis after a period of several years increased even the risk of clinical malaria. With or without chemoprophylaxis the clinical attacks of malaria continue. Diarrhoea as a cause of death was not common in Bwamanda or Kasongo areas in Zair (12, 69) but a maternal behavioural risk factor for severe childhood diarrhoeal diseases was observed by Dikassa in Kinshasa (70).

In a study in the North Sudan (30), on 29.615 children age 0-72 months, about 17% had diarrhoea, >20% cough and 0,3% measles. Following Rozov (71), in a 1 month to 1 year old age group, the leading cause of mortality in Sudan (52%) is diarrhoea. According to NCHS standards, 38% were considered as stunted, 6% as wasted, another 6% as stunted and wasted and 50% as normal. Bayoumi (72) described a high prevalence of lactose malabsorption among the Nilotic

The most frequent diseases and symptoms are shown in figure 3.1.

FIGURE 3.1. The most frequent diseases and symptoms

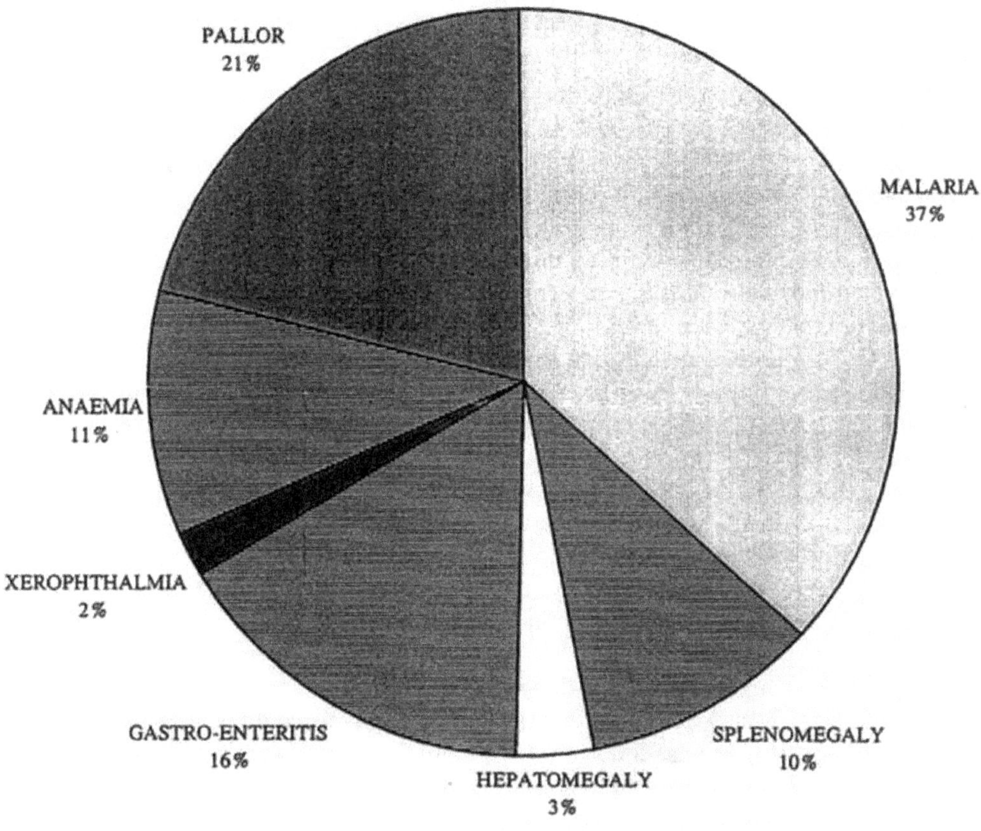

4. BIOLOGICAL DATA

by Z. L. Ostrowski, P. Aymard*, M. Pressac*, M.-Ch. Josse, J. v. Rooij, G. I. Suliman,

Because of difficulties to get blood samples in the studied population a limited number of data was available. A sample of 132 persons from the cross-sectional study (218 cases), and a sample of 74 persons from the longitudinal study (948 cases) were submitted for biological analyses. The longitudinal study covered a period of 3 years but blood samples have been taken during the last year of the study and only once for each person. The blood samples of 206 people were divided into three sub-groups. The repartition by age and sexes, in each studies cohort, is shown in table 4.1.

The biological values were compared with French, American and some available data of African Masai population. The comparison between the Shilluk and Nuer population is given by age and sexes groups.

4.1. SERUM PROTEIN PATTERN

In both ethnic groups of adults, the total serum protein level (73,95±5,74 and 79,55±8,24) was higher than common mean values observed in temperate climates due primarily to a very high gamma globulin level (table 4.2).

In Nuer adults and children the level of protein and gamma-globulin are significantly higher ($p<0.001$) than in Shilluk (table 4.2 and 4.3). The distribution is also significantly skewed in Nuer. These high levels could be explained partially by dehydration because the study in the Nuer area has been carried out at the end of the dry season, when water was hardly available.

In Shilluk elderly children the values are significantly higher than in infants ($p<0.001$) (table 4.5). Between Shilluk men and women there are no differences (respectively 74,00±5,52 for men and 73,95±6,22 for women) (table 4.4).

In Shilluk pregnant women, the values of protein and albumin were in the range, but significantly ($p<0.0001$) lower than in non pregnant or lactating women. The albumin values increase normally (32,25 mmol/l) (table 4.6).
The histogram (figure 4.1) shows the value of protein in age and sexe groups. The histogram (figure 4.2) shows the distribution of albumin, gamma-, alfa1-, alfa2- and beta-globulin in age and sexe groups.

* *Hôpital Armand Trousseau, Laboratoire de Biochimie, Paris*

TABLE 4.1. Number of cases for the biological analyses of the crossectional and longitudinal studies

STUDIES	Ethnicity	Class	Total number	Biological sample n	%	Mean age
CROSSECTIONAL	SHILLUK	Children 4-14 years	52	22	42%	10 years
		Women > 14 years	28	19	68%	28 years
		Men > 14 years	36	30	83%	33 years
	NUER	Children 4-14 years	14	11	79%	9 years
		Women > 14 years	57	33	58%	29 years
		Men > 14 years	31	17	55%	35 years
		Sub-total	**218**	**132**	**61%**	
LONGITUDINAL	SHILLUK	Pregnant women	374	32	9%	28 years
		Lactating women	261	23	9%	28 years
		Children 1-3 years	314	19	6%	24 months
		Total	948	74	8%	
		GLOBAL	***1166***	***206***	***18%***	

TABLE 4.2. Protein values of blood serum (g/l) in the Shilluk and Nuer (adults)

		SHILLUK			NUER		
	n	Mean	sd	n	Mean	sd	p
Protein (g/l)	48	73.98	5.74	44	79.55	8.24	***
Albumin/globulin	45	1.21	.32	40	.93	.27	***
Albumin (g/l)	45	38.63	4.89	36	37.02	5.38	
Alfa 1 (g/l)	45	1.87	.63	36	2.23	.64	*
Alfa 2 (g/l)	45	5.46	1.48	36	5.35	1.44	
Beta (g/l)	45	5.60	1.55	36	6.13	1.19	
Gamma (g/l)	45	20.60	4.70	36	26.67	7.71	***
IgG (g/l)	41	18.47	3.88	31	23.60	5.44	***
IgA (g/l)	41	2.58	1.07	33	1.94	.76	**
IgM (g/l)	41	1.97	1.00	34	3.00	1.82	**
Alfa1-antitrypsin (g/l)	44	1.60	.38	14	2.13	.71	?

TABLE 4.3. Protein values of values of blood serum (g/l) in the Nuer tribe

	Children (4-14 yrs)			Women			Men			
	n	Mean	sd	n	Mean	sd	n	Mean	sd	p
Protein	9	85.89	7.94	29	80.79	7.11	15	77.13	9.89	*
Albumin/globulin	9	.75	.28	25	.95	.21	15	.89	.35	
Albumin	8	35.95	8.00	23	37.87	3.85	13	35.51	7.31	
Alfa 1	8	2.59	.50	23	2.24	.56	13	2.21	.79	
Alfa 2	8	6.79	2.16	23	5.40	1.09	13	5.27	1.96	
Beta	8	6.93	1.65	23	6.17	1.17	13	6.07	1.27	
Gamma	8	33.51	11.66	23	27.85	7.71	13	24.58	7.57	
IgG	4	20.19	4.52	17	22.90	4.18	17	25.07	5.82	
IgA	7	2.03	.57	19	1.83	.52	17	2.24	1.04	
IgM	7	2.22	.94	19	2.63	1.25	17	3.76	2.40	
Alfa1-antitrypsin	3	2.82	.80	6	2.31	.88	8	2.00	.59	

TABLE 4.4. Protein values of blood-serum (g/l) in the Shilluk tribe

	Children (4-14 yrs)			Women			Men			
	n	Mean	sd	n	Mean	sd	n	Mean	sd	p
Protein	24	71.87	6.64	19	73.95	6.22	29	74.00	5.52	
Alb/glob	24	1.10	.30	19	1.21	.30	26	1.20	.35	
Albumin	24	35.93	4.87	19	38.75	4.98	26	38.55	4.92	
Alfa 1	24	2.00	.77	19	1.98	.70	26	1.78	.57	
Alfa 2	24	6.64	2.06	19	5.72	1.46	26	5.26	1.50	*
Beta	24	5.85	2.02	19	5.89	1.55	26	4.38	1.55	
Gamma	24	19.77	5.76	19	19.48	3.78	26	21.42	5.20	
IgG	19	16.83	5.23	16	16.71	3.55	25	19.59	3.73	*
IgA	20	2.14	.98	16	2.40	1.07	25	2.69	1.08	
IgM	20	1.53	.49	16	2.07	.71	25	1.91	1.16	
Alfa1-ant	20	1.83	.46	17	1.61	.41	27	1.60	.37	

TABLE 4.5. Protein values of blood-serum (g/l) in the Shilluk children

	Children (0-12 yrs)			Children (4-14 yrs)			
	n	Mean	sd	n	Mean	sd	p
Protein	19	65.68	5.03	24	71.87	6.64	***
Albumin/globulin	18	1.28	.23	24	1.10	.30	*
Albumin	18	36.48	3.12	24	35.93	4.87	
Alfa 1	18	2.13	.53	24	2.00	.77	
Alfa 2	18	8.30	1.31	24	6.64	2.06	**
Beta	18	6.08	1.18	24	5.85	2.02	
Gamma	18	12.52	2.93	24	19.77	5.76	***
IgG	16	9.66	3.28	19	16.83	5.23	***
IgA	16	1.01	.48	20	2.14	.98	***
IgM	16	1.32	.57	20	1.53	.49	
Alfa1-antitrypsin	1	1.75		20	1.83	.46	

TABLE 4.6. Protein values of blood-serum (g/l) in the Shilluk women

	Non pregnant (N)			Pregnant (P)			Lactating (L)			p :	(t =	test)
	n	Mean	sd	n	Mean	sd	n	Mean	sd	NP	NL	PL
Protein	19	73.95	6.22	31	65.26	6.50	22	72.50	7.46	***		***
Albumin/glob	19	1.21	.30	31	1.02	.18	21	1.22	.27	*		**
Albumin	19	38.75	4.98	31	32.25	3.24	20	38.86	5.22	***		***
Alfa 1	31	2.55	.90	20	1.97	.61	20	1.97	.61	*		*
Alfa 2	19	5.72	1.46	31	6.85	1.27	20	6.11	1.43	**		
Beta	19	5.89	1.55	31	6.23	1.16	20	5.30	1.22			**
Gamma	19	19.48	3.78	31	16.88	4.41	20	19.80	4.35	*		*
IgG	16	16.71	3.55	29	13.20	4.85	14	18.88	3.58	**		***
IgA	16	2.14	1.07	30	1.74	.69	15	1.78	.48	*		
IgM	16	2.07	.71	30	2.08	1.13	15	1.97	1.28		*	
Alfa 1-antitrypsin	17	1.61	.41	16	2.02	.40	1	1.73		**		

FIGURE 4.1. Protein values of blood serum

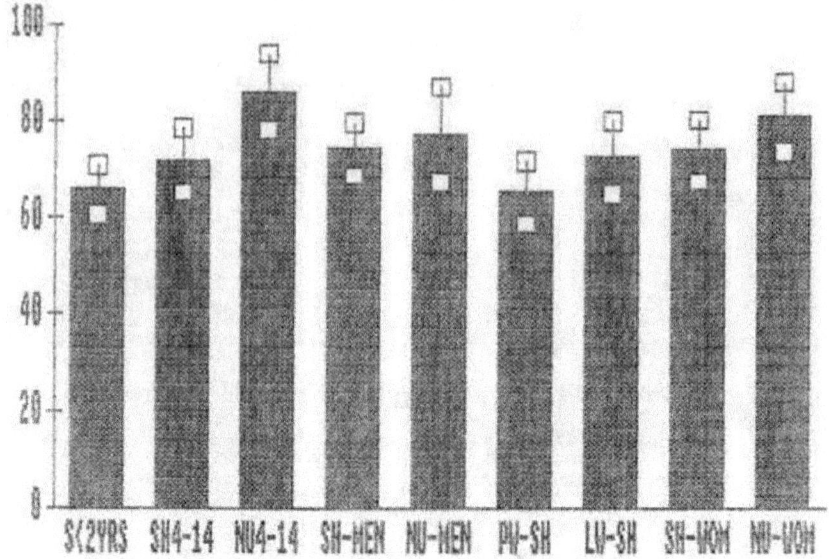

FIGURE 4.2. Distribution of Albumin, gamma-, alfa1-, alfa2- and beta-globulin

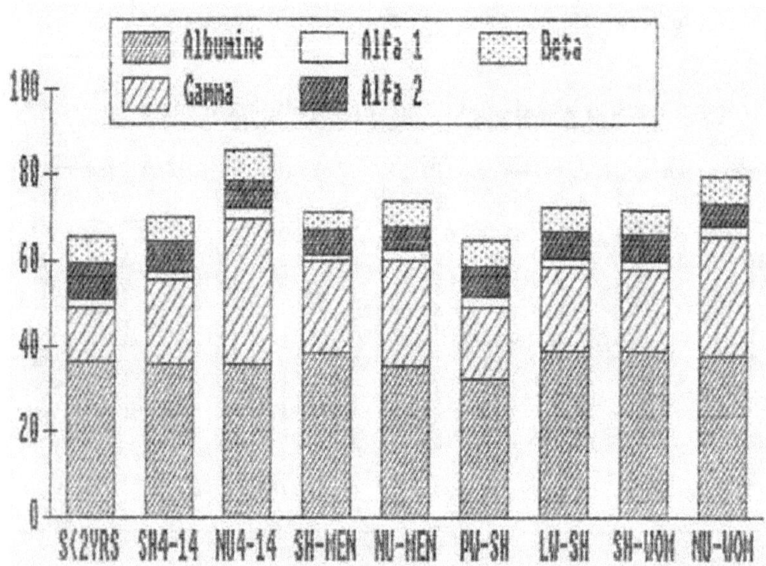

4.2. IMMUNOGLOBULINES

Since the **serum gamma-globulin** level of the studied population is high, particularly in Nuer, where for children the mean value reaches up to 33.51 g/l (table 4.3), analyses were made to determine whether this increase was due to elevation of one or more of the immunoglobulin components.

The **IgG** values are very high in both sexes, even higher than in the Masai population. The Nuer adult have a significantly higher level (26,67 ±7,71) then the Shilluk (20,60 ±4,70). The difference is significant ($p<0.001$) (table 4.2). These high values could be explained by high parasitic infections. Only in Shilluk pregnant women and in children, less than 2 years old, the IgG values are in the upper limits (table 4.5 and 4.6).

The **IgM** values are also significantly higher in Nuer than in Shilluk ($p<0.01$) especially in adult men (3.76 ±2,40 g/l).

The mean value of **IgA** are in the range, but significantly higher ($p<0.01$) in Shilluk adults (2,58 ±1,07 g/l) compared with Nuer adults (1,94 ±0,76 g/l) (table 4.2). It is interesting to mention that the mean level of Masai adults and children is also high (mean = 2.97 g/l).

The **alfa-1-antitrypsin** level is significantly higher ($p<0.01$) in pregnant women compared to non-pregnant women (table 4.6).

It is important to note that in the study area, a high level of infections has been diagnosed.

4.3. HAEMATOLOGY

The haematological values of 157 children and 359 pregnant women shows that more than one third of the population under study, were more or less anaemic. Figure 4.3 shows the mean values of Hb, MCV, RBC and MCH for the following groups: (A) all children less than 3 years, (B) all children 3-5 years, (C) pregnant women and (D) non pregnant women (F*or Hb the WHO standard for anaemia is indicated)*. Data are shown in tables 4.7 to 4.11).

The comparison between the two adult populations of Nuer and Shilluk (table 4.7) shows that:

1) The Hb level is higher in Shilluk (14,04 g/dl) as well as the hematocrit (45.07 ±1.7%). In Shilluk pregnant women, the low level of Hb (12.43 ± 1.34 g/dl) can be explained by the physiological haemo-dilution during the last months of pregnancy

(table 4.11). The pregnant women had higher iron level and transferrin level than the lactating and others women, as assessed by lower haematocrit, haemoglobin and plasma ferritin concentrations (table 4.11). In a study of 364 Nigerian pregnant women, Daouda (73) found that anaemia was observed in 46% if defined by a low haematocrit value and 47.8% if defined by iron deficiency.

The iron level is not different between the Shilluk adults (16.97 ±5.78) and the Nuer adults (15.83 ±4.34). But the transferrin level is higher in the Nuer (2.78 ±0.62) than in the Shilluk adults 2.32 ±0.5). The transferrin saturation is lower in the Nuer women. Because malaria is endemic in this region, its high frequency makes the iron status difficult to interpret but the microcytosis and the relations of haematological data with the iron status suggest the importance of iron contribution in anaemia, particular in children. But the role of folic acid as a contributing factor in anaemia has to be also considered.

A significant diminution ($p<0.01$) of haemoglobin was observed in Nuer children and adults (table 4.9). The Hb values are at the lower limits for Nuer adults (12.63 g/dl) (table 4.7) and especially in women (12.32g/dl) (table 4.9) who have a low level of haematocrite (37.33%) and low level of the saturation coefficient (0.22).

In Shilluk children under 3 years, the mean levels of Hb (10.89 ±1.5 g/dl), MCV (68.88 ±9.08fl) and MCH (22.44 ±3.93pg) are low (table 4.10). 57% of these children were anaemic with microcytosis (48%) and low transferrin saturation as main features (figure 4.4). The frequency distribution curves for haemoglobin concentration (figure 4.5 show the difference with normal Hb levels (Dallman-Siimes).

No association with Hb levels and Z-score of Weight/Height was found. It is important to underline, that children had prolonged breastfeeding with a late introduction of solid foods. Only cow's milk was often introduced in the first year of life. In children over 3 years and adults, microcytosis was rarely found with a tendency to macrocytosis. Thin blood-slides showed anisocytosis in 83%. In these groups ferritin values was in the upper level of the normal range.

TABLE 4.7. Haematological and serological values in Shilluk and Nuer (adults men and women)

	SHILLUK			NUER			
	n	Mean	sd	n	Mean	sd	p
WBC	41	6.35	1.73	21	7.23	3.42	*
RBC	41	4.79	.47	26	4.47	.64	**
Haemoglobin (g/dl)	47	14.04	1.70	28	12.63	2.24	
MCV (μ)	39	94.03	8.01	29	89.55	12.98	
MCH	41	30.07	3.16	25	28.40	3.88	
MCHC (g/dl)	39	31.78	1.97	25	32.20	2.31	
Haematocrit (%)	39	45.07	4.99	26	39.63	8.00	***
Iron (μmol/l)	42	16.97	5.78	49	15.83	4.34	
Transferrin (g/l)	46	2.32	.50	48	2.78	.62	***
Saturation coefficient	41	.30	.12	47	.25	.10	*
Serum Ferritin (ng/ml)	30	61.70	78.39				

TABLE 4.8. Biological values of blood serum in the Shilluk tribe

	Children (4-14 yrs)			Women			Men		
	n	Mean	sd	n	Mean	sd	n	Mean	sd
WBC (%)	18	8.81	3.92	15	6.83	1.52	26	6.08	1.82
RBC (%)	18	4.39	.61	15	4.80	.55	26	4.78	.43
Hemoglobine (g/dl)	21	13.00	1.42	18	13.30	1.41	29	14.49	1.72
MCV (μ)	18	88.72	6.44	15	92.00	8.53	24	95.29	7.58
Hematocrit (%)	18	38.83	5.28	15	44.07	5.15	24	45.70	4.89
Iron (μmol/l)	16	14.08	4.28	17	15.78	5.72	25	17.78	5.80
Transferrin (g/l)	22	2.31	.55	18	2.21	.55	28	2.39	.46
Saturation coeff.	15	.24	.09	17	.30	.12	24	.31	.13
Serum Ferritin (ng/ml)	11	133.64	77.18	13	138.38	80.41	17	179.53	74.22

TABLE 4.9. Biological values of blood serum in the Nuer tribe

	Children (4-14 yrs)			Women			Men		
	n	Mean	sd	n	Mean	sd	n	Mean	sd
WBC (%)	5	11.84	3.02	14	7.47	4.10	7	6.74	1.44
RBC (%)	6	4.60	.83	15	4.41	.57	11	4.54	.75
Hemoglobine (g/dl)	6	12.00	1.64	18	12.32	2.11	10	13.19	2.46
MCV (μ)	6	84.67	5.89	18	86.72	14.34	11	94.18	9.17
Hematocrit (%)	6	38.82	6.79	15	37.33	7.33	11	42.78	8.13
Iron (μmol/l)	9	16.16	7.00	32	15.40	3.98	17	16.64	4.96
Transferrin (g/l)	9	2.93	.58	32	2.92	.59	16	2.50	.60
Saturation coeff.	9	.23	.10	31	.22	.07	16	.29	.14
Serum Ferritin (ng/ml)	-			-			-		

TABLE 4.10. Haematolocical and serological values in Shilluk children

		0 – 2 years			4 – 14 years		
	n	Mean	sd	n	Mean	sd	p
WBC	17	12.20	4.05	19	8.75	3.92	*
RBC	17	4.88	.54	19	4.37	.60	*
Haemoglobin (g/dl)	17	10.89	1.50	23	12.80	1.40	***
MCV (μ)	17	68.88	9.08	19	88.37	6.45	***
MCH	17	22.44	3.93	19	29 76	3.20	***
MCHC (g/dl)	17	32.67	2.45	19	33.75	3.50	
Haematocrit (%)	17	33.30	3.65	19	38.	5.2	***
Iron (μmol/l)	17	16.11	5.83	16	14.08	4.28	
Transferrin (g/l)	19	3.33	.78	22	2.31	.55	***
Saturation coefficient	17	.20	.09	15	.24	.09	
Serum Ferritin (ng/ml)				11	133.64	77.18	

TABLE 4.11. Haematological and serological values in Shilluk women

	Non pregnant			Pregnant			Lactating			p: (t-test)		
	n	Mean	sd	n	Mean	sd	n	Mean	sd	N-P	N-L	P-L
WBC %	15	6.83	1.52	26	6.35	2.12	11	7.34	3.51			
RBC %	15	4.81	.55	26	3.91	.49	12	4.42	.41	***	*	**
Hemoglob g/dl	18	13.30	1.41	27	12.43	1.34	13	13.25	1.00	•		*
MCV (μ)	15	92.00	8.53	27	97.63	6.45	12	95.17	3.21	*		
Hematocrit %	15	44.07	5.15	26	31.92	3.03	12	42.10	4.71	***		*
MCH	15	28.43	3.40	26	37.93	4.41	12	30.10	2.14	**		*
MCHC	15	30.92	2.71	26	32.79	2.70	12	31.70	2.73	*		
Iron (μmol/l)	17	15.78	5.72	29	21.03	4.13	17	14.52	5.22	**		***
Transferrin g/l	18	2.21	.55	30	3.23	.85	17	2.35	.37	***		
Saturation coef	17	.30	.12	28	.28	.10	17	.26	.10			
SerumFerritin (ng/ml)	13	138.38	80.41	16	84.13	45.06	1	96.00		*		

TABLE 4.12. BIOLOGICAL VALUES IN DIFFERENT CATEGORIES

	Iron (µmol/l)	Transferrin (g/l)	Transferrin saturation	SF (µg/l)
Children less than 3 years	15.9 (n=16)	3.36 (n=16)	20 (n=16)	
Children 3-14 years	15.8 (n=21)	2.56 (n=19)	25 (n=19)	136 (n=9)
Non pregnant women	15.8 (n=50)	2.58 (n=64)	27 (n=50)	135 (n=14)
Men over 14 years	17.8 (n=36)	2.43 (n=43)	31 (n=34)	174 (n=18)
Pregnant women	20.1 (n=19)	3.23 (n=30)	30 (n=19)	85 (n=16)

TABLE 4.13. : Correlations between some biological parameters in children and women by Pearson Coefficient Correlation (r=0)

	Children < 3 years	Children 4-14 years	Women non pregnant	Pregnant women
Hb – Iron	*	**	*	*
Hb - Transferrin			**	
Hb-Saturation cof	**		*	
Iron - Ferritin			*	
RBC - Iron	*	**		
MCV - Iron			*	
MCV-Transferrin	**			
MCV-Saturation c	**		*	
MCV - RBC	*		*	

* = $p \leq 0.01$ ** = $p \leq 0.001$

FIGURE 4.3 : Haematological indices for children and women (Mean, S.D. and number of cases)
A=Children <3 years, B=Children 3-5 years, C=pregnant women, D=non pregnant women

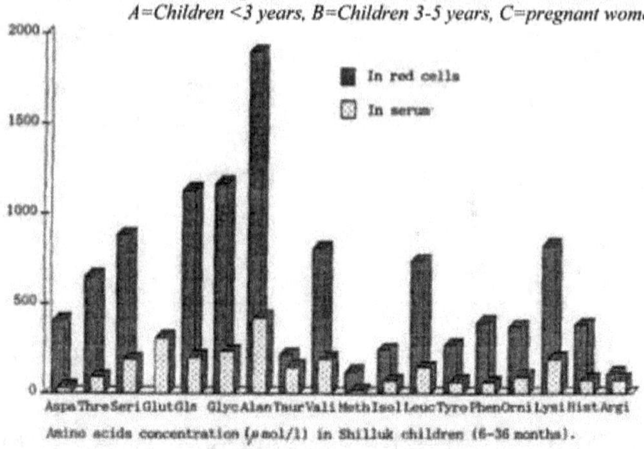

FIGURE 4.4. Hb values to transferrin saturation for 14 children under 3 years
PLOT OF HB WITH SATCOEF

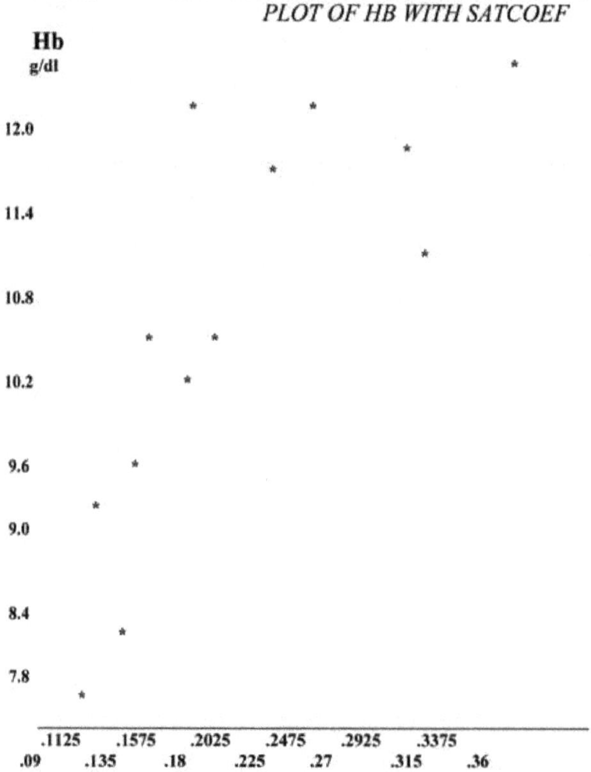

FIGURE 4.5. Frequency distribution curves for haemoglobin concentration in (A) children with normal Hb levels (based on Dallman-Siimes) and (B) children from Sudan (age 6-35 months)

```
Count  Midpoint            Histogram frequency
  2     4.30
  0     4.55 =====
  0     4.80
  0     5.05
  1     5.30
  0     5.55  ==
  1     5.80
  1     6.05  ==
  0     6.30 ===
  1     6.55
  0     6.80 ===
  3     7.05
  2     7.30 ====  ===
  2     7.55 ====  ==
  2     7.80 =====
  1     8.05 ======
  3     8.30 ===
  1     8.55 ==========
  4     8.80 ===
  2     9.05 ============  ==
  3     9.30 ========
  0     9.55 ==========
  8     9.80     A                            B
  1    10.05 ================  =============
 14    10.30 ===
  4    10.55 ================  ===========================
  5    10.80==============
  3    11.05 =================
  1    11.30 ===========
  6    11.55 ====
  6    11.80 =============  ====
  6    12.05 ===========   ======
  7    12.30 ==========  == =======
  2    12.55 =========  ===========
  5    12.80 =======
  3    13.05 =========  =======
  1    13.30 =======  ==
  2    13.55 ====
  1    13.80 =====  ==
  0    14.05 ====
  0    14.30
  0    14.55
  0    14.80
  0    15.05
  0    15.30
  0    15.55
  1    15.80
  0    16.05 ====
            ______+______I______+______I______+______I______+____I
          0       4             8             12            16
```

4.4. IONOGRAMME

The level of sodium, chloride and urea are significantly higher ($p<0.001$) in Nuer adults than in Shilluk adults (table 4.14). The value of glucose is in the lower range, especially in Nuer children (3,20 ±0,87mmol/l) (table 4.15). Only Shilluk infants (<3 years) have a higher value of glucose (4.96 ±0,92 mmol/l) due to permanent breast feeding. The significant ($p<0.001$) increase with age of CO^2, urea and creatinin is normal (table 4.15).

The significantly ($p<0.001$) higher level of urea nitrogen in Nuer (in the range of references) is probably depended to the higher level of protein (table 4.15). The higher level ($p<0.5$) of creatinin (in the range of references) could be related to muscular catabolism in the nomad Nuer population (hunters). The significant ($p<0.001$) lower level of creatinin in smaller Shilluk children can be due to a weak protein catabolism (table 4.17).

Similar lower level of urea and creatinin ($p<0.01$) in Shilluk pregnant women can be explained by the higher use of food rich in protein during pregnancy (table 4.18 and figure 4.6).

The alkaline phosphatise values are low, especially in Nuer and in pregnant women. The slightly higher level of alkaline phosphatise in children may be related with the accelerate growth and ossification at this age. In Shilluk children the alkaline phosphatise is even more important (table 4.16).

In Nuer population the triglycerides are slightly higher than in the Shilluk (table 4.21). In Shilluk women during pregnancy a significant ($p<0001$) higher level of triglycerides was observed (table 4.23). The cholesterol level is in the range of references but it is significantly lower ($p<0.01$) in Shilluk children 4-14 years old (2,49 ±0,45mmol/l) than in children 0-3 years old (3,25 ±0,73) (table 4.22), may be because the hepatic syntheses is weak. In Europe it is twice higher (4.60 to 7.00 mmol/l) (!).

The cholesterol level in pregnant women as well as in lactating women and non pregnant women was lower than those found in occidental populations. This difference can be partly due to the ethnic differences and partly to the fact that the Southern Sudanese had a low fat diet.

A significantly higher ($p<0.001$) level of SGOT, SGPT and copper was observed in the Nuer population (table 4.17) if compared with the Shilluk population (table 4.20). The transaminases are significant higher in the Nuer adults ($p<0.001$) compared to Shilluk adults (table 4.19).

TABLE 4.14. Biological values of blood-serum in Shilluk and Nuer adults

		Shilluk			Nuer			p
		n	Mean	sd	n	Mean	sd	
Sodium	(mmol/l)	45	132.73	4.74	43	138.95	4.58	***
Potassium	(mmol/l)	25	4.24	1.16	43	3.84	.48	*
Chloride	(mmol/l)	46	99.91	3.61	41	104.41	6.32	***
CO2	(mmol/l)	47	17.34	2.54	44	17.91	2.32	
Urea	(mmol/l)	47	4.09	1.38	44	5.52	2.29	***
Glucose	(mmol/l)	47	3.64	.56	44	3.53	.96	
Creatinin	(mol/l)	45	70.56	17.93	46	83.48	31.53	*
Calcium	(µmol/l)	38	2.27	.17	49	2.21	.20	
Phosphor	(mmol/l)	40	1.25	.28	48	1.16	.34	
Alc. Phosphatise	(mmol/l)	37	82.08	48.51	48	75.06	36.69	

TABLE 4.15. Biological values of blood-serum (mmol/l) in the Nuer tribe

	Children (4-14 yrs)			**Children (4-14 yrs)**			**Women**			p
	n	Mean	sd	n	Mean	sd	n	Mean	sd	
Sodium	9	137.22	3.87	28	139.18	4.25	15	138.53	5.26	
Potassium	9	3.92	.29	27	3.80	.44	16	3.91	.56	
Chloride	8	101.63	2.97	27	105.59	4.64	14	102.14	8.45	
CO2	9	18.22	3.03	28	18.00	1.74	16	17.75	3.15	
Urea	8	3.81	1.18	28	5.36	2.39	16	5.79	2.14	
Glucose	8	3.20	.87	28	3.55	.85	16	3.51	1.16	
Creatinin	10	60.80	20.14	30	80.33	29.24	16	89.38	35.66	
Calcium	9	2.26	.16	32	2.25	.14	17	2.15	.27	
Phosphor	10	1.51	.36	31	1.19	.38	17	1.09	.22	**
Alc. Phosphatise	9	146.44	50.70	31	71.29	29.51	17	81.94	47.37	***

TABLE 4.16. Biological values of blood-serum (mmol/l) in the Shilluk tribe.

	Children (4-14 yrs)			**Children (4-14 yrs)**			**Women**			p
	n	Mean	sd	n	Mean	sd	n	Mean	sd	
Sodium	22	131.68	4.83	17	132.29	5.37	28	133.00	4.40	
Potassium	10	4.74	.51	9	4.24	1.39	16	4.23	1.05	
Chloride	23	101.43	3.98	18	100.39	3.02	28	99.61	3.51	
CO2	23	16.96	2.77	18	16.06	2.60	29	18.14	2.18	*
Urea	23	4.83	1.59	18	4.39	1.48	29	3.91	1.31	*
Glucose	23	4.08	.95	18	3.66	.47	29	3.63	.62	**
Creatinin	20	52.00	12.02	17	72.00	19.93	28	69.68	16.92	***
Calcium	19	2.23	.18	12	2.23	.10	26	2.28	.19	
Phosphor	18	1.44	.31	13	1.30	.21	27	1.23	.31	*
Alc. Phosphatise	17	171.59	78.92	12	100.42	69.85	25	73.28	32.33	***

TABLE 4.17. Biological values of blood-serum in the Shilluk children.

		Children 0 – 2 years			Children 4 – 14 years			
		n	Mean	sd	n	Mean	sd	P
Sodium	(mmol/l)	19	135.21	5.11	22	131.68	4.83	*
Potassium	(mmol/l)	18	4.47	.77	10	4.74	.51	
Chloride	(mmol/l)	19	102.32	4.44	23	101.43	3.98	
CO2	(mmol/l)	19	11.68	1.67	23	16.96	2.77	***
Urea	(mmol/l)	19	2.13	.99	23	4.83	1.59	***
Glucose	(mmol/l)	19	4.96	.92	23	4.08	.95	**
Creatinin	(µmol/l)	18	32.44	7.31	20	52.00	12.02	***
Calcium	(mmol/l)	18	2.26	.24	19	2.23	.18	
Phosphor	(mmol/l)	18	1.80	.18	18	1.44	.31	***
Alc. Phosphatise	(mmol/l)	18	197.89	52.06	17	171.59	78.92	

Table 4.18. Biological values of blood-serum (mmol/l) in the Shilluk women.

	Non pregnant (N)			Pregnant (P)			Lactating (L)			p: (t-test)		
	n	Mean	sd	n	Mean	sd	n	Mean	sd	NP	NL	PL
Sodium	17	132.29	5.37	30	133.70	3.65	21	137.57	8.12		*	*
Potassium	9	4.24	1.39	20	4.54	1.16	17	4.51	.72			
Chloride	18	100.39	3.82	30	101.13	5.25	22	103.91	5.35		*	
CO2	18	16.06	2.60	30	16.03	3.18	22	18.41	3.08		*	*
Urea	18	4.39	1.48	30	3.10	.71	22	3.66	1.53	**		
Glucose	18	3.66	.47	29	3.57	.90	22	4.29	1.16		*	
Creatinin	17	72.00	19.93	24	55.46	11.50	14	55.93	6.26	**	**	
Calcium	12	2.23	.10	29	2.14	.15	14	2.20	.27	*		
Phosphor	13	1.30	2.21	30	1.09	.19	14	1.24	.18	**		*
Alc. Phosph	12	100.42	69.85	29	72.79	37.13	12	79.25	20.71			

TABLE 4.19. Biological values of blood-serum in the Shilluk and Nuer (adults)

		SHILLUK			NUER			
		n	Mean	sd	n	Mean	sd	P
Cholesterol	(mmol/l)	41	2.91	.71	46	2.88	.75	
Triglycerides	(mmol/l)	41	.88	.43	45	.90	.43	
Phospholipids	(mmol/l)	34	2.01	.65	45	1.77	.47	
SGOT	(UI/l)	40	18.27	5.27	49	26.22	12.62	***
SGPT	(UI/l)	40	9.38	3.61	49	14.06	6.89	***
Uric Acid	(µmol/l)	46	290.87	88.78	36	309.14	117.70	***

TABLE 4.20. Biological values of blood-serum in the Shilluk tribe

		Children 4-14years			Women			Men			
		n	Mean	sd	n	Mean	sd	n	Mean	sd	P
Cholesterol	(mmol/l)	19	2.49	.45	14	2.94	.66	27	2.89	.75	
Triglycerides	(mmol/l)	19	.87	.40	14	.79	.49	27	.93	.40	
Phospholipids	(mmol/l)	17	1.71	.31	15	1.94	.27	19	2.06	.84	
SGOT	(UI/l)	18	23.83	10.38	13	18.46	5.94	27	18.19	8.73	
SGPT	(UI/l)	18	12.61	5.68	13	9.69	4.71	27	9.22	3.04	*
Uric Acid	(µmol/l)	19	203.47	63.32	17	234.24	69.68	29	324.07	82.48	***

TABLE 4.21. Biological values of blood-serum in the Nuer tribe

		Children 4-14 years			Women			Men			
		n	Mean	sd	n	Mean	sd	n	Mean	sd	P
Cholesterol	(mmol/l)	10	2.59	.59	30	2.90	.79	16	2.84	.70	
Triglycerides	(mmol/l)	10	.99	.40	29	.96	.50	16	.80	.26	
Phospholipids	(mmol/l)	10	1.70	.40	29	1.84	.48	16	1.64	.42	
SGOT	(UI/l)	10	27.90	9.40	32	25.59	14.42	17	27.41	8.55	
SGPT	(UI/l)	10	13.30	6.83	32	14.44	6.84	17	13.35	7.12	
Uric Acid	(µmol/l)	9	294.44	75.84	24	207.13	116.09	12	333.17	122.31	

TABLE 4.22. Biological values of blood-serum in the Shilluk children

		Children 0 - 2 years			Children 4 - 14 years			
		n	Mean	sd	n	Mean	sd	P
Cholesterol	(mmol/l)	18	3.25	.73	19	2.49	.45	***
Triglycerides	(mmol/l)	18	1.18	.58	19	.87	.40	
Phospholipids	(mmol/l)	18	1.93	.28	17	1.71	.31	*
SGOT	(UI/l)	17	17.94	9.24	18	23.83	10.38	
SGPT	(UI/l)	18	12.06	7.27	18	12.61	5.68	
Uric Acid	(µmol/l)	15	253.93	107.44	19	203.47	63.32	

TABLE 4.23. Biological values of blood-serum in the Shilluk women

		Non pregnant (N)			Pregnant (P)			Lactating (L)			p: (t-test)		
		n	Mean	sd	n	Mean	sd	n	Mean	sd	NP	NL	PL
Cholesterol	(mmol/l)	14	2.94	.66	28	3.42	.90	15	2.97	.79			
Triglycerides	(mmol/l)	14	.79	.49	28	1.37	.70	16	.63	.27	**		***
Phospholipids	(mmol/l)	15	1.94	.27	28	2.05	.40	16	1.74	.37			*
SGOT	(UI/l)	13	18.46	5.94	25	18.72	8.13	14	19.64	10.99			
SGPT	(UI/l)	13	9.69	4.71	26	10.50	8.65	15	12.93	5.55			
Uric Acid	(µmol/l)	17	234.24	69.68	26	239.15	91.63	15	230.60	100.35			

FIGURE 4.6. Differences between non-prenant, pregnant and lactating women for ionogramme

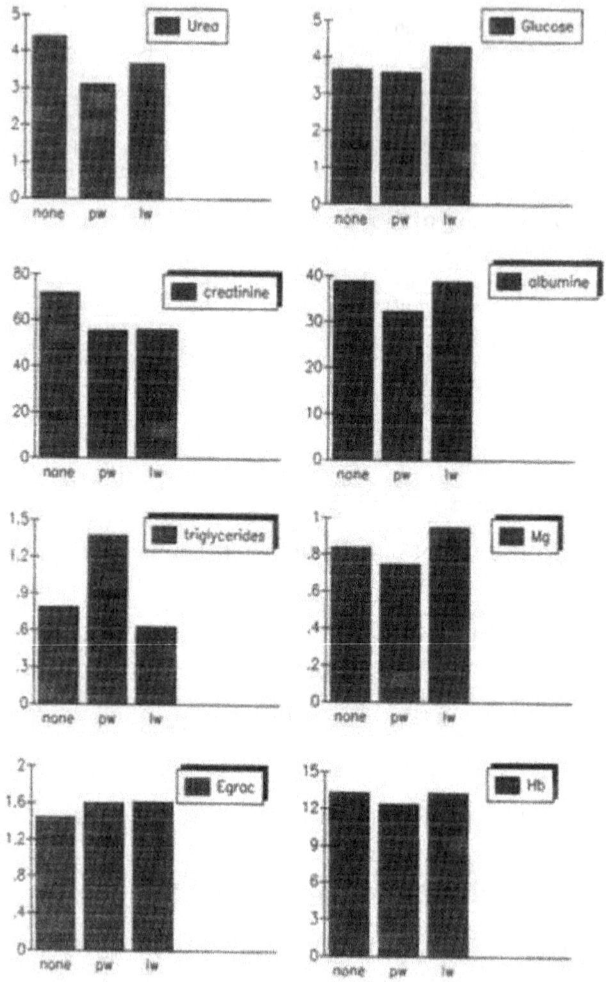

4.5. VITAMINS AND MINERALS

4.5.1. Vitamin A

The vitamin A analysis were performed on 43 Nuer adult, 32 Shilluk adult, 31 Shilluk children, 14 pregnant and 9 lactating women.

The results (Tables 4.24, 4.25 and 4.26) suggest that if the collective means of serum vitamin A are «adequate» (>20 μg/dl) in all groups, there are following points to take into consideration:

1- In the Shilluk adult population serum retinol levels are significantly higher than in the Nuer adult population;
2- Serum retinol levels decrease during gestation;
3 - There are subjects «at high risk» (< 20μg/dl) in children 4-14 years old pregnant women and lactating women as well as in all Nuer groups. The number and percentage of subjects classified as very low, low, acceptaband high according to the IVACG criteria are shown in table 4.24.

In this sub-sample, 8.5% have serum retinol inferior 20μg/dl. One 14 years old child and two pregnant women have a value inferior 10μg/dl strongly suggestive of deficiency and below which xerophthalmia is imminent; none of them showed clinical signs of vitamin A deficiency. For one child with retinol=19.8 μg/dl we found a history of night blindness. Compared to Heese study in Namibia (74), the mean value of serum retinol in infants is similar (34-36 μg/dl).

Association between infection diseases and low levels of serum vitamin A was evident: at the time of examine, the subjects presented malaria and hepato-splenomegalia. An adequate consumption of vegetables and fruits can reduce or eliminate *vitamin A deficiency (VAD)* and limit the risk of infection, including diarrhoea and other febrile illnesses such as measles (75). It is particularly the case when physiological needs are greatest, especially in infancy, early childhood and pregnancy (periods of rapid growth and development) as well as during lactation when breast milk carries vitamin A in highly absorbable form.

Xerophthalmia, xerosis and Bitot's spots are the most obvious health consequences of severe *VAD* which involve the visual system. But vitamin A deficiency contributes also to impaired growth and development and to in-efficient utilization of iron for haemoglobin production (74).

4.5.2. Other vitamins and minerals

The serum **vitamin E** level is low in all sub-groups. However, in the Nuer adults the mean level is higher than in the Shilluk (Tables 4.25 to 4.29). **Egrac** values are similar in both sub-groups (above 1.20 indicate riboflavin deficiency).

Assessment of **vitamins B1, B2** and **B6** status of a pregnant women sub-sample showed a relative deficiency in all three vitamins when compared with non-pregnant women from the north Sudan.

The **copper** level is also higher in the Nuer adults ($p < 0.001$) than in Shilluk adults. It is also higher then reference values (11-22 µmol/l) (table 4.23). Data concerning vitamins and minerals (tables 4.25 to 4.29) may have only indicative values because of small number, possible technical errors or rich in copper soil.

DATA FROM THE PILOT STUDIES

During the previous pilot studies in the same area (Ostrowski & Suliman – 76), the haematological analysis of a subsample of 75 cases (1978-9) showed that mainly women and children are anaemic (table 4.30).

From the pilot study (1981), the biological values, analysed by Feldmann and coll (77), were similar: a high levels of IgG (18,54mmol/l) and IgM (2,37mmol/l) but a lower level of alkaline phosphatise (61,62 mmol/l) (table 4.31). The results confirmed the correct way of taken blood samples as well as transport.

When compared with results of trace elements in pregnant women from Northern Sudan (table 4.32) it was noticed that no significant differences exists regarding calcium, magnesium or cooper. The same rise in copper level is observed both in pregnant women from Southern and Northern Sudan (Bayoumi – 78).

The vitamin status of a sub-sample (1981) of pregnant women from Jonglei in South Sudan was compared with a control group of adult non-pregnant women from northern Sudan (table 4.33). It is obvious that the degree of activation of all three enzymes is higher in the southern Sudanese women. This reflects a relative deficiency in all three vitamins when compared with adult non-pregnant women from the North Sudan (Bayoumi – 79, 80).

In another sub-sample (1981) of red cells from southern Sudanese pregnant women (figure 4.7), Turnham (81, 82) found, that only two of these subjects gave results within normal range for riboflavin. Seven subjects were marginally deficient. Four subjects were moderately so and six subjects were markedly deficient. It means that the six subjects get probably less than 0.5 mg riboflavin per day.

Table 4.34 shows the concentrations of the 2 metabolites of niacin expressed in mmol/l creatinin which were measured by Bender (83). The methods used were for N1-methyl nicotinamide modification (84) of the fluorimetric technique of Carpenter & Kodicek (85) and for N1-methyl pyridone carboxamide of Holman (86). Values which are equal to or less than 1 are taken as indicative of deficiency. 17 samples of urine from southern Sudanese pregnant women were analysed. By this measure, over half the results shown in table 4.32 may indicate niacin deficiency, probably due to the food habits. The main cereal staple food of the population living in the South Sudan was a form of sorghum known as durra. Sorghum and maize are the two cereals which are commonly associated with niacin deficiencies for several reasons. The first is that the actual concentration of niacin is lower in maize and sorghum than in the other major cereals, the second reason is that the tryptophan concentration is also low (table 4.35) (87, 88), thirdly, niacin present in maize and sorghum tends to be present in a bound form and lastly it is suggested that the high quantity of leucine relative to isoleucine present in these cereals, may interfere with tryptophan utilisation and the metabolism of niacin.

Plasma from 15 southern Sudanese pregnant women and the red blood cells from 23 were analysed by gas liquid chromatography for their fatty acid profile. Dodge (89) found that no eicosapentaenoic acid was measurable in any of the red cell samples (table 4.36) and a small trace only in four of the plasmas (table 4.37). On the other hand, the levels of docosahexaenoic acid were normal. An unidentified acid was present in the red cells of these women but not in the controls (25 healthy European males).

Cholesterol levels were measured by Bertier and Apfelbaum (90) in southern Sudanese pregnant women. Lipoprotein fractions A (HDL) and B (VLDL, LDL and LPA) were separated by precipitation using concanavaline. Cholesterol was estimated by an enzymatic technique. The mean serum cholesterol was 1.39 g/l in plasma, 0.43 g/l and 0.95 g/l in fractions A and B respectively. Cholesterol A to cholesterol B ratio was 0.46. No significant correlation was found between cholesterol levels versus uterine height or women's age or weight.

TABLE 4.24. Number and percentage of subjects with different serum Vitamin A levels (µg/dl)

GROUPS	ETHNICITY	RETINOL LEVELS (g/dl) < 10	10 – 19	20 – 39	> 40	Mean sd
Children < 2 years	***Shilluk***			6 54.5%	5 45.5%	
Children 4-14 years	***Shilluk***		1 8.3%	6 50.0%	5 41.7%	39.36 14.30
Children 4-14 years	***Nuer***	1 12.5%	1 12.5%	3 37.5%	3 37.5%	28.44 13.90
Men	***Shilluk***			8 38.1%	13 61.9%	53.20 17.30
Men	***Nuer***		3 20.0%	5 33.3%	7 46.7%	38.31 17.50
Women	***Shilluk***			4 36.4%	7 63.6%	56.12 26.10
Women	***Nuer***		1 3.6%	15 53.6%	12 42.9%	37.84 14.40
Pregnant	***Shilluk***	2 14.3%	1 7.1%	6 42.9%	5 35.7%	35.61 16.83
Lactating	***Shilluk***		1 11.1%	3 33.3%	5 55.6%	46.92 20.30
TOTAL %		3 2.3%	8 6.2%	56 43.4%	62 48.1%	

TABLE 4.25. Minerals and vitamins in blood serum (μmol/l) in Shilluk and Nuer adults

		SHILLUK			NUER			
		n	Mean	sd	n	Mean	sd	P
Zinc	(μmol/l)	41	12.77	7.38	6	15.55	5.08	
Copper	(μmol/l)	31	14.48	6.17	14	24.52	4.99	***
Magnesium	(mmol/l)	42	.83	.16	46	.85	.08	
Vitamin A	(μg/l)	32	542.03	203.94	42	380.02	153.38	***
Vitamin E	(μg/l)	18	3.78	1.25	43	4.94	1.82	*
EGRAC		42	1.43	.15	43	1.51	.42	

TABLE 4.26. Minerals and vitamins in blood serum in the Shilluk tribe

		Children 4-14 years			Women			Men			
		n	Mean	sd	n	Mean	sd	n	Mean	sd	P
Zinc	μmol/l	16	10.26	2.97	17	11.58	4.25	24	13.60	8.97	
Copper	μmol/l	17	14.95	6.16	12	14.08	4.79	19	14.73	7.02	
Magnesium	mmol/l	18	.80	.12	15	.84	.14	27	.82	.17	
Vitamin A	μg/l	12	393.42	171.37	11	561.18	261.08	21	532.00	173.44	*
Vitamin E	μg/l	3	4.33	.61	6	3.43	1.62	12	3.96	1.07	
EGRAC		21	1.27	.12	17	1.44	.11	25	1.43	.18	***

TABLE 4.27. Minerals and vitamins in blood serum in the Nuer tribe

		Children 4-14 years			Women			Men			
		n	Mean	sd	n	Mean	sd	n	Mean	sd	P
Zinc	μmol/l	3	18.07	3.29	2	12.60	2.69	4	17.03	5.65	
Copper	μmol/l	2	30.60	7.64	9	24.19	4.90	5	25.12	5.69	
Magnesium	mmol/l	9	.93	.08	29	.88	.06	17	.81	.09	***
Vitamin A	μg/l)	8	284.38	139.05	28	378.36	143.90	15	383.13	175.00	
Vitamin E	μg/l)	8	4.88	.97	28	5.07	2.11	15	4.71	1.13	
EGRAC		9	1.52	.15	28	1.53	.11	15	1.49	.19	

TABLE 4.28. Minerals and vitamins in blood serum in the Shilluk children

		Children 0 – 2 years			Children 4 – 14 years		
		n	Mean	sd	n	Mean	sd
Zinc	(µmol/l)	-			16	10.26	2.97
Copper	(µmol/l)	-			17	14.95	6.16
Magnesium	(mmol/l)	14	.86	.11	18	.80	.12
Vitamin A	(µg/l)	11	393.64	143.04	12	393.42	171.37
Vitamin E	(µg/l)	10	4.57	1.31	3	4.33	.61
EGRAC		15	1.21	.09	21	1.27	.22

Table 4.29. Minerals and vitamins in blood serum in the Shilluk women

		Children 4 - 14 years			Women			Men			
		n	Mean	sd	n	Mean	sd	n	Mean	sd	P
Zinc	(µmol/l)	16	10.26	2.97	17	11.58	4.25	24	13.60	8.97	
Copper	(µmol/l)	17	14.95	6.16	12	14.08	4.79	19	14.73	7.02	
Magnesium	(mmol/l)	18	.80	.12	15	.84	.14	27	.82	.17	
Vitamin A	(µg/l)	12	393.42	171.37	11	561.18	261.08	21	532.00	173.44	*
Vitamin E	(µg/l)	3	4.33	.61	6	3.43	1.62	12	3.96	1.07	
EGRAC		21	1.27	.12	17	1.44	.11	25	1.43	.18	***

TABLE 4.30. Haematological values in a pilot study of 75 men, women and children in South Sudan (1978-9) (63)

	Women	Men	Children
Hcte	29.0 %	35.0 %	21.0 %
Hb	8.3 g	11.0 g	8.6 g
RBC	2.9	3.5	3.1
MCV	100 u3	100 u3	68 u3

TABLE 4.31. Biological values of blood serum in the Shilluk pregnant women in 1981 and 1983

	1981			1983		
	n	Mean	sd	n	Mean	sd
Protein (g/l)	53	62.09	1.14	31	65.26	6.50
Albumin/globulin	53	.85	.03	31	.	
Albumin (%)	53	45.85	.79	31		
Alfa 1 (%)	53	4.59	.15	31		
Alfa 2 (%)	53	8.75	.22	31		
Beta (%)	53	10.98	.22	31		
Gamma (%)	53	29.78	.79	31		
IgG (g/l)	53	18.54	.97	29	14.17	5.20
IgA (g/l)	53	1.55	.08	30	1.74	.69
IgM (g/l)	53	2.37	.11	30	2.08	1.13
AAT (g/l)	53	2.24	.07	16	2.02	.40
Sodium (mmol/l)	53	135.00	1.53	30	133.70	3.65
Potassium (mmol/l)	53	3.96	.09	20	4.54	1.16
Chloride (mmol/l)	53	101.26	1.08	30	101.13	5.25
Urea (mmol/l)	53	2.98	.40	30	3.10	.71
Glucose (mmol/l)	53	4.59	.12	29	3.57	.90
Creatinin (µmol/l)	53	48.78	3.10	24	55.46	11.50
Calcium (mmol/l)	53	2.42	.04	29	2.14	.15
Phosphor (mmol/l)	53	1.19	.03	30	1.09	.19
Alc. Phosph. (UI/l)	53	61.62	5.70	29	72.79	37.13
Cholesterol (mmol/l)	53	3.91	.20	28	3.42	.90
Triglycerides (mmol/l)	53	1.55	.12	28	1.37	.70
Phospholipids (mmol/l)	53	2.34	.10	28	2.05	.40
SGOT (UI/l)	53	19.70	1.09	25	18.72	8.13
SGPT (UI/l)	53	15.50	1.80	26	10.50	8.65
Zinc (µmol/l)	17	30.00	10.00 *	11	10.39	2.75
Copper (µmol/l)	27	20.20	4.60 *	9	21.18	7.00
Magnesium (mmol/l)	32	.80	.14 *	29	.75	.08
Vitamin A (µg/l)	53	425.00	26.00	14	356.07	168.31
Vitamin E (mg/l)	10	4.20	.23	12	4.33	2.38

TABLE 4.32. Trace elements in serum pregnant women from North Sudan and South Sudan (*)

ELEMENTS	NORTH SUDAN			SOUTH SUDAN		
	n	**Mean**	**sd**	**n**	**Mean**	**sd**
Magnesium (mg/100 ml)	30	2.3	0.5	32	1.92	0.35
Calcium (mg/100 ml)	30	8.8	1.2	25	8.66	1.39
Cooper (μg/100 ml)	30	127	25	27	129.1	29.8
Zinc (μg/100 ml)	30	136	32	17	194.4	64.5

(*) Bayoumi (78)

TABLE 4.33. Vitamin B1, B2 and B6 status of pregnant women assessed by in vitro activation of transketolase, glutathione reductase and aspartate amino-transferase by cofactors (*)

ENZYME	VITAMIN	ACTIVITY without enzyme		ACTIVITY with enzyme		% ACTIVATION
		Mean	sd	Mean	sd	
Transketolase	**B 1** n=25	0.38	0.16	0.54	0.23	45
control	n=30	0.39	0.08	0.44	0.10	27
Glutathione reductase	**B 2** n=28	3.17	2.04	5.26	2.87	74
control	n=30	3.31	1.68	4.41	1.97	45
sparatate Amino Transferase	**B 6** n=33	2.50	0.99	4.44	1.75	90
control	n=30	3.06	1.11	5.89	2.01	66

(*) Bayoumi (79)

FIGURE 4.7. Riboflavin Status (Vitamin B2) in Pregnant women (*)

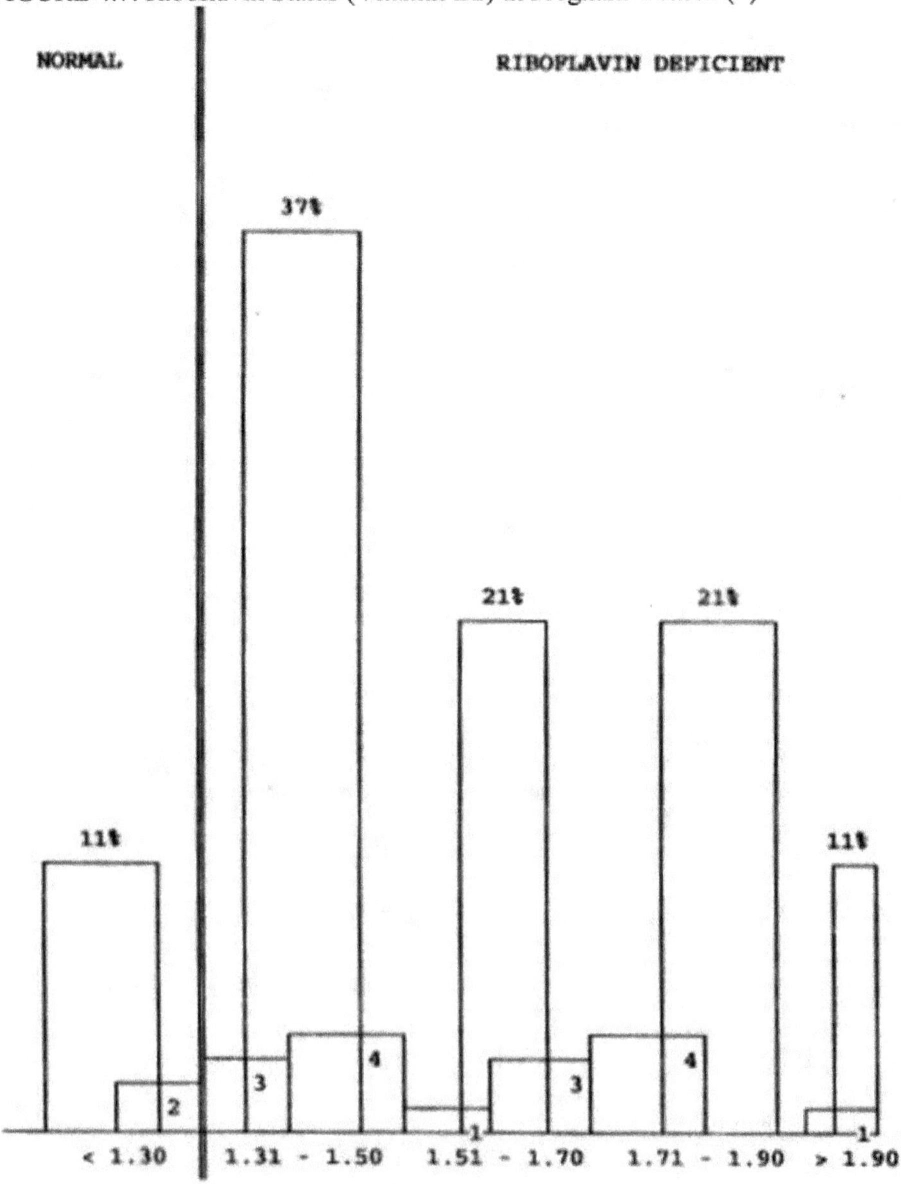

EGR-AC (Erythrocyte glutathione reductase Activity Coefficient)
(*) Turnham (81)

TABLE 4.34. Urinary niacin metabolites in Shilluk pregnant women (Bender (83)

CODE N°	NMN 1	MPCX 2	MXPCX : NMN 3
108	O.78*	1.98	2.54
125	6.80	1.39	0.20*
191	0.19*	2.09	11.00
232	0.49*	1.26	2.57
242	1.58	1.76	1.11
243	1.87	1.73	0.93*
244	3.28	2.46	0.75*
251	2.03	1.13*	0.56*
252	0.40*	1.38	3.37
260	2.65	2.64	1.00
298	5.83	2.01	0.35*
318	1.77	1.72	0.97*
323	1.11*	1.49	1.34
324	5.84	0.79*	0.14*
325	1.54	1.09	0.71*
333	0.92*	1.97	2.14*
334	2.82	1.34	0.48*
Mean (sd)	2.3 (1.96)	1.64 (0.49)	1.7 (2.5)

(*) Sub-clinical deficiency :

1. NMN (N1-methyl nicotinamide) < 1.5 mmole/mol creatinin
2. MPCX (N-methyl pyridone carboxamide) < 1.0 mmole/mol creatinin
3. MPCX:NMN ratio < 1.0

TABLE 4.35. Concentrations of niacin and tryptophan in cereals

	Wheat	rice	maize	sorghum	millet
Niavin Mg/100g (1)	4.3	4.7	1.7	3.9	2.3
Tryptophan Mg/100g (2)	142	98	181	105	164

Sources: (87) Composition of Foods. B.K. Watt & A.L. Merrill, Agric. Handbk no 8. U.S. Dept. Agric., Washington 1963

(88) Amino Acid Content of Foods. Food & Agric. Org., 1968 (Microbiological Assay).

TABLE 4.36. Erythrocyte fatty acids content in Shilluk pregnant women

FATTY Acides	14.0	16.0	16.1	18.0	18.1	18.2	20.4	20.5	22.6	20.0 22.5
SHILLUK n=25 Mean sd	1.70 0.94	33.48 3.36	2.37 1.37	11.43 2.24	23.10 5.79	11.67 1.96	8.39 2.50	0 0	2.11 1.48	1.67 1.51
Control n=25 Mean sd	0.56 0.12	25.90 2.10	0.91 0.25	10.80 1.51	19.70 1.34	13.10 1.23	11.60 1.75	1.05 0.43	2.60 0.87	* *

TABLE 4.37. Plasma fatty acids content in Shilluk pregnant women

FATTY Acides	14.0	16.0	16.1	18.0	18.1	18.2	20.4	20.5	22.6
SHILLUK n=15 Mean sd	2.10 1.00	27.59 4.15	4.27 2.24	5.56 1.28	25.26 3.98	21.70 5.41	6.31 1.65	0 0	1.63 0.79
Control n=25 Mean sd	0.92 0.96	24.01 4.90	3.14 1.77	9.32 3.05	27.04 5.20	26.86 5.18	4.73 2.14	NK NK	NK NK

4.6. AMINO ACIDS CONCENTRATION

The amino acids concentration in blood serum of 120 Shilluk (33 children, 23 men, 64 women) and 57 Nuer have been analysed for 18 amino acids by chromatography method. The obtained values have been compared with usual reference values (91, 92).

Figure 4.8 shows a histogram of amino acids concentration in the Shilluk and Nuer population, compared to normal values. Lower values are for glutamine, threonine, valine and lysine. Higher values are for glutamic acid.

Compared to Norma, the mean values of the population under study is similar to reference values except for four amino acids (taurine, asparagine, citrulline and proline) (table 4.38 to 4.42). The increase of the mean value of aspartic acid and glutamic acid (in all age groups) can be related to the instability of asparagine and glutamine. A transformation of these amino acids may occur before analysis (91). In the Shilluk population an increase of phenylalanine and of some other values are still in the upper range of reference values (table 4.36 - 4.39). It was observed a lower value of valine only in Shilluk adults. There is a slight difference in amino acids levels between the two ethnic groups. The values of taurine (table 4.43), aspartic acid and phenylalanine are higher in Nuer adults (table 4.42) then in Shilluk. Contrary the values of glutamic acid are higher in Shilluk adults (table 4.38)

The values of amino acids are similar in both sexes. Only for aspartic acid, alanine and phenylalanine the values are slightly higher in Shilluk men (table 4.38) the values of aspartic acid and glutamic acid are slightly higher in Nuer women (table 4.39). Most values of amino acids are respectively lower in pregnant and lactating women than in non-pregnant Shilluk women (aspartic acid, glutamic acid and taurine). The values of glycine are lower only in pregnant women (table 4.40). In Shilluk children (age 0-2), the values are increased for the majority of amino acids, especially for alanine, serine, aspartic acid and leucine (table 4.41). Figure 4.9 shows the amino acids concentration in Shilluk children (6-36 months) in serum and red cells. The low serum threonine level can be related with PEM in lactating women. The higher alanine level is probably the expression of an adaptation to the extremely high intake of carbohydrates that represents about 90% of the calories with a low protein intake.

A statistical analysis was carried out to check if there are correlations between biological values and some food consumed by adults in the Shilluk and Nuer population. The main food items have been taken into consideration: milk, fish, meat, durra (cereal) and beer. The food intake data have been obtained by a 24 hour recall method (R) and by description of habits (H). Some correlations are shown in table 4.44. The differences are not statistically significant.

FIGURE 4.8. Histogram of amino acids concentration in the Shilluk and Nuer population, compared to normal values.

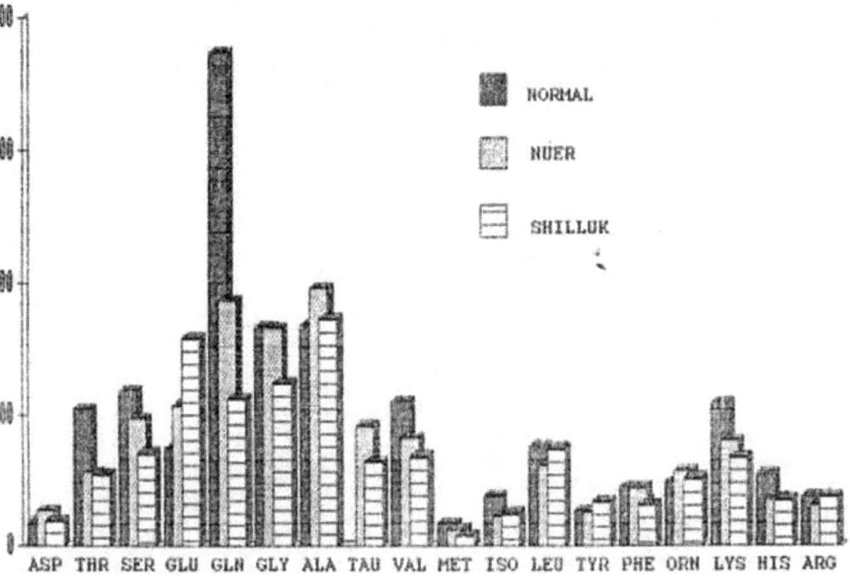

FIGURE 4.9. Histogram of amino acids concentration in Shilluk children (6-36 months) in serum and red cells.

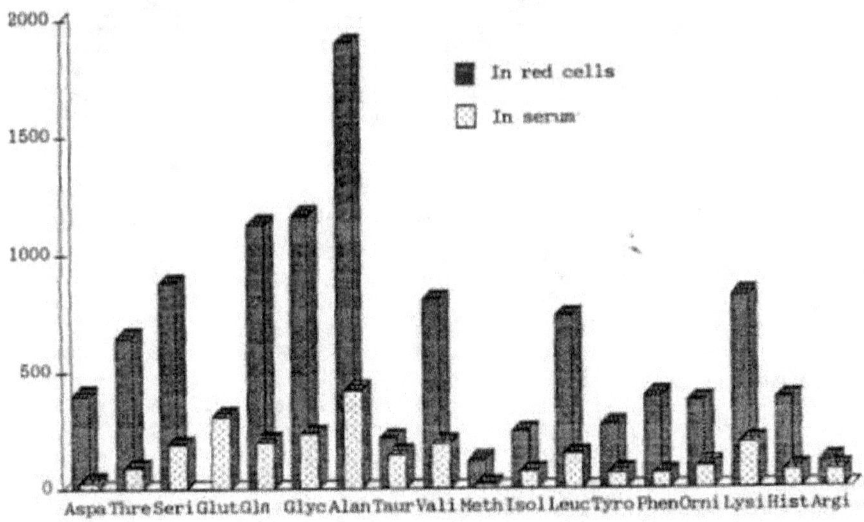

TABLE 4.38. Amino Acids concentration in blood-serum (μmol/l) in the Shilluk tribe

	Children (4-14 yrs)			Women			Men		
	n	Mean	sd	n	Mean	sd	n	Mean	sd
Aspartic-Acid	17	41.05	14.87	17	47.49	16.66	23	42.54	22.05
Threonine	17	102.49	42.38	17	107.39	32.74	23	107.97	33.24
Serine	17	143.45	39.72	17	149.58	37.58	23	135.86	33.94
Glutamic-Acid	17	222.13	101.14	17	338.31	173.90	23	330.40	114.84
Glutamine	17	218.28	132.88	17	223.02	147.06	23	255.05	171.39
Glycine	17	215.15	60.39	17	266.99	90.60	23	251.18	72.35
Alanine	17	351.33	113.06	17	393.15	107.67	23	330.79	96.85
Valine	17	201.91	64.80	17	148.25	39.97	23	147.90	38.59
Methionine	17	18.70	6.10	17	19.63	6.95	23	18.82	4.61
Isoleucine	17	60.85	19.73	17	50.09	12.22	23	53.17	16.51
Leucine	17	156.78	40.53	17	152.60	38.80	23	140.77	46.51
Tyrosine	17	71.78	23.65	17	66.71	20.80	23	71.72	17.82
Phenylalanine	17	76.88	34.89	17	70.49	21.30	23	62.86	15.95
Ornithine	17	92.84	38.59	17	107.49	60.12	23	96.22	33.15
Lysine	17	155.91	50.90	17	150.71	47.22	23	142.01	42.38
Histidine	17	68.11	11.57	17	74.96	13.02	23	72.30	13.28
Arginine	17	50.12	31.32	17	70.42	28.72	23	82.60	23.46
NON ESS/ESS	17	1.24	.35	17	1.53	.23	23	1.40	.29

TABLE 4.39. Amino Acids concentration (μmol/l) in blood-serum in Nuer tribe

	Children (4-14 yrs)			Women			Men		
	n	Mean	sd	n	Mean	sd	n	Mean	sd
Aspartic Acid	10	54.45	23.63	30	56.52	27.87	17	85.58	120.81
Threonine	10	191.46	59.52	30	118.83	52.08	17	134.87	75.29
Serine	10	111.65	46.51	30	195.82	62.15	17	208.21	43.34
GlutamicAcid	10	222.71	122.56	30	245.37	151.88	17	244.39	90.10
Glutamine	10	366.75	196.10	30	352.52	158.72	17	428.86	211.74
Glycine	10	344.72	102.13	30	342.54	130.37	17	348.45	79.72
Alanine	10	441.28	117.39	30	416.33	141.34	17	443.45	110.00
Valine	10	175.77	64.92	30	178.48	87.76	17	217.95	99.91
Methionine	10	27.49	15.73	30	26.42	14.66	17	39.38	25.48
Isoleucine	10	54.47	27.57	30	48.24	30.75	17	67.15	37.84
Leucine	10	143.71	51.17	30	131.74	61.37	17	158.14	61.81
Tyrosine	10	62.35	27.93	30	58.60	28.49	17	73.49	35.40
Phenylalanine	10	99.18	20.84	30	91.76	32.77	17	100.74	29.25
Ornithine	10	108.99	44.69	30	120.74	43.88	17	124.02	41.95
Lysine	10	176.58	99.60	30	160.80	65.24	17	202.53	92.59
Histidine	10	75.97	21.88	30	71.95	19.06	17	81.45	18.01
Arginine	10	102.35	52.58	30	70.32	61.76	17	86.87	56.88
NON ESS/ESS	10	1.72	.48	30	1.75	.44	17	1.68	.83

TABLE 4.40. Amino Acids concentration in blood-serum (μmol/l) in the Shilluk women

	Non pregnant			Pregnant			Lactating		
	n	Mean	sd	n	Mean	sd	n	Mean	sd
Aspartic-Acid	17	47.49	16.66	30	35.20	12.19	17	28.88	22.18
Threonine	17	107.39	32.74	30	121.11	39.30	17	87.11	36.70
Serine	17	149.58	37.58	30	131.37	64.40	17	146.08	48.96
Glutamic-Acid	17	338.31	173.90	30	225.33	161.63	17	212.54	107.61
Glutamine	17	223.02	147.06	30	260.47	172.25	17	473.00	205.16
Glycine	17	266.99	90.60	30	163.82	56.05	17	270.57	62.21
Alanine	17	393.15	17.67	30	308.67	109.08	17	318.27	97.94
Valine	17	148.25	39.97	30	133.57	40.06	17	138.24	47.25
Methionine	17	19.63	6.95	30	17.28	5.92	17	17.30	3.12
Isoleucine	17	50.09	12.22	30	46.32	12.65	17	43.21	14.70
Leucine	17	152.60	38.80	30	20.84	57.75	17	102.27	26.51
Tyrosine	17	66.71	20.80	30	49.33	23.53	17	45.34	14.82
Phenylalanine	17	70.49	21.30	30	64.67	23.98	17	51.34	19.94
Ornithine	17	107.49	60.12	30	78.07	42.90	17	95.46	49.11
Lysine	17	150.71	47.22	30	144.13	52.71	17	134.04	33.16
Histidine	17	74.96	13.02	30	71.13	23.98	17	67.38	14.97
Arginine	17	70.42	28.72	30	68.68	70.96	17	54.55	26.50
NON ESS/ESS	17	1.53	.23	30	1.28	.23	17	1.79	.45

TABLE 4.41. Amino Acids concentration in blood-serum (μmol/l) in the Shilluk children

	0 – 2 years			4 – 14 years		
	n	Mean	sd	n	Mean	sd
Aspartic Acid	16	51.18	36.56	17	41.05	14.87
Threonine	16	104.93	45.70	17	102.49	42.38
Serine	16	198.24	63.48	17	143.45	39.72
Glutamic Acid	16	330.82	136.80	17	222.13	101.14
Glutamine	16	248.08	126.71	17	218.28	132.88
Glycine	16	246.71	88.18	17	215.15	60.39
Alanine	16	449.57	152.63	17	351.33	113.06
Valine	16	213.56	83.00	17	201.91	64.80
Methionine	16	22.01	13.59	17	18.70	6.10
Isoleucine	16	87.19	35.70	17	60.85	19.73
Leucine	16	169.65	75.38	17	156.78	40.53
Tyrosine	16	74.18	25.97	17	71.78	23.65
Phenylalanine	16	71.06	30.40	17	76.88	34.89
Ornithine	16	102.22	52.56	17	92.84	38.59
Lysine	16	226.92	89.20	17	155.91	50.90
Histidine	16	78.54	21.46	17	68.11	11.57
Arginine	16	73.98	49.49	17	50.12	31.32
NON ESS/ESS	16	1.59	.63	17	1.24	.35

TABLE 4.42. Amino Acids concentration in blood-serum (µmol/l) in the Shilluk and the Nuer

	SHILLUK n	SHILLUK Mean	SHILLUK sd	NUER n	NUER Mean	NUER sd
Aspartic Acid	40	44.64	19.86	47	67.03	75.93
Threonine	40	107.72	32.60	47	124.63	61.17
Serine	40	141.69	35.73	47	200.30	55.90
Glutamic Acid	40	333.76	140.93	47	245.01	131.78
Glutamine	40	241.44	160.31	47	380.13	181.25
Glycine	40	257.90	79.89	47	344.68	113.73
Alanine	40	357.30	104.98	47	426.14	130.29
Valine	40	148.05	38.67	47	192.76	93.25
Methionine	40	19.16	5.65	47	31.11	20.02
Isoleucine	40	51.86	14.74	47	55.08	34.33
Leucine	40	145.80	43.28	47	141.29	62.19
Tyrosine	40	69.59	19.05	47	63.99	31.62
Phenylalanine	40	66.10	18.55	47	95.01	31.52
Ornithine	40	101.01	46.20	47	121.93	42.76
Lysine	40	145.71	44.12	47	175.90	77.94
Histidine	40	73.43	13.07	47	75.38	19.05
Arginine	40	77.43	26.20	47	76.31	59.95
NON ESS/ESS	40	1.46	.27	47	1.72	.60

TABLE 4.43. Taurine concentration (µmol/l) in blood-serum

	Children 4 – 14 years n = 17			**Women n = 17**			**Men n = 23**		
	P 25	**Median**	**P 75**	**P 25**	**Median**	**P 75**	**P 25**	**Median**	**P 75**
Shilluk	116	155	172	115	133	196	84	127	179
Nuer	192	229	264	141	181	215	165	184	210

	Non-pregnant n = 17			**Pregnant n = 30**			**Lactating n = 17**		
	P 25	**Median**	**P 75**	**P 25**	**Median**	**P 75**	**P 25**	**Median**	**P 75**
Shilluk women	115	133	196	63	85	119	44	65	123

	Children 4 – 14 years n = 17			**Children 0 – 3 years n = 16**		
	P 25	**Median**	**P 75**	**P 25**	**Median**	**P 75**
Shilluk children	116	155	172	125	151	210
	Shilluk n = 40			**Nuer n = 47**		
	P 25	**Median**	**P 75**	**P 25**	**Median**	**P 75**
Adults	99	130	180	146	184	215

TABLE 4.44. Biological values in relation with food consumption in adults depend of habits (H) or recall (R)

	BEER H	BEER R	FISH H	FISH R	MILK H	MILK R	MEAT R	MEAT/FISH R	DURRA R	VEGETABLE R
Protein g/l										
Album/glob	**	*							*	
Albumin %	*									
Alfa 1 %	*					*			*	
Alfa 2 %	**					*				
Beta %							*			
Gamma %										
IgG g/l										
IgA g/l							*	*	*	
IgM g/l			**		*	*				
AAT g/l						*				
Iron µmol/l										
Transferrin g/l					*	*			*	
Satur coef g/l										
SerFerritin ng/ml				*						
Sodium mmol/l										
Potassium mmol/l									*	
Chloride mmol/l										
Urea mmol/l					*					
Glucose mmol/l	**	*			*	*	*	*		*
Creatinin µmol/l									**	
Calcium mmol/l	*									
Phosph mmol/l	***	**			**	***		*	*	
Alc. Phosph UI/l		*		*	*			*		
Cholest mmol/l										
Triglyce mmol/l				*				*		
Phos.lip mmol/l	*									
SGOT UI/l	*	*						*	*	
SGPT UI/l								*	*	
Zinc µmol/l										
Copper µmol/l			*							
Magnes mmol/l	**	**	*			*		*		
Vitamin A µg/l				*						
Vit. E mg/l										

4.7. BLOOD GROUPS AMONGST THE SHILLUK WOMEN
by Dr. J. REVIRON *

The objective of this study was to identify the frequency of the blood group antigens in the Southern-Sudan population.

Material and methods: Twenty four samples of blood, from pregnant women were obtained from the A.D.E. longitudinal study. Eight blood group systems were investigated.

A B O System : The prevalence of **O** group was similar (41.67%) to that reported by Ikin and Mourant (88). The percentage of **B** phenotype (33.34%) was twice the percentage observed by Roberts & all, but, because of the small number of samples in the present work, the difference is not statistically significant.

Rhesus system : **D c c e e** is the most frequent phenotype among the Shilluk (79.16%) in the southern part of Sudan. On the contrary, this phenotype is seldom seen in the northern part. In other respects, the frequency of the **C** antigen (8.34%) is higher than usually observed in the South.

M N S s system : The distribution of **M** (79.16%) and **N** (62.51%) antigens is similar. The **s** antigen (79.16%) is more frequent than the **S** one (29.18%).

Duffy system : 100% of the samples are **Fy** (a-b-). This phenotype is the commonest in black population. Such red cells are resistant to penetration by Plasmodium vivax but are sensitive to infection by Plasmodium falciparum.

Kell system : All samples are **K** negative. **(P1, P** : All samples are **P1)**

Lewis system : 75% of the women are $\mathbf{Le}^{\mathbf{a}}$ or $\mathbf{Le}^{\mathbf{b}}$ positive. 25% are **Le (a- b-**).

I antigen : None of these adults is deficient.

In conclusion: The frequency of the blood group antigens in the Shilluk population appears close to the expected frequency in that area of Central Africa; except for the **C** antigen of the Rhesus system (more samples are necessary to calculate the accurate frequencies).

** Dr. REVIRON, Centre de Secteur d'Hémobiologie-Transfusion, Hôpital Saint-Louis, Paris*

4.8. HAEMATOLOGICAL INDICES IN SUDAN WITH REFERENCE TO IRON STATUS

by Hans von Rooij (*)

The objective of this particularly study was to identify anaemia and determine the iron status in the Southern-Sudan population.

Iron deficiency anaemia (*IDA*) is the most prevalent nutritional deficiency worldwide (99). It is a major public health problem with adverse consequences especially for women of reproductive age and for young children. Over 90% of affected individuals live in developing countries. Severe anaemia may be a contributory factor in up to 50% of maternal death. The majority of children in Premji (61) study in Bagamoyo in Tanzania were iron deficient.

The iron deficiency develops in three stages:

- The first stage refers to a reduction in iron stores without reduced serum iron levels. Biologically this stage is characterized by the decrease of serum ferritin.
- The second stage consists of a decrease in transport iron. In this stage the biochemical abnormalities usually detected are decease of concentration of serum iron, a decrease of transferrin saturation and an increase of free erythrocyte protoporphyrin.
- The third stage develops when the amount of iron transport decreases sufficiently to restrict the haemoglobin synthesis and iron-deficiency anaemia is evident with the concentrations of haemoglobin below the lower limit of normal (table 4.45).

TABLE 4.45. Haemoglobin levels, indicative of anaemia

Age/sexes group	Haemoglobin level (g/dl)
Children 6 months - 5 years	< 11
Children 6 years _ 14 years	< 12
Adults males	< 13
Adults females (non pregnant)	< 12
Adults females (pregnant)	< 11

Source: Nutritional Anaemia : Report of WHO scientific group. Technical Report Series N°405, WHO, Geneve, 1968

* *Hans von Rooij, A.D.E. Research Centre, Paris and Sobat*

A sample of 803 blood samples from children and adults (including pregnant women) from the A.D.E. longitudinal study was taken into consideration. The haematological data was obtained by electronic counter (Coultronics S5). From a subsample, iron, ferritin and transferrin were determined by micro-method. Thin blood films were prepared. Food intake was evaluated by interrogation of nutritional habits.

One third (30-35%) of the whole population, except children under 3 years, was anaemic (figure 4.1). In children under 3 years 57% were anaemic with microcytosis (48%) and low transferrin saturation as main features (figures 4.2 and 4.3). No association with Hb levels and Z-score of Weight/Height was found. It is important to underline that children had prolonged breastfeeding with a late introduction of solid foods; cow's milk was often introduced in the first year of life.

In children over 3 years and adults, microcytosis was rarely found. There was a tendency to macrocytosis. Thin blood slides showed anisocytosis in 83%. In these groups ferritin values was in the upper level of the normal range. Significant associations of haematological data with iron, transferrin and ferritin were found in some groups of the population under study (table 4.12 and 4.13). Rougereau (106) underlined that the very low serum ferritin levels (<20 ng/ml) encountered in 75.6% of Senegalese women demonstrate the small size of their iron stores.

Because malaria is endemic in this region, its high frequency makes the iron status difficult to interpret but the microcytosis and the relations of haematological data with the iron status suggests the importance of iron contribution in anaemia, particularly in children. But the role of folic acid as a contributing factor in anaemia has to be also considered. N'Diaye (107) found in his study of 76 women and 56 children (age 3-7 years) in Senegal that the haemoglobin level was lower than WHO references (52,3% of the population had a level <11g/dl and 31,8% <10g/dl). In another study of 172 women in Senegal, N'Diaye (108) found that 37% were anaemic (Hb level <11 g/dl) and 18% had an Hb level <10%. But when taking into consideration plasma iron only 5,8% women were anaemic. According to N'Diaye, the plasmatic level do not relate directly to anaemia. Bushra and coll. (109) in a study in Wad Medani hospital fund that 52.5% of pregnant women had anaemia (Hb<11gm/dl) and 1.5% had severe anaemia (Hb<%%7gl/dl).

4.9. DISCUSSION

Very few studies on health and nutritional status are available in the remote areas in Africa where people still live in a very traditional way. Especially biological data are rare due to the difficulties of obtaining blood samples and the procedure to analyse them in high qualified laboratories. The principal limitations to this study are the permanent movement of the population and the climatic conditions which do not allowed a programmed follow up of children from birth until three years old as well as destruction of some blood samples by accident.

Mean values of 56 biochemical parameters have been analysed in a population living in the South Sudan. These parameters can be considered for references in adults (male and female, pregnant and lactating women) as well as in children (in two age groups: 0-3 and 4-14 years old) in nutritional studies in other rural communities in Africa. Data from small samples can be only indicative.

As compared with references from studies in other African rural areas, some biological data can be discussed. The majority of biological data are in the range of normal values; i.e. we didn't observe a relation between mortality risk and albumin level as described by Dramaix (94), who suggested that mortality level, can be defined in terms of values of less than 16g/l of albumin.

Change in the concentration of **serum proteins** during pregnancy and lactation in temperate climates are reported by many investigators. According to N'Diaye study in Senegal (95), there was no difference in serum protein levels between pregnant and non-pregnant women as well as between pregnant women with or without anaemia. Generally the levels of albumin and gamma-globulins fall, while alfa-1, alfa-2 and beta globulins rise add the mean period of lactation.

Some cholesteremia cases were observed in pregnant Masai women (Mann – 96) also atherosclerosis in Masai population (Biss - 97) were reported which is not confirmed in our study, where low level of lipids was due to low fat diet. Noseda (98) also reported similar observations.

Epidemiological criteria can be used to define severe (>40%), moderate (10-39%) or mild (<10%) prevalence of anaemia within populations. In Africa the prevalence of anaemia for the whole population was 37, 9%; in pregnant women 46,9%, in men 28%, in children (< 4 years) 33,1% and in children (5-14 years) 52% (Walker - 99).

In our study, children under 3 years with a low level of haemoglobin (<8g/dl) had similar signs of anaemia like indicated by Luby and coll. (100) who considered pallor of the conjunctive, tongue, palm and nail beds as main clinical signs to diagnose anaemia in African children. They distinguished children between moderate anaemia (Hb concentration 5-8g/dl) and severe anaemia (Hb concentration <5g/dl). I n our study, children were not iron deficient, but 57% were anaemic with microcytosis (48%) and low transferrin saturation, contrary to Premji and coll. (61) who found that the majority of children 6-40 months old under study in Tanzania were iron deficient followed by normochromic macrocytic anaemia. There was also strong evidence in this age group that anaemia was associated with malaria (fever and parasitaemia were mostly observed). In Sudanese children under 7 years old, anaemia, mostly hypochromic, was detected in 79% by Hag and Karrar (101).

Anaemia was less present in adults, especially in Shilluk population, even that malaria and parasitaemia was very high in the study area. This low number of anaemia can be explained by the high consumption of local beer. Gordeuk and coll. (102) described that iron overload in Africa is purely due to excessive iron in traditional beer but recent hypothesis of Moyo and coll. (103), showed that an iron-loading gene may also be implicated in pathogenesis.

The major causes of iron deficiency anaemia are intestinal helminths (hookworm infections) which cause gastrointestinal blood loss. In pregnancy an inadequate iron intake reduced bioavailability of dietary iron (3). Other then iron deficiency anaemia was malaria (Weatherall – 104), thalassaemia and other micro-nutrient deficiency (eg vitamin A deficiency) (Suharno – 105, Underwood - 75).

Dietary diversification is the most effective impact to combat IDA. In megablastic anaemia, following Walker (99), folic acid plays also an important role.

5. NUTRITIONAL STATUS

by Z. L. Ostrowski and E. Ojaba

This cross-sectional study was conducted on three tribal groups: Shilluk, Nuer and Dinka covered a period of eight months including one rainy and one dry season. The Nuer and Dinka groups were surveyed during the dry period and the Shilluk group during the wet one.

The sample was constituted of 77 men, 103 women and 94 children from the three ethnic groups: 137 Shilluk, 196 Nuer and 31 Dinka. 274 food recalls were analysed (table 5.1) and 261 habits were registered (table 5.2). The population was categorized under four groups by age, sex and ethnicity as indicated in table 5.1. Two out of the 276 cases were dropped as their ages and sex was not specified. Due to seasonal migration of the Nuer at the time of survey, this sample was constituted mostly by adults. In the Dinka village only 31 persons were present due to local fightings at the time of the study.

Among the three ethnic groups, only the Shilluk and Nuer groups have been further analysed for comparison. The Dinka group, surveyed by 24-hours recall method, being very small in numbers (31 cases) could not be sub-grouped to give a significant indication. There also was a low coverage on the Nuer children which has some effect on the present results.

The 24 hours recall method was applied to obtain dietary intake. For better assessment, a questionnaire was used to get additional information on the general food habits. Since the recall alone gives only the current status of feeding, general food habits provide supportive information about the mean feeding habits regardless of seasonal variability.

5.1. FOOD INTAKE

Food items and frequency of consumption by recall is expressed in percentages by age and sex (table 5.3). Breast feeding was a habit practiced by all mothers. About half of the children under 5 years were breast-fed on demand (as often as they cry or reach out for the breast).

Cow's milk was consumed mostly by children (young and older at the same proportion, but younger ones received it frequently). Nuer adult men and women had very low milk intake. Meat consumption was fairly low. The mean meat intake was once a day. Adults ate more than children (younger children even rarely). Fish was more widely and frequently eaten than meat. The consumption was the same for all age groups except younger children. Vegetable consumption was fairly low. It was hardly eaten by younger children and very few adults and older children consumed it once a day. Fruits (only wild), usually eaten with staple foodstuffs when fish, meat, milk and vegetables are lacking were extremely rarely consumed by adults and never by younger children.

Beer *(merissa)* which was brewed locally from sorghum and sometimes maize, was generally consumed by adults mostly men (very few children drank it occasionally). The main source of energy was carbohydrate derived from sorghum. The consumption was high as it was the staple food. However, younger children had lower intake since their basic diet was milk.

TABLE 5.1. NUMBER OF CASES SURVEYED BY 24 HOURS FOOD RECALL METHOD

Ethnicity	Children 0-5 years	Children 6-14 years	Men	Women	Pregnant	Total
Shilluk	29	33	38	29	8	137
Dinka	8	11	29	58	-	106
Nuer	7	6	10	8	-	31
Total	44	50	77	95	8	274

TABLE 5.2. NUMBER OF CASES SURVEYED FOR FOOD INTAKE BY HABITS

Ethnicity	Children 0-5 years	Children 6-14 years	Men	Women	Total
Shilluk	33	38	38	38	147
Nuer	9	11	33	61	114
Total	42	49	71	99	261

No answers from 13 persons

TABLE 5.3. FOOD INTAKE BY 24 HOURS RECALL METHOD :
FREQUENCY OF CONSUMPTION BY SEX AND AGE GROUPS
(expressed in percentage)

Food items	Children 0-5 years			Children 6-14 years			Men > 14 years			Women > 14 years		
	Never	Once	Twice	Never	Once	Twice	Never	Once	Twice	Never	Once	Twice
Brest milk	59	0	41	-	-	-	-	-	-	-	-	-
Cow milk	32	18	50	36	30	34	79	12	10	75	14	10
Meat	91	5	5	82	14	4	68	27	5	71	19	9
Fish	75	20	5	66	32	2	67	26	7	62	31	6
Vegetables	96	5	0	76	18	6	81	16	4	83	16	1
Fruits	100	0	0	96	4	0	91	7	2	91	5	4
Sorghum	37	11	57	2	12	86	1	18	81	3	27	70
Beer	93	7	0	94	4	2	63	35	2	40	49	10

5.2. COMPARISON BETWEEN SHILLUK AND NUER FOOD INTAKE BY TWO METHODS: HABITS AND RECALL

Food consumption pattern studies by 24 hours recall and habits were carried out at the time of survey. For both methods, there was less coverage of 391 Nuer than of 512 Shilluk. Significant relationship between recall and habits is expressed by cross tabulation (chi-squares).

Comparison was only made for positive answers. Table 5.4 shows the consumption of breast milk, cow's milk, meat, fish and beer expressed in percentages according to sex and age-group by the two methods of estimation : «24 hours recall» (RE) and «general food habits» (HB).

Booth Shilluk and Nuer give higher responses for breast-feeding by questionnaire (HB) than by recall (RE). By recall (RE) they indicated that only half of Shilluk breast fed their children.

Milk consumption was much higher in Shilluk than Nuer communities. Most Nuer young children often had more milk by habit than recall. The Shilluk group showed no much variation in intake by the two methods. Because the nomadic Nuer had their cattle in the grazing lands at the time of the survey, milk was not easily available for younger children (at recall time) who usually follow the cattle to the grazing areas and therefore had better access to milk. Shilluk adults consumed more milk than Nuer. Shilluk men consumed much more than women: a clear indication of their tradition.

For both ethnic groups, meat consumption was highly responded by «habits» while «recall» evaluation indicated that mostly they consumed once a day.

Most people had fish more than once a day, except Nuer young children. By recall (RE), fish consumption was significantly higher in Shilluk than in Nuer. Beer *(Merissa)* was consumed only by adults. Nuer men and women drank beer at the same rate while Shilluk men drank much more than their women. By custom, children do not take beer.

5.3. WAY OF EATING

Generally adult men do not take meals with their wives or children (table 5.5). 76% of Shilluk and 61% of Nuer men ate with other men and 13% of Shilluk and 33% of Nuer ate alone. By Nuer, Dinka and Shilluk custom, men usually do not eat together with women. Nevertheless, three Shilluk men had meals with women (those who live close to the French CCI camp). 62% of Nuer women and only 32% of Shilluk women ate with other women. 42% of Shilluk women ate with children and very rarely alone. Children generally share meals among themselves. Nuer older children never ate with adults whereas it was possible for the Shilluk to eat with women (16%).

5.4. FREQUENCY OF MEAL CONSUMPTION PER DAY

261 Nuer and Shilluk surveyed by food habits, and 243 by food recall were evaluated for the number of meals eaten per day (table 5.6). Nuer and Shilluk usually eat twice a day. However, the Nuer showed greater tendency to eat less. Data are similar by both methods. One third of Nuer had only one meal per day. One Shilluk man had eaten nothing the whole day as there was no food. Also one Nuer woman did not take any meal because she drank only beer (*merissa*) for the whole day. Both Shilluk and Nuer young children frequently eat more than twice a day, 20 % of children had even 3-4 meals per day (by HB).

5.5. FREQUENCY OF FOOD CONSUMPTION

5.5.1. Shilluk community feeding pattern

More Nuer children got breast milk between ages 0-5 years, than Shilluk children (table 5.7). Generally, milk consumption was very high in children. Younger children drank it more frequently: 3 to 5 times a day. With age, the consumption decreased: older children (73%) and adults (34%). Among adults, women drank less milk (16%) than men; pregnant women not at all due to a customary milk taboo associated with their physiological status. Meat consumption was generally poor. Only 7 % younger and 12 % older children had meat dishes. Adults ate twice as much as children. Women ate less except during pregnancy. Contrary, fish, being the first source of protein, was more consumed by all groups, especially by men. Vegetables (a rare food in this area) were mostly consumed by women especially during pregnancy. Men and older children ate it occasionally. Fruits were rarely consumed by Shilluk, while wild fruits more often by Nuer. The consumption of cereals (sorghum) was very high, often consumed twice a day. It was the mean food for adults and older children (97 % - 100 %), while younger children consumed less frequently (62 %). Beer was drank twice as much by men than by women. Children drank beer occasionally with their parents (6-10 %).

5.5.2. Nuer community feeding pattern

Half of the Nuer children aged 0-5 years were being breast-fed at the time of the survey. Generally, milk consumption was very poor for Nuer. Older children drank milk more frequently (36%), women less (24%) and only very few men (7%) drank milk. Meat constitutes the basic source of protein in the Nuer diet during the dry season. The consumption was relatively high in adults (30%): *women (45%), men 38% and children without age distinction only 26%.* The Nuer consumed less fish than meat, while younger children did not consumed fish. Apparently, there was no variation in the rate of consumption of fish and meat for older children. Vegetable consumption was not observed in the Nuer community (probably because the survey was conducted during the dry season). Fruits (wild) were consumed often by adults and older children. The consumption of cereals was very high in the whole Nuer population, except by younger children (62%). Men and women consumed often beer (40%), while children never!

TABLE 5.4. COMPARISON BETWEEN SHILLUK AND NUER FOR HABIT AND RECALL FOOD INTAKE ACCORDING TO SEX AND AGE GROUPS EXPRESSED IN PERCENTAGES

	Ethnicity	Brest milk		Cow milk		Meat		Fish		Beer	
		HB	RB	HB	RB	HB	RB	HB	RB	HB	RB
Children 0-5 years	Shilluk	76	38	82	83	84	7	63	18	42	0
	Nuer	56	50	89	26	78	25	67	0	0	0
Children 0-5 years	Shilluk			68	72	89	12	89	42	58	6
	Nuer			18	36	100	27	72	27	36	0
Men > 14 years	Shilluk			53	34	95	24	92	55	94	66
	Nuer			3	6	88	38	97	27	73	41
Women > 14 years	Shilluk			42	16	87	19	90	40	82	30
	Nuer			13	24	92	45	89	33	72	40

TABLE 5.5. WAY OF EATING IN SHILLUK AND NUER FAMILIES ACCORDING TO SEX AND AGE GROUPS (IN %)

	Ethnicity	Alone	With children	With men	With family	Unknown
Children 0-5 years	Shilluk	39 %	36 %	9 %	0	16 %
	Nuer	11 %	56 %	22 %	0	11 %
Children 0-5 years	Shilluk	5 %	63 %	16 %	5 %	11 %
	Nuer	18 %	82 %	0	0	0
Men >14 years	Shilluk	13 %	3 %	8 %	0	0
	Nuer	33 %	3 %	0	0	3 %
Women >14 years	Shilluk	3 %	42 %	32 %	8 %	15 %
	Nuer	15 %	15 %	62 %	2 %	6 %

TABLE 5.6. COMPARISON BETWEEN SHILLUK (Sh) AND NUER (Nr) FOR FREQUENCY OF MEAL INTAKE/DAY (IN %) by Recall *«RE»* (243 cases) and by Habits *«HB»* (261 cases) according to age and sex

Frequency meals/day	Ethnicity	Once/day HB	Once/day RB	Twice/day HB	Twice/day RB	Three/day HB	Three/day RB	Four/day HB	Four/day RB	Unknown HB	Unknown RB
Children 0-5 years	Shilluk	0	38	48	76	18	14	18	0	15	3*
	Nuer	0	50	56	75	11	0	22	0	11	13*
Children 0-5 years	Shilluk	3	6	87	82	3	12	0	0	8	0
	Nuer	27	18	73	82	0	0	0	0	0	0
Men >14 years	Shilluk	5	21	92	76	3	0	0	0	0	3**
	Nuer	27	31	67	69	3	0	0	0	3	0
Women >14 years	Shilluk	13	16	76	84	0	0	0	0	11	0
	Nuer	26	16	66	83	0	0	0	0	8	2***

* = Breast fed only, ** = No food to cook, *** = Drank beer only

TABLE 5.7. FREQUENCY OF FOOD CONSUMPTION BY 137 SHILLUK AND 106 NUER ACCORDING TO AGE GROUPS

	Ethnicity	Brest milk	Cow milk	Meat	Fish	Vegetabl	Fruit	Beer	Sorghum
Children 0-5 years	Shilluk	38	83	7	38	3	0	10	62
	Nuer	50	25	25	0	0	0	0	88
Children 0-5 years	Shilluk	0	73	12	42	24	0	6	97
	Nuer	0	36	27	27	0	18	0	100
Men >14 years	Shilluk	0	34	24	55	24	0	66	100
	Nuer	0	7	38	28	0	24	41	96
Women >14 years	Shilluk	0	16	19	40	43	0	30	100
	Nuer	0	24	45	30	0	16	40	98

5.6. DISCUSSION

Children are breast-fed already from the first hours after delivery. The duration of breast-feeding was until 2-3 years. In the first year of life the beneficial effect of breast feeding has been reported by many authors. Salih (110) observed in the Sudan that almost all mothers (99.9%) initiated breast-feeding on the first hours after delivery. In the same study it was found that in the rural communities it was delayed of 6 hours. The breast-feeding rate was 92% at 7 months, 65% at one year and 4% still breast-fed at 2 years. The majority of mothers stopped it if the baby had diarrhoea or they wanted another child. For Nur (111) the length of birth interval appears to be primarily a result of the interruption of lactation. Fawzi (1) reported that breast feeding was a strong modifier of the association between weight-for-height and mortality. It can be explained by the fact that breast fed babies receive antibodies and other immunologic substances from their mother's milk and this may provide some protection even against death from infections (7, 9). For Victoria (112) the risk of death from infections other then diarrhoea or respiratory infection was less clearly associated with breast-feeding. For de Vries (113) feeding practices were factors influencing survival. The author disagreed with western studies suggesting that infants with difficult temperaments are at greater risk for behavioural and physical disorders. Our study showed that the Nilotic population, as well as the Masai (*), is genetically prepared to the lifestyle in the specific environment. Their health status and survive is in a great part due to the protective breast-feeding practices.

In our study, the priority food for children until 13 years in this population was milk. The other main sources of protein are fish and meat. Sorghum (durra) was the staple food easily available and most frequently consumed by all except the youngest children. Vegetable and fruits are extremely rare consumed. Beer which provides a secondary source of energy and occasionally acts as a meal-substitute where there was no food was consumed largely by adults: 59 % by men and 37 % by women. Between the two ethnicities, the Nuer consumed more meat, while the Shilluk more fish. Women had more protein rich foods (milk, meat, and fish) than men. Among all age groups, the only fair consumption of vegetables was observed in older children. Dietary vitamin A intake was very poor, however it is very protective especially among children who were wasting and stunted. Fawzi (114) concluded that it has an important role in reducing childhood mortality in developing countries (probably because vegetables and fruits contain also other vital nutrients which can reduce childhood morbidity).

The main source of energy was sorghum for both Shilluk and Nuer populations and its consumption was in the same proportion for children, men and women.

While the Shilluk consumed more milk, fish, vegetables and beer; the Nuer ate twice more meat, lot of fruits but no vegetables. This difference in the type of foods eaten basically results from the nature of their local environment.

* *Masai belongs to the same Nilotic population as Dinka, Nuer and Shilluk.*

The nutritional value of food consumed by pregnant women was low caloric (about 1200 cal). The fat content was very small and provides about 19.8% of energy. The intake of carbohydrate (sorghum) was relatively large and provides about 62% of total caloric intake. The contribution of protein was relatively high (approximate about 18.4%) due to high fish and meat consumption.

Because indications obtained by «food habits» are always higher than data obtained by «24-hour recall» method, it is important to confirm data obtained by the first method.

6. INFANT AND CHILD FEEDING PRACTICES AMONG THE SHILLUK TRIBE

by E. Ojaba and Z. L. Ostrowski

Feeding habits and practices were based on 261 children age 0 to 30 months. Dietary information was obtained through direct interview of mothers, observations, and 1392 food recalls treated as cross-sectional survey.

The main objective of this study was to reveal the habits and patterns of child feeding from birth to weaning and after. Table 6.1 shows a gradual progression from breast feeding, supplementary feeding to total weaning. It also shows that all children are breastfed at least for one year. At the same time, more than half are given supplementary food which was mostly milk at this stage. A few children are weaned by the beginning of the second year (7%) and, about a third (28%), by the end of the second year. To make detailed description easier, information was further subjected to four classifications as follows:

1° - Pre-breast milk feeding practices.
2° - Breast-feeding practices.
3° - Supplementary feeding practices.
4° - Weaning and post-weaning feeding practices.

6.1. PRE-BREAST MILK FEEDING PRACTICES

During the immediate period after birth, it is a customary practice that all mothers offer their babies the breast as soon as they have recovered well enough from labour (from few minutes to one day). As breast milk was not usually available immediately after birth, several liquid preparations are being given to neonates during this period. Some like water and salt solutions have no nutrition value; others like cow milk, sheep milk and goat milk have a nutritional value (Table 6.2a). A few mothers even continue to give these «feeds» much longer after the breast milk was available. Some of these are mixed with sugar. Moreover, there was a high tendency for mothers to give those preparations to their babies without first boiling (65%) (Table 6.2b). Such attitudes may possibly have traditional implication. Day-to-day observations and proceeding food recalls of the same babies seem to support this finding. The indication is that some of those mothers, who had been giving un-boiled milk during the pre-breast milk period, continued to give un-boiled milk supplements and started boiling it once the supplementation period was over.

TABLE 6.1. Progression of breast and supplementary feeding to total weaning by age

Age groups / Feeding status	0 – 6		7 – 12		13 – 18		19 – 24		25 – 30		Total	
	n	%	n	%	n	%	n	%	n	%	n	%
Brest-fed only	163	41	48	14	32	9	22	9	2	3	267	19
Brest-fed and supplementar	233	59	29	85	28	84	14	63	23	30	984	71
Food only	1	0	2	1	22	7	65	28	51	67	141	10
Total	397		344		340		235		76		1392	

TABLE 6.2a. Feeding preparation given to infants during the pre-breast milk periods

Values	Feeding preparations	n	%
Nourishments	Water, sugar, salt	69	47 %
	Water, sugar	9	6 %
	Milk, sugar, salt	5	3 %
	Cow milk	11	7 %
	Sheep milk	16	11 %
	Goat milk	6	4 %
	Powder milk	1	1 %
	Total	117	79 %
Non nourishments		16	11 %
		12	8 %
		3	2 %
	Total	31	21 %
	GENERAL TOTAL	148	100 %

TABLE 6.2b. Infants given boiled and unboiled feeds During the pre-breast milk periods

Feeding praparation	Boiled		Unboild		Total	
	n	%	n	%	n	%
Cow milk	5	10 %	6	12 %	11	22 %
Sheep milk	7	14 %	9	19 %	16	33 %
Goat milk	1	2 %	5	10 %	6	12 %
Water	4	8%	12	25 %	16	33 %
Total	**17**	**35 %**	**32**	**65 %**	**49**	**100 %**

6.2. BREAST FEEDING PRACTICES

As mentioned previously, breast feeding was a common tradition practiced by all mothers in this community. Children are breast fed on demand or when they cry, usually interpreted by most mothers as sign or expression of hunger.

Mothers preferably breast-feed in a sitting position apart from night feeding which was usually done lying down. The position of feeding was however modified during long journeys walking on foot; mothers suckle while walking, holding their children by one hand supported on their hips and/or chests, whichever of the two breasts taken first is given to the child. In this way, children have good chance of suckling from both breasts alternatively at every feed. This however was not always the case. Where there are twins, the custom is that each suckles from one breast only: the first sucks only from the right breast and the second only from the left. Under no circumstance would the mother alternate the breasts during the same feed. During another feed, the mother puts them to different breasts from the previous feed.

Table 6.3 and figure 6.1 shows the proportion and rate of decline in breast feeding practices on 1251 recalls at various ages. One important indication is that a few children were still breast fed even after the second year. This by itself is not surprising since in the past, it was not unusual to find children over 3 years still suckling. Such customs are sometimes common among other tribes of the Southern Sudan. An example of prolonged breast feeding is that which practiced by the Madi tribe of Eastern Equatorial was. Children suckled until 4 to 5 years old. This age factor is further stressed by the story that «*those children actually went away all day attending sheep and goats with older children: on arriving home in the evening, they first rushed to their mothers for breast milk*».

TABLE 6.3. Breast feeding and the rate of decline (by 6 months age groups)

Age groups	**n**	**%**
0 - 6	396	31,7%
7 - 12	342	27,3%
13 -18	318	25,4%
19 - 24	170	13,6%
25 - 30	25	2,0%
TOTAL	1251	

However, prolonged breast-feeding in the case of the Shilluk may have some direct link with the old tradition. This concerns the practice that all food supplements other than milk were with-held until such a time when children are able to pick and actually eat food by themselves. A reason a few mothers mentioned for with-holding was that the stool of their children would develop a strong offensive smell if they gave cereals and other foods earlier. As children often soil themselves with stool when small, mothers try to avoid this by late introduction of food, especially cereals.

If we consider the conclusions of Mata (115) and Jelliffe (116) that breast milk has unique anti-infective properties, the results of our study are satisfactory since almost 100 % of infants are breast-fed at least one year. Moreover, for Victoria (112) no breast feeding increase the risk of death from diarrhoea 14,2 times and from respiratory diseases 3,6 times.

6.3. SUPPLEMENTARY FEEDING

Supplementary food in this context means «*any additional food given to a child besides breast milk*» (figure 6.2). For all children studied from 0 - 30 months, the following food items have been recorded as supplements: milk constitutes 42%, cereals 22%, sugar and fish 11-12%, soup 6% and vegetables 3%. Meat, oil, beverage and egg were rarely consumed (table 6.4. and figure 6.3).

Milk, being the major supplementary diet, is also the first to be introduced to children. Many infants take milk supplements during the first months. 96 % were already receiving milk by the age of 6 months. As children grow older, the frequency of milk consumption decreases (table 6.4). On the other hand, the quantity of milk consumed increases from 135g during the first 6 months to 339g by the end of the second year. This important amount of milk consumed by the children provides protection at this stage of life.

a) Different types of milk consumed

The different types of milk recorded as consumed by children were: cows, goats, sheep and mixed (*). Cow's milk being the most frequently consumed constituted 84 % of the total milk diet. Goats, sheep and mixed milk were rarely (Table 6.5) consumed by children of poor families, who have no cows or when family cows become non-lactating. The consumption of powder milk was recorded rarely only in the Sobat-Nile area, due to the Jonglei Canal construction.

* *A mixture of more than one type of milk: usually prepared when cow's milk is in shortage, or purposely given as it is believed to prevent or stop diarrhoea.*

b) Different ways of milk preparation

Milk supplements are prepared in 5 different ways (table 6.6). Most mothers boil milk before giving to children. This practice remains fairly constant throughout the different stages. However, those who do not boil it do so under the mistaken belief that «boiled milk causes diarrhoea». Compared to the total milk consumption, figure 6.4 shows the percentage of boiled diluted milk and powder milk (after reconstitution) in the first 3 years.

FIGURE 6.1. Breast feeding and the rate of decline

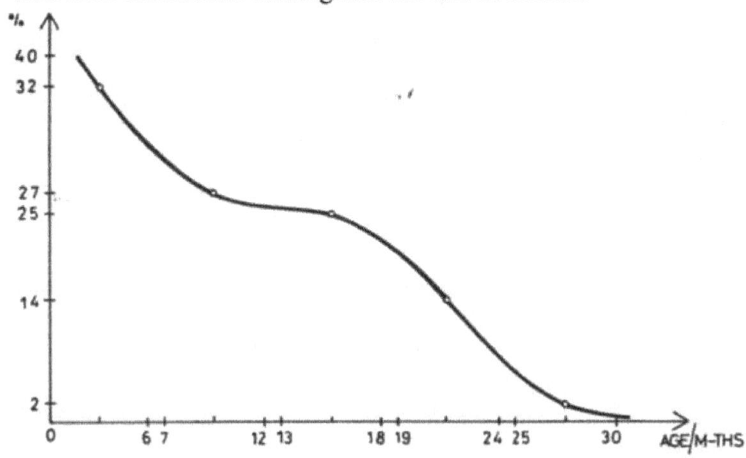

TABLE 6.4. Age of introduction of foods and frequency of consumption by age

Age groups / Food grups	0 – 6 n	0 – 6 %	7 – 12 n	7 – 12 %	13 – 18 n	13 – 18 %	19 – 24 n	19 – 24 %	25 – 30 n	25 – 30 %	Total n	Total %
Meat	0	-	0	-	8	1	18	3	3	1	29	1
Fish	0	-	39	9	112	16	71	12	29	12	251	11
Soup	0	-	15	3	43	6	52	8	23	10	133	6
Oil	0	-	1	0	4	1	6	1	5	2	16	1
Egg	0	-	3	1	3	1	2	0	0	-	8	0
Milk	234		269	62	229	32	150	25	49	21	931	42
Cereals	96		65	12	193	27	171	28	61	26	901	22
Vegetables	0	-	0	-	10	1	30	5	15	6	55	3
Beverages	0	-	0	-	13	2	20	3	19	8	52	2
Sugar	0	-	41	10	93	13	89	15	32	14	266	12
	1											
		4										
Total	245		433		708		609		236		2231	

Dilution of milk is a very common practice, particularly during the first 6 months. Diluted milk was gradually replaced by undiluted milk as children approach the end of their first year. The administration of sour milk follows a different pattern. While sour milk was rarely given to children during the earlier months, it was consumed more often during the second and third years (table 6.6 and figure 6.6). This is also under the mistaken belief that sour milk causes diarrhoea when given to infants but provides protection against diarrhoea when given to older children.

c) Mode of administration of milk feeds

The mode of administration of milk feeds during the first year was variable. While some mothers fed their children with spoon, others gave with calabash, cups, tins or bottles (table 6.7). Spoon feeding however is applied only when children are still small.

Bottle feeding was observed in 80 cases (30%). Bottles used for feeding were "*normal feeding bottles*" purchased from local shops or from a pharmacy in Malakal about 40 km away. Others were thrown-away empty beer bottles or any kind of bottles that mothers could lay hands on. Normal teats were rarely later purchased or obtained from neighbours and fitted on to those collected bottles.

Table 6.7 shows the age of introduction and discontinuation of bottle-feeding. No information has been obtained from 6 % of the sample about the time of introduction and 21 % of the sample for the time of discontinuation.

50 % of infants were introduced to bottle-feeding at the age of 1-2 months, 30 % at 3-4 months, 10 % at 5-6 months and 4 % at 7-8 months. What is strange is «*why mothers should still want to start bottle feeding as late as 7-8 months*».

Possible reasons for such attitudes and practices are:

1) The inabilities of mothers to find feeding bottles earlier, on gathering enough money, they could buy bottles and introduce their children to bottle feeding at any time.

2) The inadequacy of fresh milk drives mothers to alternatively buy rarely powder milk, consequently feeding bottles. The latter was confirmed by the fact that a few mothers have actually indicated the availability of powder milk as their main reason for bottle feeding.

Duration of bottle feeding was calculated from the time difference between age at introduction and age at discontinuation. Consequently, for children who were bottle-fed for a certain period, the most frequent duration was 1-2 months (35%) and 3-4 months (45%). A few children continued to receive milk by bottles even after the ninth month. It was not however possible to determine the duration of bottle-feeding for some children (27%) as their mothers knew neither when they started, stopped nor both.

Some reasons given for bottle feeding were:

- When mothers go away to the fields or some far places, it was easier for older children to feed younger children with bottles.
- Bottle-feeding was very good: «It is like the breast».
- Children refused to drink from a cup.

TABLE 6.5. Different types of milks given to children by age

Age groups	0 – 6		7 – 12		13 – 18		19 – 24		25 – 30		Total	
Food items	n	%	n	%	n	%	n	%	n	%	n	%
Cow milk	182	78	250	91	201	83	138	84	55	90	826	84
Goat milk	19	8	7	3	12	5	9	6	2	3	49	5
Sheep milk	6	3	0	-	7	3	2	1	1	2	16	2
Mixed milk	0	-	4	1	1	0	0	-	0	-	5	1
Powder milk	27	11	15	5	22	9	15	9	3	5	82	8
Total	234		276		243		164		61		978	

TABLE 6.6. Mode of milk preparation for children by age

Age groups	0 – 6		7 – 12		13 – 18		19 – 24		25 – 30		Total	
Preparations	n	%	n	%	n	%	n	%	n	%	n	%
Raw whole	4	2	18	7	16	7	10	7	7	12	55	6
Raw diluated	3	1	0	-	2	1	0	-	0	-	5	1
Boiled whole	65	31	153	60	121	56	81	56	26	45	466	51
Boiled diluated	135	65	42	16	9	5	1	1	0	-	187	21
Souer milk	1	1	43	17	67	31	53	36	25	43	189	21
Total	208		256		215		145		58		882	

TABLE 6.7. Age at begging and stoping of bottle feeding (*)

Age groups	1 – 2	3 – 4	5 – 6	7 – 8	9 – 10	11 – 12	No data	Total
Age of beginning Bootle feeding	40 50 %	24 30 %	8 10 %	3 4 %	-	-	5 6 %	80
Age of stopping Bootle feeding	4 5 %	19 24 %	25 31 %	9 11 %	4 5 %	2 3 %	17 21 %	80
Duration of Bootle feeding	20 25 %	26 33 %	7 9 %	3 4 %	2 3 %	-	22 27 %	80

(*) These bottles were available in this area because of the CCI Jonglei Canal camp.

6.4. WEANING AND POST WEANING FEEDING PRACTICES

SUGAR is the first food item introduced to the newborn. By sugar we are referring generally to normal sugar, sugar cane and sorghum stalks. Table 6.4 shows sugar as the second food item introduced during the first 6 months. Normal sugar was always consumed incorporated into other foods:

(a) with milk during the first 6 months,
(b) with milk and cereals between 7 and 12 months,
(c) with milk, cereals or beverages from second year onwards.

Sugar cane and sorghum stalk were also chewed during the second year. Sometimes, it was initially chewed by either mother or bigger child and put into the month of the child to press out its sweet liquid. Sugar started to play a greater role with the development of the Jonglei Canal in the study area.

OTHER FOODS like cereals, fish, soup and eggs were introduced between 7-12 months. Later, from 13-18 months, meat, vegetables, beverages and oil (rarely) were also introduced (table 6.4 and figure 6.3).

By the age of 2 years most children were able to eat from all the above 10 groups of food, who have been further categorized in two sub-groups (table 6.8):

Sub-group I - «<u>Infant and child foods</u>». This group comprises mostly of liquid and semi-liquid food which is usually regarded by the community as suitable for infants and young children. They are milk, soup, egg, beverage, sugar and semi-liquid cereal preparations such as porridge, custard,...

Sub-group II - «<u>Adult food</u>» or «<u>Family food</u>» comprises mainly of solid items. This is food normally prepared for consumption by the entire house-hold such as: meat, fish, oil, vegetables and solid cereal preparations like stiff-porridge, «kisra», «akelo» and maize.

The mean age at introduction of sub-group I food item was 7 months and of sub-group II food items was 12 months. Fish was a common family diet, because of its soft texture and palatability; it was given to children as early as 7 months. On the other hand, beverages, mostly sweetened water (or tea) and fresh fruit juice (if available) are introduced at 13 months and above. The importance of fish and meat in children's diet is shown in figure 6.5. If fish consumption increase rapidly between the 7th and 15th month, meat consumption in the second year of life remains at a low level. The place of vegetables in the first 3 years of life was very poor. If the total consumption of vegetables at age 30 months is 100%, figure 6.6 shows the part of vegetables between 12 and 27 months. Compared to milk consumption (figure 6.7) or to cereal consumption (figure 7.8), vegetables are consumed in a very small amount.

Other food items like soup, oil and eggs, compared to different milk consumption, present a very low percentage (table 6.4 and figure 6.9.).

The mean nutritional value of supplementary food par day, **in a sub-sample of infants**, was calculated based on the adapted to the South Sudan Food Tables (Ostrowski and Josse - 117). The results were compared between infants receiving still breast milk and infants without breast milk. The nutritional value of the supplementary food was very low: for infants without breast milk: 489 Cal with a higher carbohydrate value (62,7%). Those who were still breast-fed get only 219 Cal and three times less iron (Table 6.9).

TABLE 6.8. Age of introduction of infant and adult food

FOOD GROUPS	AGE OF INTRODUCTION
INFANT FOOD	
Milk	1 month
Soup	9 month
Egg	8 month
Beverage	13 month
Sugars	2 month
Cereals semi-liquid	7 month
FAMILY FOOD	
Meat	13 month
Fish	7 month
Oil	15 month
Vegetables	14 month
Cereals solid	10 month

TABLE 6.9. Mean nutritional value of supplementary food received by infants/day

Nutritional value	**Still Brest-fed**		**Without Brest milk**	
Calories	219 Cal		489 Cal	
Proteines	9,3 g	17,0%	19,5 g	16,0%
Lipides	7,4 g	30,4%	11,6 g	21,3%
Carbohydrates	28,8 g	52,6%	76,7 g	62,7%
Iron	0,9 mg		2,7 mg	
Vitamin C	1,0 mg		1,3 mg	

FIGURE 6.2. Relative importance of breast milk only (B), breast and supplementary food (BS) and other food (OF)

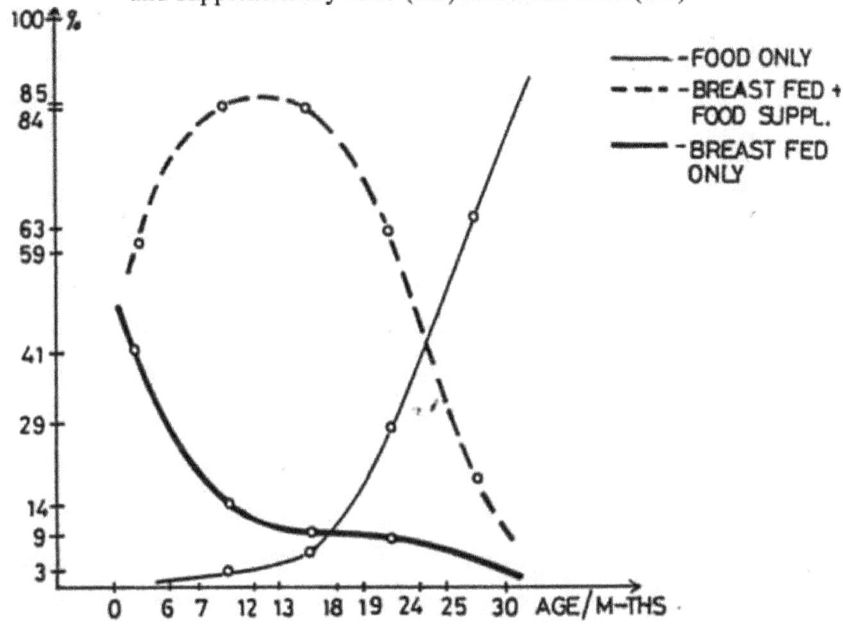

FIGURE 6.3. Age of introduction and frequency of consumption of different food items

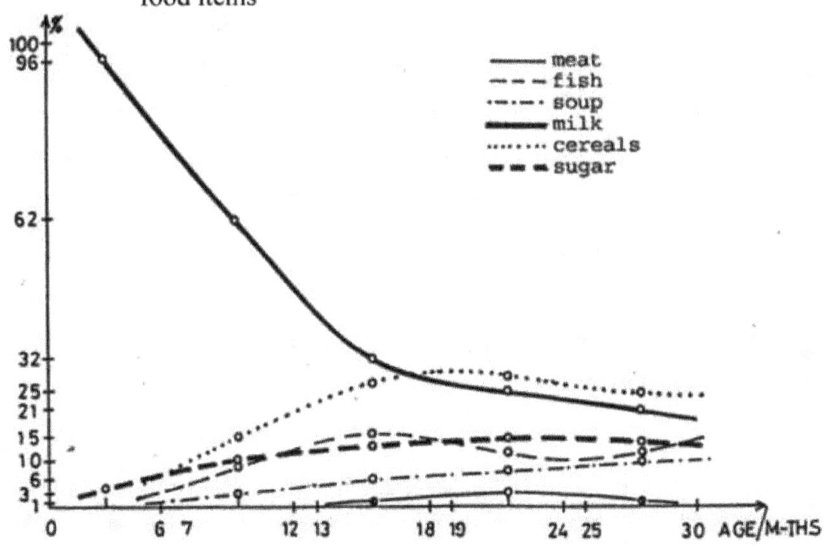

FIGURE 6.4. Pourcentage of powder milk and boild diluated milk in the first 3 years

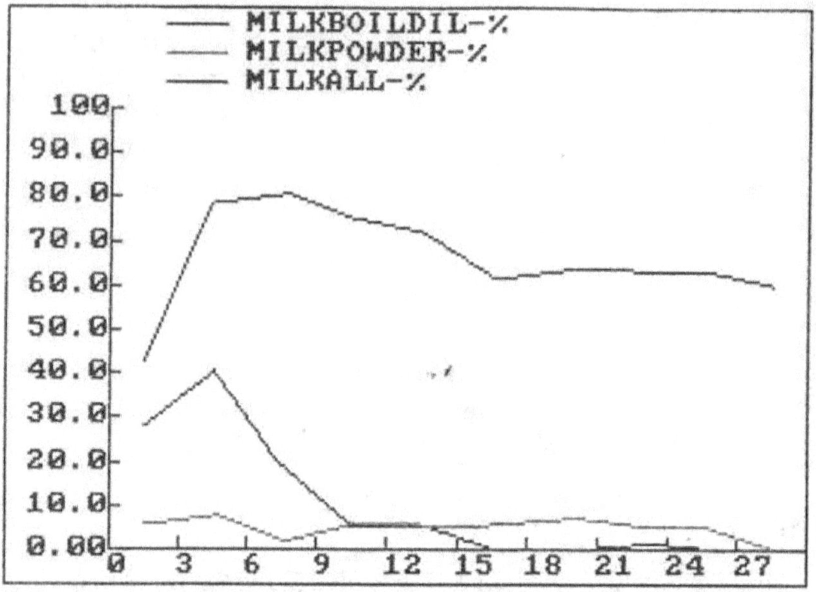

FIGURE 6.5. The importance of fish and meat in children's diet

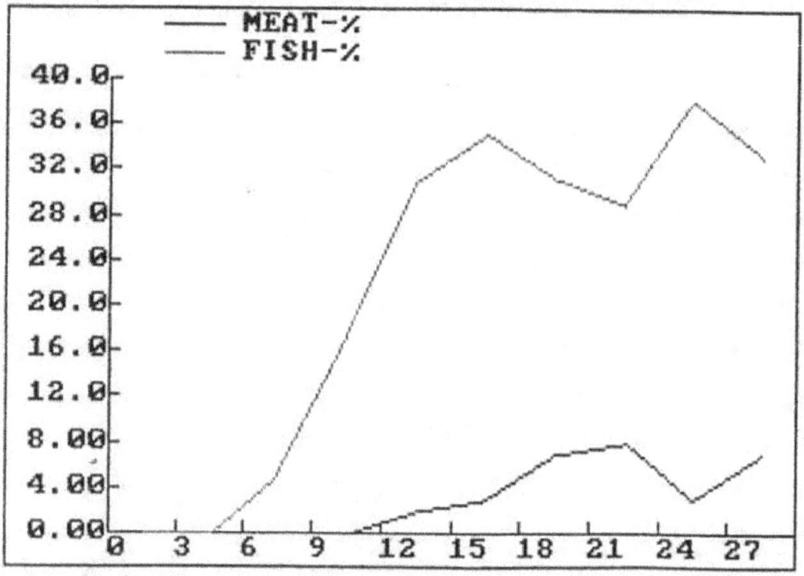

FIGURE 6.6. Part of vegetables between 12 and 27 months

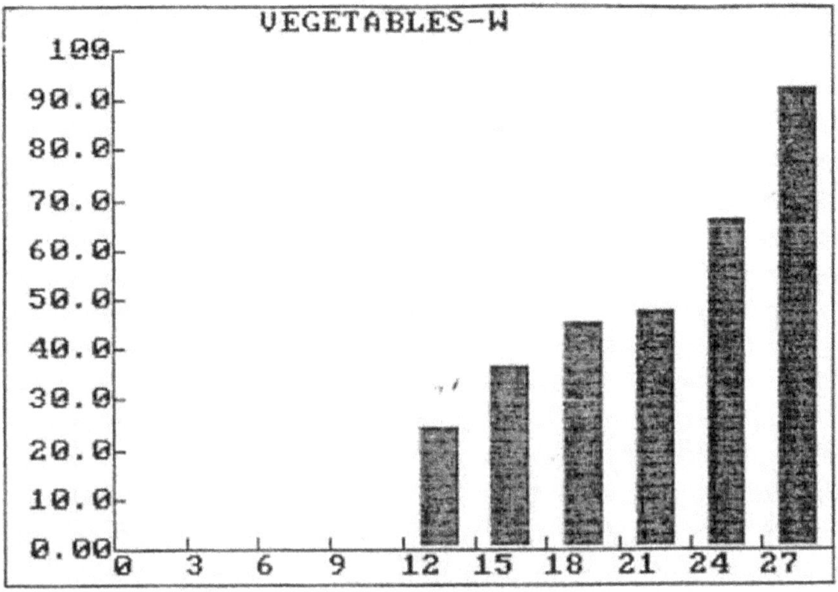

FIGURE 6.7. Milk and vegetables consumption

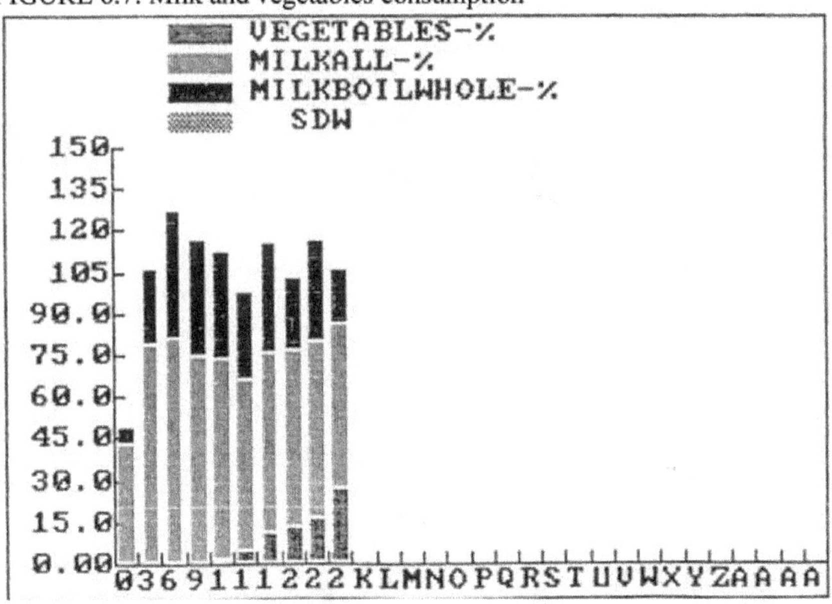

FIGURE 6.8. Milk and cereals consumption

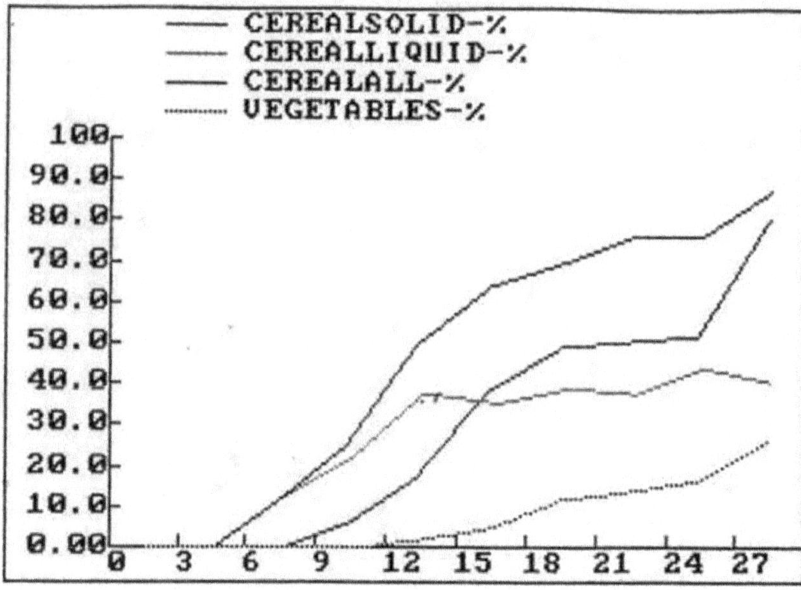

FIGURE 6.9. Other food items like soup, oil and eggs, compared to milk consumption

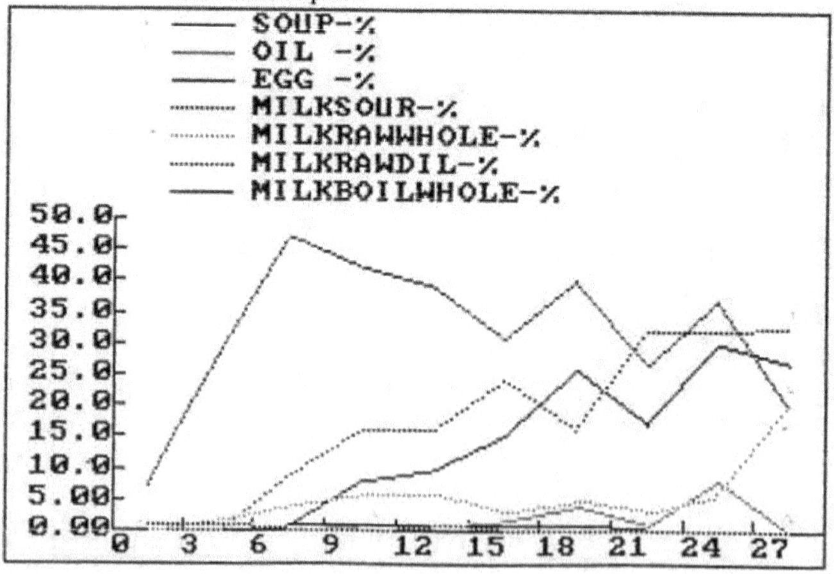

7. CULTURAL ATTITUDES TOWARDS FEEDING PRACTICES

by E. Ojaba and Z. L. Ostrowski

Each society and especially those living still in a traditional way have own food habits. Because some difference appeared between the three main ethnic groups, it was of interest to study the frequency and pattern of meal consumption per day, the weaning practices and the cultural attitudes towards infants and child feeding practices.

7.1. FREQUENCY OF CONSUMPTION OF FOOD/DAY

Frequency of consumption was expressed in terms of the number of times a child had eaten a certain food item per day (table 7.1). Some foods were mostly consumed once a day: meat (97%), vegetables (93%), soup (88%), oil (81%) or eggs (62%). Occasionally it was consumed twice a day, and never three times per day. Fish and beverages were consumed often once (87% and 83%), occasionally twice (12% and 9%) and rarely three times (1% and 8%). The frequency of sugar consumption was evenly distributed. Unlike other items, milk was consumed often three times or twice (40%) and rarely once a day (22%).

7.2. FREQUENCY AND PATTERN OF MEAL CONSUMPTION/DAY

The number of times children were fed per day is indicated in table 7.2. 51 % of children had 3 meals per day, 32 % twice and 17 % only once.

The most frequent pattern of meal was breakfast, lunch and dinner (52%). This was followed by breakfast and lunch (20%), breakfast alone (13%) and breakfast and dinner (11%). Other patterns of meals occurred very rarely (table 7.3). The breakfast and lunch pattern applies often to children less than 15 months. This gradually shifts to breakfast and dinner as children grow older.

The change to the latter pattern is a result of some mothers resorting to providing only breakfast before going to the fields for cultivation, guard or harvest of the crops. These children are then left for the whole day without food until the mothers return home to prepare the evening meal.

The important meal of the day was breakfast (40 %), then lunch (32 %) and dinner (28 %). It should be noted that breakfast was usually eaten between 10-11 am; lunch between 2-3 pm and dinner between 6-8 pm (always in darkness to avoid flies and termites).

7.3. WEANING PRACTICES

Many nutrition and health publications describe the term «**weaning**» as the time of introduction of foods other than mother's milk. «Weaning» interpreted as such may be quite misleading and less meaningful. Since in the Shilluk community, milk supplement was introduced as early as the first week or month, it would thus seem quite improper to consider this time as a weaning period. The term weaning in our study therefore is intended to carry the meaning as the period when children are completely stopped feeding from the breasts.

The consequent **progression of weaning** along with age shows that breast feeding decreases rapidly at the end of the first year, remaining until the 3rd year at 10% (table 7.4 and figure 6.1). For 144 food recalls of children who were not having breast milk, 16% were weaned between 13 and 18 months, 45% between 19 and 24 months and 37% after 2 years. 2% had no breast milk during the first year. These were: 2 children visited only during the first day after birth before breast milk was available and one child whose mother had died earlier.

It used to be customary (tradition) among the Shilluk that children were not weaned until they were 3 years or over. This coincided with the prolonged period of breast-feeding. It also has a link with the old custom that a woman must not practice sex as long as she is lactating. It is believed that the mother's milk becomes contaminated and poisonous for the child after having sexual relationship (*). The prolonged breast feeding encouraged delayed weaning. Naturally, it would not be very easy or pratical neither for the man with one wife or for the woman to abstain from sexual relationship for 3 years.

From direct interview of a sub-sample of 23 mothers, **the appropriate age for child weaning** was indicated as ranging from 1-3 years with a mean age of 2 years. Data from longitudinal recalls of 261 mothers however revealed a much earlier weaning age, varying within localities. For example in Obang village, near the base of a French camp (construction of the Jonglei Canal), and easy accessibility to Malakal town, the mean age for weaning was found to be 16 months. In two other villages Obai and Doleib Hill, about 7 km away on either sides of Obang, the mean weaning age was 18 months. In Pajur village 20 km

** As example of lack of knowledge is the death at age 13 months of a strong and healthy baby. During one of our regular visit to a village far in the bush, the mother said that the magician sends death of the family because they didn't offer a bull for the magic ceremony. This poor family having no cows could not effort this demand. Following the tradition to give only breast milk at this stage of age, the child suckled, but there was no milk. The child died by starvation. The mother was pregnant!*

further away, the mean weaning age extended to over 20 months. In the Dinka and Nuer villages, the mean weaning age was found to be 24 months and above.

These findings simply point out the fact that the more people are exposed to new external factors that cause environmental change, the more readily are the tendencies for change in socio-cultural habits and practices. As for people living in more remote areas, these tendencies are less remarkable since they do not experience much external influence.

The actual time of weaning was predominantly determined by husbands. However, a woman has the right to refuse her husband's demand if she thinks that her child was still too young to be weaned, or if she has no enough food for the child after weaning. She also has the right to appeal to elders when unable to arrive at a compromise with her husband. After the weaning time is finally determined, weaning follows very suddenly. Most mothers send their children to stay with the grand mothers or relatives for 2 weeks to 1 month; a few spend more than 2 months. This is done to make children forget about the breast. A few mothers who have no 'relatives', weaned children at home. The latter keep their breasts wrapped with some clothes to prevent the child from reaching them. Some paint the breasts with irritating smells or taste (spices) so that the child does not like them.

Some reasons given for weaning are apart from the husband's demand:

a) - child refused breast milk because of illness,

b) - illness of the mother,

c) - mother decided to stop breast feeding because she wanted to have another baby,

d) - to motivate child to eat other foods because it was not interested in them while suckling,

e) - «*Mother thought that the breast milk caused diarrhoea and vomiting*», so must avoided through weaning.

The composition of diet for children already weaned (age 13-30 months) was milk alone or with a combination of other food items mostly cereals and fish. Milk accounts for 75% of diet and 16% constitutes other foods. These are mainly the adult foods previously referred to. Only 7% of children depend entirely on milk diet. 2% had not eaten at all for the whole day, because of illness at the time of food recall (table 7.5).

7.4. REMARKS RELATED TO CULTURAL ATTITUDES TOWARDS INFANT AND CHILD FEEDING PRACTICES

To illustrate the traditional and cultural attitudes, some examples of expressions have been noted:

- Some mothers think that cow milk is better than own milk.
- Some mothers believe that breast milk causes diarrhoea.
- Some mothers believe that boiled milk causes diarrhoea.
- Some mothers say that a mixture of sour and fresh un-boiled milk is better. It causes no diarrhoea but even stops diarrhoea.
- Some grandmothers say that only sour milk is best for a child. It prevents diarrhoea and vomiting. They believe that diarrhoea comes from bad weather and sudden change of wind currents.
- Some mothers believe that sour milk causes gum and mouth sores and delays teething.
- Some mothers believe that vegetables are bad for children.
- Some mothers would not introduce cereals early for fear that the child may develop bad bowl habits in terms of having offensive stools.
- Some mothers believe that it is not good to give food other than milk to child until it can pick and eat by them self.
- Some mothers believe that it is good to send child away to grandmother for weaning.
- The custom about twin suckling demands that each twin only suckles from one breast and then alternate the breasts in the next feeding.
- The majority of the population believes in magic and follows still the Witch doctors advices.

Because of lack of dispensaries and/or health centres as well of schools in the study area, no nutritional or hygiene education was available to this population.

7.5. DISCUSSION

Almost all mothers put their babies to the breast, even before mother's milk is available. This ensures that at least most infants will have the protection from the colostrums. It equally ensures that lactation starts.

After the second year, the major food supplement was milk. 10 % of children had cow's milk introduced into their diet during the first month. Cereals and fish were introduced at 7 months. Meat, very rarely consumed (1%), between 13 and 18 months. This late introduction of foods other than milk may have a negative impact on child development. Milk alone cannot provide all the necessary nutrients after the first 6 months of live.

The traditional practice of giving un-boiled feeds during the pre-breast milk period and boiled supplements after this period is most likely to have negative effect on health status.

The sad observation during weaning is the fact that most women seemed to favour sending children away to stay with relatives to forget breastfeeding. The sudden change of environment, separation from the mother and the sudden weaning may torment a child from the psychological point of view, affecting his whole well being.

Some deviations from the customary child feeding patterns were: declining duration of breast feeding, increasing bottle-feeding practices and the decrease in the age at weaning. These are attributes of the progressive external influences and are bound to produce some socio-cultural impact by time should these influences continue to exist.

TABLE 7.1. Frequency of food consumption per day

FREQUENCY	Once		Twice		Three times		Total
	n	%	n	%	n	%	n
Meat	28	97	1	3	0	-	29
Fish	218	87	31	12	2	1	251
Soup	117	88	16	12	0	-	133
Oil	13	81	3	19	0	-	16
Egg	5	62	3	38	0	-	8
Milk	207	22	344	38	371	40	931
Cereals	220	45	193	40	73	15	901
Vegetables	51	93	4	7	0	-	55
Beverages	43	83	5	9	6	8	52
Sugar	87	33	88	33	91	34	266

TABLE 7.2. Frequency of meal consumption per day

FREQUENCY OF MEALS	n	%
No food	3	
Once	188	17 %
Twice	359	32 %
Three times	578	51 %
Total	1128	

TABLE 7.3. Pattern of meal consumption per day (in percentages)

Age group	Breakfast	Lunch	Diner	Breakfast and lunch	Breakfast and diner	Lunch and diner	Breakfast lunch + diner
0 – 3	30 %	9 %	-	42 %	2 %	2 %	17 %
4 – 6	17 %	1 %	1 %	42 %	4 %	1 %	14 %
7 – 9	13 %	1 %	1 %	32 %	6 %	1 %	46 %
10 – 12	12 %	1 %	2 %	17 %	6 %	1 %	61 %
13 – 15	6 %	1 %	2 %	16 %	13 %	3 %	54 %
16 – 18	14 %	3 %	1 %	7 %	12 %	1 %	62%
19 – 21	11 %	7 %	3 %	3 %	20 %	1 %	60 %
22 – 24	8 %	-	1 %	7 %	25 %	1 %	58 %
25 – 27	13 %	2 %	-	2 %	20 %	-	63 %
28 – 30	-	7 %	-	14 %	22 %	7 %	50 %
Means	13 %	2 %	1 %	20 %	11 %	1 %	52 %

TABLE 7.4. Total weaning and the rate of progression

AGE GROUPS IN MONTHS	n	%
0 - 6	7	1 %
7 - 12	7	1 %
13 - 18	22	16 %
19 – 24	65	45 %
25 – 30	53	37 %
Total	144	

TABLE 7.5. Children completely weaned depend of types of diet

AGE GROUPS	13 - 18		19 - 24		25 - 30		Total	
	n	%	n	%	n	%	n	%
Milk only	3	14 %	4	6 %	3	6 %	10	7 %
Milk and other food	18	82 %	53	82 %	34	64 %	105	75 %
Other food	1	4 %	8	12 %	14	26 %	23	16 %
Nothing to eat	0	-	0	-	2	4 %	2	2 %
Total	22		65		53		140	

FIGURE 7.1. Breast feeding and the rate of decline

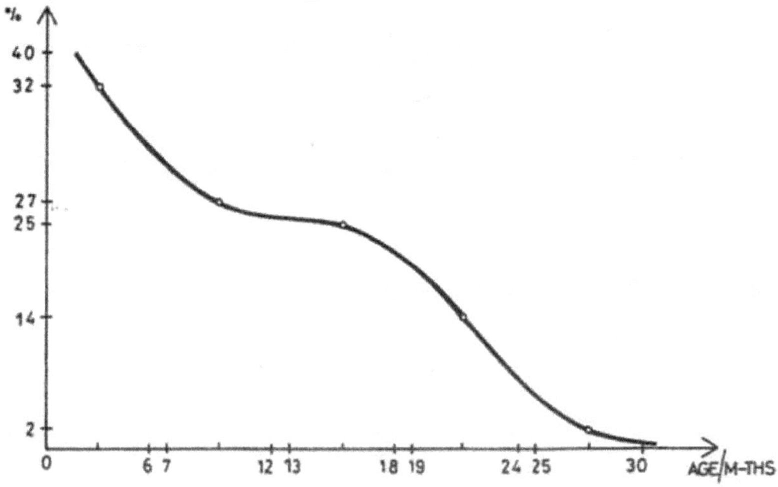

FIGURE 7.2. Relative importance of breast milk only, breast milk and supplementary food and other food.

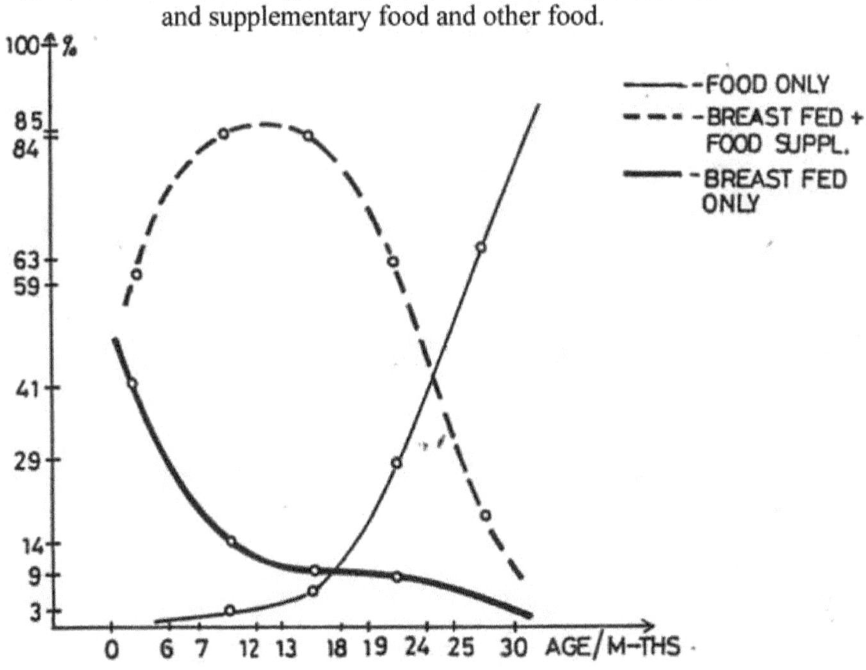

FIGURE 7.3. Age of introduction and frequency of consumption of different food items

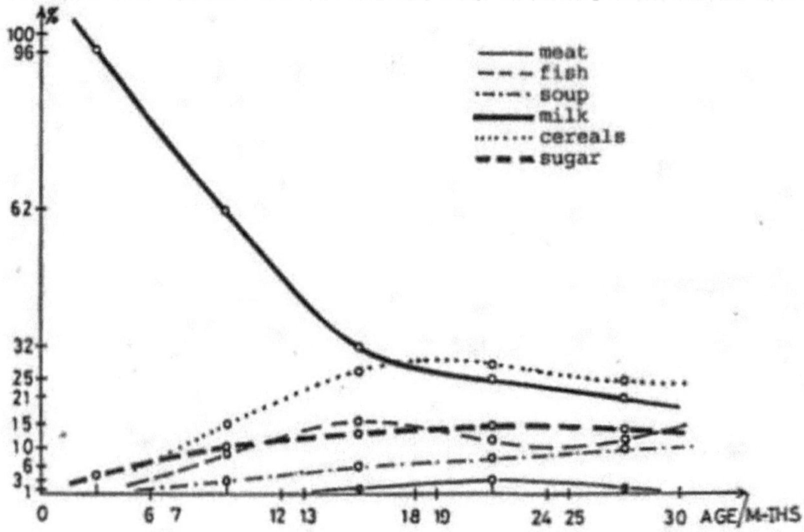

FIGURE 7.4. Percentage of powder milk and boiled diluted milk in the first three years

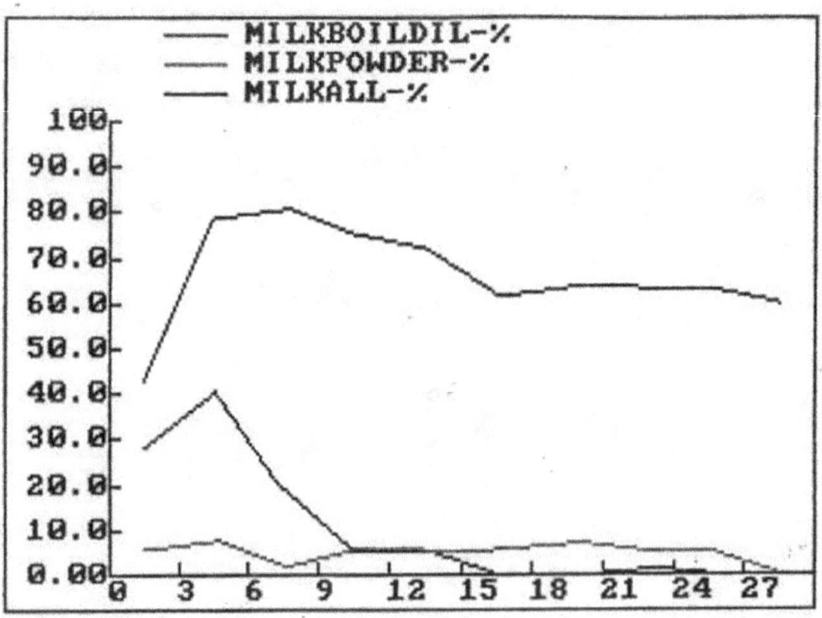

FIGURE 7.5. The importance of fish and meat in children's diet

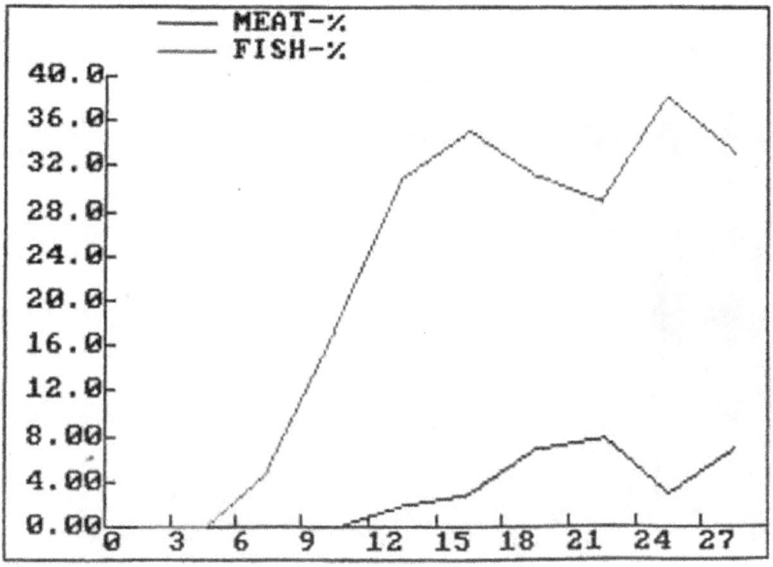

FIGURE 7.6. Part of vegetables between 12 and 27 months

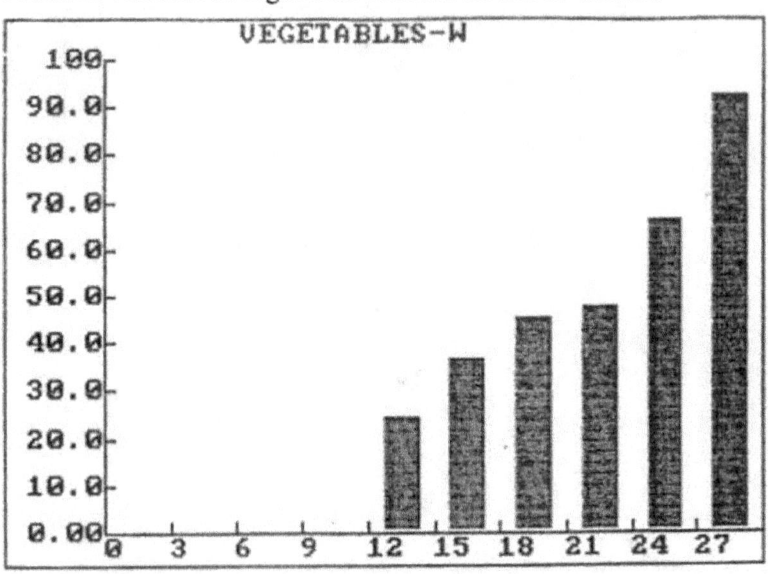

FIGURE 7.7. Milk and vegetables consumption

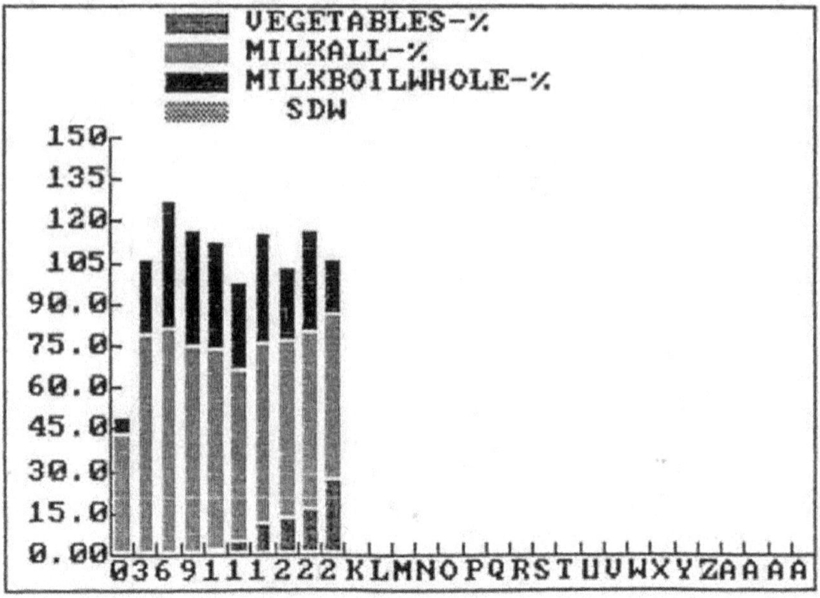

FIGURE 7.8. Milk and cereals consumption

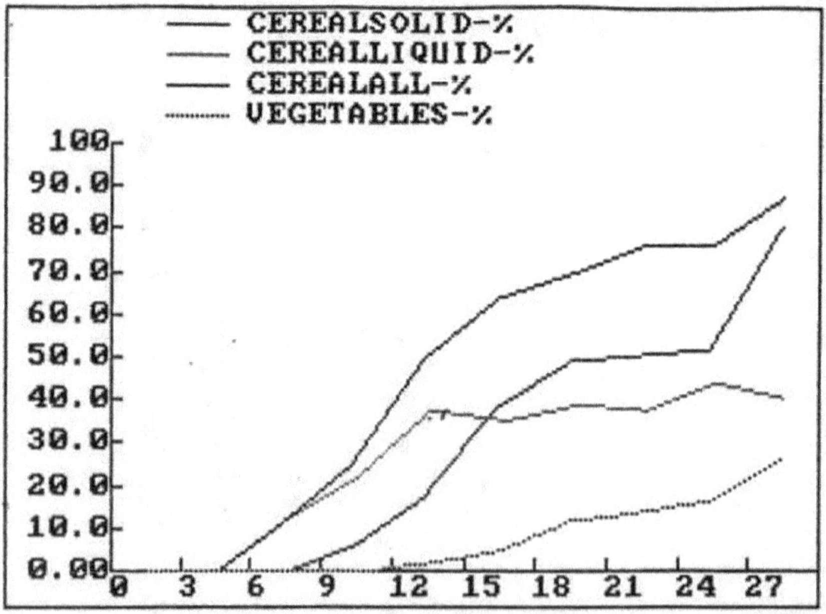

FIGURE 7.9. Other food items like soup, oil and eggs, compared to different milk consumption.

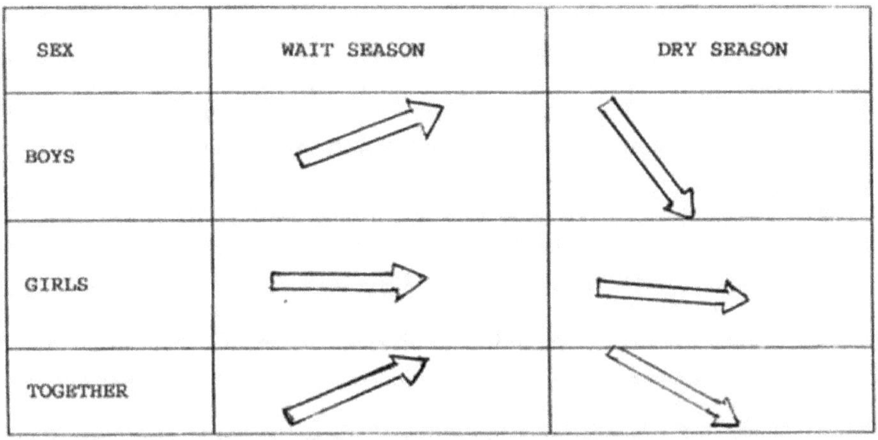

8. CORRELATION BETWEEN SEASONAL VARIATIONS OF FOOD AVAILABILITY AND GROWTH PATTERN

by Z. L. Ostrowski and E. Ojaba

This part of the study was carried out in the Shilluk area, living around the confluence of the Sobat and the White Nile rivers. The whole population in the studied area was homogenous and lives still in a traditional way (photo 1 to 4). The Shilluk are traditionally pastoralists. It appeared that they may change from a predominantly migratory to an almost sedentary mode of life. Consequently, cattle are still socially very important, though economically there was more reliance on crop production and fishing than animal production.

This area has only two seasons in a year: rainy and dry. The wet season, starting from May and ending in October, is characterized by heavy rains in July and August with mean monthly rainfalls of 169.6 mm and 182.0 mm respectively. During this period most people are preoccupied with small scale subsistence agriculture cultivating mainly durra (sorghum) and maize. Vegetable crops like tomatoes, jute, okra and cow peas are grown on very small quantities around the huts mainly for sale. On average, most of the families can only cultivate a small plot of 1.5 feddans. Harvesting of the main crops (sorghum, maize) is in September/October period. The dry season from November to April is characterized by reduced general activities. During this period, men spend their time mostly fishing or occasionally hunting, women on brewing local beer while youth and older boys take care of cattle at the dry season grazing areas.

The objective of this study was to find out if there is correlation between seasonal food availability and growth pattern in the second year of life.

A sub-sample of 49 children (19 boys and 30 girls) were selected from the A.D.E. longitudinal study of 261 Shilluk children aged 0-30 months. The criteria for selection were based on all children ages 15-22 months who had two or more consecutive routine examinations and had complete information on food intake, anthropometric measurements and health status.

Food intake was assessed by 24 hours recall method. Quantitatively figures were obtained from mothers using local household measures to obtain the grams of food eaten/day. These data were then transformed into qualitative values for the determination of mean nutrient intake per day. The nutrient values have been calculated using a special adapted Sudanese food composition table (Ostrowski and Josse- 110) which had been adjusted to contain all recently encountered indigenous food items in their right composition and circumstances.

To scrutinize the effects of seasonal fluctuation of foods on seasonal intake an analysis of data from 135 recalls were processed (9 cases were excluded because they were only breast-fed). The remaining 126 recalls were categorized in two groups:

I - 88 recalls of children breast-fed and taking supplementary food,
II - 38 recalls of already weaned children, eating food only.

Anthropometric measurements of weight, height and Z-score for weight to height (40, 41) were used to determine the pattern of growth.

Health status was evaluated by a medical doctor from clinical diagnosis as «good», «moderate» or «poor» based on past and present illness. Diseases and illnesses were codified using W.H.O. codes (56).

Biostatistics analysis was performed on IBM 5110 and IBM PC XT computer using Josse (23) and SPSS PC programs.

All studied children had been examined at least twice; 49 children during both seasons. 39% had only two examinations, 47% three and 14% four or more. Among all examinations, 65 have been done during wet seasons and 70 during dry season. The mean interval between the first and the last examination for both seasons was three months.

The mean age of all children examined is 18 months (at the «rainy season» children are 1 month older than at the «wet season» ones). During the rainy season, the mean age at the first examination is 17 months and 20 months at the last, while in the dry season they are 16 and 19 months respectively.

52% of the first examination during dry season was done between December/January and 61% of the last examination in April. In the rainy season, 65% of the first examination was done in May/June and 81% of the last examination in September/October.

The evolution of the three analysed parameters, using data obtained from two or more routine visits during each season, are the following: nutrition status, growth and health status.

8.1. Nutritional status

Food intake by 24 hours recall method indicated that 7 % of children were entirely breast-fed, 65 % taking food supplements and 28 % were weaned with solid foods only.

Nine different food items had been recorded (Table 8.1). The most frequently consumed during both seasons were milk, cereals, sugar and fish. Milk, mostly cow's and very rarely sheep's, goat's, and/or powder milk constituted about 30 % of the diet in both seasons. Cereals (sorghum and occasionally maize) are consumed about 27 %. Eggs and fruits were rarely consumed.

Sugar (14%) has been always incorporated into other foods such as milk, cereals and beverages. Fish, the basic source of animal protein in this area, contributed to 11 % of children's diet during rains and 13 % during dry season. Meat (cow and game), vegetables (wild and cultivated), beverages (tea and lime juice), oil (local milk-fat and commercial-fat) as well as soup were rarely consumed.

No statistically significant variation in the frequency of consumption of various food items was found except in vegetables which were rarely eaten during the dry season. Vegetables consumed during wet season (13g/day) were mostly wild plants gathered along the river banks. Rarely cultivated vegetables were grown in back-yard gardens on a very small-scale.

On the other hand, fish and soup were consumed in slightly higher amounts during dry season, 36 g/day and 17 g/day respectively (table 8.1).

Intake values of 6 basic nutrients: protein, lipids, carbohydrates, calcium, iron and vitamin C have been compared during wet and dry seasons for two patterns of feeding recalls:

Group I - children breast-fed and also eating solid foods.

Group II - children eating solid food only.

While group I showed a tendency for higher intake of iron and vitamin C during rainy season, group II had a tendency for higher intake of protein and lipid during the dry season.

During wet season vitamin C intake remained higher for both groups. Obvious significant differences in nutrient intake exist between group I and II during the same season. However, because of undetermined values of breast milk in group I valid assessment could not be made.

For all children eating solid food (Group I and II), the contribution of proteins, lipids and carbohydrates in the caloric value of the diet during rainy and dry seasons was compared with W.H.O. standards.

The contribution of protein in energy intake was higher during rainy (18%) and dry seasons (16 %) than the recommended reference. Carbohydrates contribution was at reference value during the rainy (54 %), and even more during the dry season (59 %). Lipids contribution during wet season (28 %) was slightly more than in a dry season (26 %). However lipids contribution did not meet the WHO recommended standard in both seasons.

8.2. Growth patterns

The two parameters used for assessment of growth are weight and height. Weight to height Z-score (of first and last examination in each season) shows an increase during rainy season and a decline during dry season. There is a significant difference between the two seasons (P= 0.003, t-test). More children lose weight during the dry season (30%) than during wet season (19%). The height is more difficult to evaluate due to the short period of observation. It increases in a similar way. However, about 40% of the children in each season seemed to have an increase in height rather slowly and 60% much faster (figure 8.1).

TABLE 8.1. Frequency of food consumption during rainy and dry season

FREQUENCY	**Rainy season**		**Dry season**	
	n	%	n	%
Milk	49	30 %	49	29 %
Cereals	45	27 %	45	26 %
Sugar	23	14 %	28	16 %
Fish	18	11 %	23	13 %
Soup	8	5 %	11	6 %
Vegetable	9	5 %	3	2 %
Beverage	5	3 %	5	3 %
Meat	6	4 %	6	4 %
Oil	2	1 %	1	1 %

FIGURE 8.1. FLUCTUATION OF GROWTH (W/H)
DEPENDING OF SEX AND SEASON

Sexes	WAIT SEASON	DRY SEASON
BOYS	oooo→ oooo oooo	ooo ooo ooo ooo ooo→
GIRLS	oooooooooooo→	oooooo ooooooo→
TOGETHER	ooo→ oooo oooo oooo	oooo oooo oooo oooo→

8.3. Health Status

Health status was expressed in terms «good», «medium» and «bad» on the basis of illnesses and symptoms. The evaluation of the health status between the first and the last medical examination showed deterioration during the dry season: upper respiratory tract infections and gastroenteritis was more frequent (table 8.2).

TABLE 8.2. HEALTH (H) AND NUTRITIONAL (N) STATUS
DEPENDING OF WAIT AND DRY SEASON
(for boys and girls)

STATUS	WAIT	SEASON			DRY	SEASON		
	Boys		Girls		Boys		Girls	
	H	N	H	N	H	N	H	N
GOOD	14%	53%	46%	25%	16%	55%	66%	42%
MEAN	72%	25%	35%	64%	79%	20%	29%	55%
BAD	14%	22%	19%	11%	5%	25%	5%	2%

8.4. DISCUSSION

In many rural communities of the developing countries where modern technologies are inexistent and food preservation methods not present or up-to-date, seasonal food variations and shortages of food have an important impact on the levels of nutrient intake by the population.

The staple diet of the Shilluk was durra (sorghum). Fish provides the major protein source followed by milk. Vegetables and fruits generally play a minor role in the diet. Seasonal availability and shortages are very variable and specific. It means, that while some foods are lacking during a certain period, others are abundant at the same time.

Fish consumption was very low and less frequent during the rains due to the following factors:

- seasonal migration of fish into streams and connecting pools for breeding (June-November),
- general migration of fish into flooded areas to feed on abundant natural food,
- periodic upstream migration of some fish when river levels become high, deep water fish was difficult to catch by nets when water level was higher,
- because of farming activities, there was less time left for fishing,
- high fish market prices and free availability of wild vegetables cause most women to prepare durra only with vegetable.

Milk was consumed in slightly more quantities during dry season than in the rainy one. This is because the longest and highest calf production period of the year occurs in dry season (December-March). The wet season production period (May-June) was rather short and poor in grazing for the cattle, resulting in less milk production.

Low intake and low frequency of consumption of **vegetables** during dry season is attributed to lack of interest in vegetable preservation methods as well as to lack of vegetables.

Cereals being the staple food remain relatively available throughout the year, although the quantity consumed may be different by seasons.

The variation in the level of **nutrient intake** is affected by both seasonal availability of food and the difference in their feeding status. The tendency for higher intake of iron during the rains is probably due to the frequent large amounts of cereal and vegetables consumed. Higher intake of vitamin C during this period is due to consumption of green vegetables. The high protein intake during dry season, by children eating only solid food, may be attributed to frequent and high amount of fish consumed at this time. The higher source of lipid is not certain but may be provided also by fish.

Weight and height measurements showed an increase in height and decrease in weight. A study of normal gain in height is a better index of development than is weight gain. Children who are growing (in height) may be generally healthy, even though they are thin and their weight may be below normal. According to Richtey (118), failure to gain height is a signal of a potential problem in childhood.

According to Pagezy (119) the subsequent favourable dry seasons resulted in a catch-up growth in Zaire babies aged 0 to 4 years, essentially due to the abundance of animal food. Seasonal changes in growth and nutritional status were also observed by Brown (50) during the monsoon in Bangladesh.

The aggravation of the **health status** in the dry season due to URTI and gastroenteritis can be explained with the increase of flies and bad hygiene. Jelliffe (38) have noted that outbreaks of infectious diarrhoea which occur during the dry season when houseflies are more numerous, are followed 3-4 weeks later by Kwashiorkor (*Protein-Calorie Malnutrition*) and/or marasmus.

9. FOOD TABOOS AMONG SHILLUK, DINKA AND NUER
by E. Ojaba

By food taboos we are specifically referring to those food items that are regarded as normal foods by some communities but are prohibited or avoided by others. Eating of those traditionally forbidden items by any member of a particular society or clan is believed to bring undesirable effects, sometimes fatal on the individual or his/her family. The information about food taboos has been exacted from a cross-sectional survey of 299 Shilluk, Dinka and Nuer. 274 individuals have been interviewed for taboos.

Table 9.1 shows the number and percentages of positive and negative responses concerning taboos. Because of the small sample size of the Dinka the data are only indicative. The presence of food taboos was indicated by 99 % Nuer and 93 % Dinka. For Shilluk, it appears that only half of this community has food taboos. In all the three ethnic groups, no much difference were observed either by age group or sex, except in Shilluk women who seem to have less taboos (table 9.2).

The food taboos among the Shilluk, Dinka and Nuer societies tend to be associated with the consumption of certain animals, reptiles, wild fowls, fish or their products (table 9.3).

Classified as such, certain variations were noted. Shilluk avoidance includes all the above four groups. Nuer indicated three: animals, reptiles and wild fowls. Dinka only two: wild fowls and animals. Table 6.3 indicated that certain food items can be a common taboo for all while others are tribes specific. For instance, Dinka and Shilluk share a common taboo against crocodiles and hyenas while Dinka and Nuer share that against lions. On the other hand, the three communities seem to share a general taboo against ostrich.

A good example of a tribe specific taboo was that of fish which applies only to Shilluk. As the Shilluk live along the Nile and the Sobat river banks, it is quite natural that they have acquired some taboos against certain fish. However, certain Dinka also share similar taboos, probably those living near the Nile River.

The reasons for avoidance of foods were split into three major sub-headings as:

1° - reasons related to religious or psychological prohibition (60 %)
2° - reasons related to health problem (27%)
3° - reasons related to distaste (13%) (Table 9.4).

Religious prohibitions arise mainly from the fact that certain animals are considered to be God, or sacred. Their flesh should not be consumed by/or in the presence of those who regards it sacred. It is interesting to note, that those animals considered as God are often the ones strong, fierce, man-eating, or harmful reptiles such as crocodiles and pythons. It is believed that the punishment from the God for eating the flesh of such origin is «immediate death».

Similarly, psychological reasons for avoidance concern man eating animals and apes. It is believed that since those creatures eat man, eating their flesh is same as eating human flesh, hence death results. As for apes, because of their strong resemblance to man, they are considered almost as humans (!).

Concerning health related reasons, the undesirable effects or punishments for disregarding tabooed foods range from general illness, respiratory tract infections, and digestive tract diseases to deaths.

Traditional linking of tabooed foods to illnesses and deaths may sound scientifically absurd. However lack of health services in those areas with high frequency of diseases and inadequate treatment which often cause death certainly plays a big role. Although many of these people are ignorant of the actual causes of their illness, they have their own explanations. Since long ago, they identify the cause of their illness by relating it to what they eat. To many people these beliefs, transmitted from their ancestors, remain a mystery which they must simply follow to satisfy the demands of their social norms.

Some foods are found not tasting good. Many members of these communities refuse eating them on the grounds of their taste. This is so despite the value the body can actually benefit from eating them.

In conclusion: Since foods regarded as taboo by Shilluk, Dinka and Nuer consists mainly of rare animal's meat, they do not contribute actively to affecting the nutritional status of the population. On the other hand, the frequent and strong reasons for food avoidance often associated with some symptoms and diseases may indirectly affect the well being of the people. In other words, it is important that people are made aware of the actual causes of such disease which may be due to some nutritional deficiencies, poor hygiene, etc.

TABLE 9.1. FOOD TABOOS IN SHILLUK, DINKA AND NUER POPULATION

Taboos	**Shilluk**		**Dinka**		**Nuer**		**Total**	
	n	**%**	**n**	**%**	**n**	**%**	**n**	**%**
Yes	62	45.3	29	93.5	104	99.1	195	71.4
No	75	54.7	2	6.5	1	0.9	78	28.6
Total	137	100	31	100	105	100	273	100

No answer from one person

TABLE 9.2. FOOD TABOOS BY AGE, SEX AND ETHNICITY (%)

Taboos	**Shilluk**	**Dinka**	**Nuer**
Children < 5 yrs	45 %	71 %	100 %
Children > 5 yrs	51 %	100 %	90 %
Men	53 %	91 %	100 %
Women	33 %	100 %	100 %

TABLE 9.3. FOOD TABOOS FOR SHILLUK, DINKA AND NUER (%)

	Taboos	**Shilluk**	**Dinka**	**Nuer**
ANIMALS	Giraffe	1	-	-
	Hyena	13	8	1
	Jaddle	11	-	-
	Leopard	-	10	-
	Lion	1	14	12
	Monkey	-	17	-
	Wild cat	-	2	-
REPTILLES	Crocodile	23	44	-
	Monitor lizard	1	2	-
	Python snakes	23	-	-
BIRDS	Ostrich	7	3	68
	Owan	1	-	-
	Wild fowls	-	-	19
FISH	Curo	17	-	-
	Caro	1	-	-

TABLE 9.4. REASON FOR AVOIDANCE OF SOME FOOD ITEMS AMONG SHILLUK, DINKA AND NUER (IN %)

REASONS	Gire	Hyen	Jack	Leop	Lion	Monk	Wcat	Croc	Tiza	Snak	Ostr	Owan	Foul	Curo	Caro	Total
Death	-	3	-	-	2	-	-	4	-	4	-	-	-	2	1	**16**
Illness	-	-	2	-	-	-	-	-	-	1	-	-	-	-	-	**3**
Chest infec.	1	-	5	-	-	-	-	3	1	3	3	-	-	4	-	**20**
Symptoms #	-	1	-	-	-	-	-	-	-	-	-	-	-	2	-	**3**
Nausea	-	1	-	-	-	-	-	-	-	-	-	-	-	-	-	**1**
Diarrhoea	-	-	-	-	-	-	-	1	-	-	-	-	-	1	-	**2**
Teeth loose	-	-	-	-	-	-	-	-	-	-	1	-	-	1	-	**2**
Lips red	-	-	-	-	-	-	-	-	-	-	-	-	-	4	-	**4**
Bad smells	-	2	-	-	1	-	-	1	-	-	-	-	-	-	-	**4**
Looks ugly	-	4	1	4	1	8	-	-	1	2	-	-	1	-	-	**21**
Eats people	-	1	-	-	-	-	-	4	-	-	-	-	-	-	-	**5**
Eats dogs	-	-	-	1	-	-	-	-	-	-	-	-	-	-	-	**1**
Like human	-	-	-	-	-	1	-	-	-	-	-	-	-	-	-	**1**
It's GOD	-	2	-	-	5	-	1	23	-	-	-	-	-	-	-	**31**
Forbidden	-	-	-	-	-	-	-	1	-	-	-	-	-	-	-	**1**
Tradition	-	3	-	1	21	1	-	6	-	8	3	1	30	1	-	**75**

10. SUMMARY

A "cross-sectional nutrition study" was carried out among the Shilluk, Nuer and Dinka ethnicities of the Southern Sudan covering a total of 276 cases: adults and children.

Two methods of estimation of dietary intake were used: 24 hours recall and general food habits to evaluate nutritional status and consumption patterns.

The population was sub-divided into four groups according to age and sex. The frequency of meals and the family way of eating were also described.

Since the main source of energy was sorghum for both Shilluk and Nuer populations its consumption was basically the same. While the Shilluk had more milk, fish, vegetables and beer; the Nuer ate more meat and fruits. Hence, the Shilluk's diet was more varied and richer than the Nuer's whose food was composed of only one major source of protein supply. This difference results from the nature of their local environment.

Food taboos among the Shilluk, Dinka and Nuer appear to affect all members of these societies irrespective of age or sex differences. These taboos are generally associated with consumption of certain animal's meat, reptiles, wild birds and fish. Animal meat is prohibited if these animals are considered God or sacred. Others are avoided because they are believed to cause diseases or death, and a few, like monkeys, because they bear strong resemblance to man.

From the A.D.E. "**Longitudinal Study of Growth and nutrition**", 261 children age 0-30 months have been studied. From these, 1935 24-hr food recalls have been used as basis for description of food habits and feeding patterns of children in this community.

Type of food, mode of preparation and administration as well as frequency of consumption have been analysed following four major sequences of feeding patterns: pre-breast milk feeding, breast-feeding, supplementary feeding and the feeding during and after weaning. The latter refers to that time when a child was stopped feeding from the breast. The diet after this period was basically the same.

The findings in this study indicate that the traditional practice of prolonged breast-feeding of 3-5 years has presently declined to 16-20 months. This change of practice from late weaning to early weaning is attributed to the rapid change in life style such as the progressive adoption of monogamous type of family and some socio-economic development in the last two years of this study, due to the construction of the Jonglei Canal.

Milk was the major and first supplementary food. 10% of infants were consuming milk during the first month and 96% by the end of 6 months. Cereals, introduced at 7 months constituted 15% of the diet by 1 year. Fish was introduced at 7 months and meat never before the second year. Liquid and semi-liquid foods are generally regarded as better for young children than solid food which was prepared for consumption by the entire family. The mean age at introduction of the above two groups of food is 7 months and 12 months respectively.

The general frequency of meals was two per day (83%). A half of the child population received 3 meals per day and 17% one meal only. The most important meal was breakfast (40%) followed by lunch and/or dinner (30%).

It is known that in rural areas in Africa, the nutritional value of available food depends on seasonal variation. In the study area of the South Sudan, the staple food was dura. The protein support came mainly from fish and/or milk. To determine the nutritional value of food consumed, special food tables were created for all food items consumed in the study area. This food tables can be used also in other similar regions in Africa.

The seasonal variation in food consumption is not very great. In the rainy season vegetables are more available. In the dry season fish is more consumed. The nutritional value in early childhood is more difficult to evaluate due to the prolonged breast feeding practice. There are seasonal differences in the subsample of children without breast milk: higher protein and lipid intake in the dry season. The nutrition and health status was better in rainy than in the dry season.

The health and nutritional status in Africa is not very good. According to Maletnlema (120), malnutrition was reported in all 13 countries of east Africa where a study was carry out in 1983-4. PEM tops the list and affects 20-70% of the under fives. This followed by goiter (90%), anaemia (78%), avitaminose B (72%) and avitaminose A (48%). Measles was reported in 10 countries, respiratory infections in 8 countries, intestinal parasites and malaria in 6 countries. For analysing the growth of children in the first period of life in remote areas, some aspects have to be taken into consideration: the difficulties to carry out anthropometrical, clinical and nutritional examinations in regular intervals («target times»); difficulties of determination of maturity, due to missing values of birth date, birth weight and height; problems of choice and application of existing models.

It seems that the Jenss-Bayley model, modified to this particular study, may be the best fitting model to the irregularity of data and time intervals of examinations. However this model can be applied to children having a minimum of 5 measurements in the first 15 months of life and that the first measurement has to be performed before the age of 4 months. Some aspects and methods for tackling nutritional problems in early childhood in Africa have been discussed at the A.D.E. Workshop in Seoul (Korea) in 1985 (113).

PART IV

PSYCHO-SOCIAL AND CULTURAL ASPECTS

by Dr Zygmunt L.OSTROWSKI

...No one is free unless he is dead...

1. INTRODUCTION

The socio-psychological status of a population is mostly determined by the environmental and economical conditions as well as by evolution or changes due to cataclysms, war, invasions or discoveries (gold, petrol...). Rare scientific descriptions are available on living populations before such changes occurred. In order to analyse the impact of those environmental changes in the Sudan, due to the construction of a 400 km long Jonglei Canal, a study was carried out on the three main tribes (Dinka, Nuer and Shilluk) living in this remote area near the future canal between the Sobat-Nile Mouth and Ayoud (see map 6).

This population still has many mystical beliefs. As described by John Wuol Makec (19), "...along with the fear of God, numerous mystical beliefs have been developed to induce obedience to law". For example, the belief which has been developed to combat the offence of adultery. It is believed that adultery produces a kind of "impurity" which exacerbates sickness, so that an adulterer or adulteress must never go near sick people..., because "sickness" is suspected to be in his or her body although there are no obvious signs of it. If he or she attends the sick or passes near the sick, purification rites have to be performed after his or her departure. To do this a flame of fire is passed over his or her foot-steps or over any piece of ground which came into contact with any part of his or her body. Fire, as the belief goes, removes the ingredient of impurity. Whether this belief is rational or not, it has served a useful purpose in controlling the incidence of adultery in Dinka society.

Another illustration is the belief developed to combat the evil of sexual cohabitation between blood relatives. Sexual cohabitation between blood relations, whatsoever the degree of cohabitation, is strictly prohibited. The evil by such a relationship is known as "akeeth" (i.e. incest). "Akeeth" is believed to be fatal to the offspring of this kind of sexual union and purification rites have to be performed by the elders to avert the evil. However, no purification rites can be conducted until the woman has publicly confessed the name of the man, or all the male relatives, who have had sexual intercourse with her. The children of "akeeth", if they survive are generally believed to be weak physically.

A further illustration concerns the offence of homicide. It is wrong or "sinful" to kill a person "in cold blood" or to kill a person and then deny it. It is believed that God punishes such a killer. The killer must still confess it somehow to his very close elderly relatives in order for them to perform (secretly) purification rites. The soul of the deceased is appeased when "apuk" (i.e. compensation) has been paid by the relatives of the killer. "Apuk" also prevents revenge. Also the effect of insult (something false) is that it merely tends to provoke the other or to cause a breach of the peace....

Following to Robert Cameron Mitchell (121) "...in case of the African primal religions, they are this-worldly, and their ultimate explanation of evil is that it is the work of witches and sorcerers (*)... Most events are not believed to happen by chance especially if they involve "unnatural" misfortune".

Because many of these mystical beliefs were probably still present in the population under study it was important to describe them in a scientific way. For example, Francis Mading Deng (122, 123) gives interesting descriptions of the challenge for law among the Dinka in Sudan and the set of principles governing the life of the Dinka, which are the aesthetics of pride, honour and dignity "dheeng". Aside from being a riveting, exciting story "In desert and Wilderness", Sienkiewicz (124) reflects the sense of honour in the southern Sudanese people (even though the author has never been there!). These values are inculcated in a child at an early age.

To study the development of this population in connection with the psychic health status it was important to determine a mean type of comportment at individual and at community level. Concerning an individual, it was required to recall personal beliefs (conscientious); dreams and their interpretation (in conscientious); sexual behaviour and their harmony (libido) as well as psychosomatic diseases (anguish, distress...). Concerning the community, it was necessary to research aggressive drives and their sublimation; filiations and their symbolic function (father-son); ritual of death and different united beliefs as well as what belongs to "I" individual, and what belongs to "I" communal.

To follow up such a population for a period of time, it was of interest to measure the intellectual and cultural progress (elimination of illiteracy); capacity to control and to sublimate the various new drives which appear with progress as well as the persistence or absence of community identity

To describe the traditional way of life in a remote area in the South Sudan, a study of a sample of this southern Sudanese population, living near the Canal between the Sobat-Nile mouth and Ayod (see map 6), was carried out from April 1982 to February 1983.

A pilot survey was carried out on 52 adults (**), heads of family or villages, by a local social worker during a one to two day interview. After a preliminary analysis of 18 questions of this first survey formula (Annexe 1) by a team of experts (medical doctors, psychologists, psychiatrists, sociologists and

* *Sorcerers are people who have the ability to work harmful magic against others photo 20). They do this in much the same way that healers work curative magic, using various materials, actions, and a formula of words in a ritual..*

** *48 Shilluk and 4 Dinka, amongst them 20 Christians, 23 Idolists, 7 mixed believers «Idolists-Christians"and 2 Muslims.*

anthropologists), a second survey formula was developed with 50 questions (Annexe 2), based on the advice of this Committee of Experts. This second survey was carried out between November 1982 - February 1983 on 37 adults (9 Shilluk and 28 Nuer). All responses were accompanied by remarks and a detailed map of villages (map 7).

To collect the exact data, James Gadluak (photo 27) a local social worker was selected because of his intellectual capacities and knowledge of English, Arabic and the three tribal languages: Nuer, Dinka and Shilluk. James was especially trained to obtain exact information according to a pre-prepared survey formula. He spent whole days within the village, sitting inside the tukul (local made hut) of the interviewed person.

The questionnaires of 88 adults (56 Shilluk, 28 Nuer and 4 Dinka), were subject to individual analyses. The frequency of answers has been given in percentage to show the priority given to the subject (sometimes more than one). The description and comments were personalised by Dr Akec Khoc's (*) remarks (indicated as "AK") or by the author (indicated as "ZLO").

* *Dr Akec Khoc, a medical doctor from the Dinka Bor ethnic group, followed a stage in the A.D.E. Centre in Paris.*

MAP 6. Study area between Sobat-Nile mouth and Ayoud

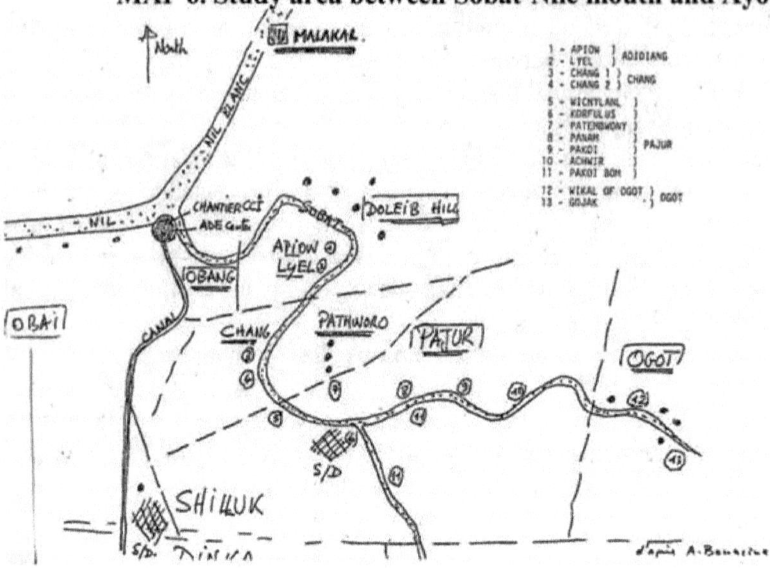

MAP 7 Gojak village

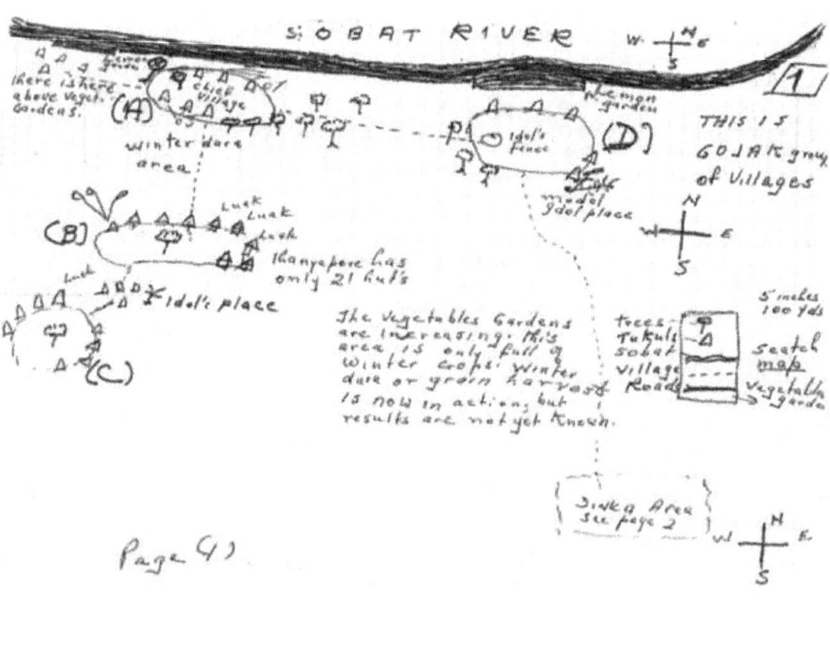

2. THE TRADITIONAL WAY OF LIFE

The objective of the first survey was to obtain some information about the way of life of the population, their households and their idols.

HOUSEHOLD AND DOWRY

52 households have been described: 48 were Shilluk (one young woman not legally married did not have her own house and didn't reply to questions) and 4 Dinka (one Muslim police and one Christian camp worker) didn't reply. The analysis of household and dowry was based only for 47 Shilluk divided in three subgroups: Idolists (20), Idolists and/or Christians (8) and Christians (19)

The observations and memories showed that, at the time of survey, the population still lived in a very traditional way (photo 1 to 4). In the majority of tukuls only traditional objects have been found (21,3%). Only in 10,6% tukuls some artificial objects have been described (these tukuls belong to Christians).

Between all objects described, 85% were recipients, 53% plates and rarely spoons (17%) or tables (13%) Between those who had clothes (47%), beds (45%), tables (13%) and boxes (11%) the majority were Christians. It's interesting to mention, that in four tukuls some wall-designs were registered (photo 23 and 24) and only in one tukul a mosquito net was present (table 1).

The marriage dowry, very important in the Nilotic society, was similar in the three subgroups. The bases of dowry are cows (6 – 22), goats (8 – 30), rarely sheep (5). In seven cases an amount of 100 - 300 £ in cash was added. Generally, cows are the base of dowry: in 42% only cows have been given, in another 42% cows and goats and in 15% cash has been added (table 2).

IDOLS

The impact of traditional beliefs in this population was still very strong. Five of the 19 Christians said, they still believe in idols and worship them (mostly inside the tukul). Only one Christian denied believing in idols. Between the remaining 28 idolists, 8 mentioned to be also Christians. All of them placed their idols outside and/or inside the tukul (photo 18) of a «witch doctor» during the ceremony). Two of them placed only inside the tukul (those said to be Christians) (table 3).

The following description concerns only the 28 believers in idols. Between the 27 who described the form of idols, 17 described as non-material (63%), 6 as non-material and non-alive (22%), 3 as non-alive (11%) and one as ghost (4%).

Those who consider idols as non-material added that it's a merciful God or ghost called «Nyikango» («man believed to be under water») or «Deng Dit».

Between the 18 persons who described additional the idols (10 did not answer), 11 view it as a man, 5 as a ghost and 2 as others (animal, reptile... without specification).

In a following question, 70% consider God as sacred, non-alive (19 cases), 11% as sacred, alive (3) and 18% as God (3) or Nyikango (2). Again some mentioned additionally that Nyikango can be like a man (3), Mohammed (3) or Jesus Christ (1). One person, (witch doctor), said he had his own idols: a Deng model and a Nyikango model (photo 19).

All, except one, agreed that God is good to the owner of idols. («Ayuin» is considered as a spiritual God). HE has power on health and peace, on man (to increase strength and vitality) and on animals (increase of reproduction). HE doesn't have power on tukuls and objects.

If God is called for help, 6 (21%) answered it gives power to the owner alone and 19 (68%) to the owner and to another man. 3 answered that it can act only on another person.

God can send calamity: burn tukuls (89%), kill animals (46%), kill children (37%) or all people (17%). Only in 11% God keep care and prevent children and animals from disease.

Generally idols help owners, mostly (81%) in war (to prevent) and threaten others (enemies). In one case «it doesn't threaten and can't be asked to revenge the owner against other people».

All people under study sacrificed to their God: 93% sacrificed a cow, three persons sacrificed a sheep, a goat or a chicken (because being alone) and 64% additional brew a «holy beer». Some sacrificed a fruit called «kuol». One person answered: «every one of the family is called and feast once a year» and another one: «she can go to a magician should she fail to realise a disease». In each case the witch doctor was present. He was asked to help to sacrifice and he was paid for that.

For 24 persons (86%) there is no other powerful God besides their idols. For 3 persons (11%) Nyikango is the only God they believe is powerful; three persons were themselves «witch doctors».

Some additional remarks explained the ritual. The Nyikango cow was usually killed by night and the Deng's cow was killed by day. One person claimed even to be descendant of Nyikango «from the king's side». The Shilluk God is so merciful that no man can use his name to threaten people but he is always prayed to make peace». For the four Dinka who have been involved in this study, only two persons answered all questions. Their answers are similar to the above

Shilluk population.

According to Jacob Jeremiah Kuany Ayon (*), almost every family has idols at home. People believe that these idols have power to make a person sick and die and to heal a sick person. People also believe that these idols eat. These idols talk and are situated in different ways. Some of these idols have their houses alone and some of these idols exist in the wall of the house where people stay. When talking, some of these idols talk through some of the people and others talk in the wall and what they say can be heard.

When someone is seriously sick, people can gather and ask the idol to tell them what made that person sick. The idol itself can say: «If you will not kill for me a bull, I will not tell you». The father of that sick person will promise a bull somewhere either in cattle camp (photo 26) or in another area and say: «Please tell me and I will bring the bull in the mentioned days». And if he fails to bring that bull this idol may kill him. The promise has to be exactly executed.

After promising the bull (or other offering), if the person will not kill a bull of a specified colour, that person will not live. If it is specified white and black he must bring white and black and if it is white only, he must bring white only. When he has brought the bull, people will gather again and ask the idol to leave the sick person and come to take his bull. People gather around the bull and the idol. If the idol has accepted it, and the bull urinates then people will know that the idol accepts the bull. Sometimes the sick person will cured and sometimes the sick person will die.

The description of the items, used by the population inside their tukul is shown in table 1. At the time of the survey, the population still lived in a traditional way. Some external influence was observed in the household tools (clothes, beds, tables or boxes). Even if some of the surveyed population mentioned are Christians, the majority still believe in idols and worship them. Strong traditional beliefs united this population.

* *Jacob Jeremiah Kuany Ayon, a young student from Dinka Bor, following his education in the A.D.E. School of Arts «POLATAKA», 1997.*

Table 1 : Tools in the household

Sub-groups	Recipient	Plate	Bed	Spoon	Table	Clothes	Boxesn	Design	Total
20 Animists	17	9	3	5	1	8	1	1	45
8Anim/Chris	5	7	1	2	-	3	2	1	21
19 Christians	18	9	4	14	5	11	2	1	64
TOTAL 47 *	40	25	8	21	6	22	5	3	130

Table 2 : Dowry in different sub-groups

Sub-groups	Cows		Goats		Sheep	Cash		Total Animals	
	N°	total	N°	total	N°	£	total		
20 Animists	6-15	187	10-30	170	5	150-200	750	362	42 %
8Anim/Chris	6-13	74	10-20	110	-	100	100	184	21 %
19 Christians	6-22	213	8-25	107	5	200-300	750	325	37 %
TOTAL 47 *	6-22	474	8-30	387	5	150-300	1600	871	100 %

Table 3 : Placement of idols

Sub-groups	Inside		Outside		Inside/Outside		No answer	Total
20 Animists	---		7	35 %	13	65 %	-----	20
8Anim/Chris	2	25 %	1	13 %	5	62 %	-----	8
19 Christians	3		1		1		(14)	5
TOTAL 47 *	5	15 %	9	58 %	19	58 %	(14)	33

(*) Four incomplete

3. THE SOCIO-CULTURAL ASPECTS

The objective of the second survey was to get some information about the socio - cultural aspects: customs, social activities, existence of magic, belief in dreams and "life after death", the relationship between an individual and his child, the importance of marriage and sexual desires, the meaning of freedom, life's obligation and ego and their collective life.

This survey started in November 1982 and was interrupted in February 1983 by the civil war. Only 37 adults (28 Nuer and 9 Shilluk) have been interviewed by the same social worker, James Gatluak, who spent many hours or days with the interviewed person. Thanks to his capacities the precious data could be collected.

The analysis of data, comments and remarks have been given by Dr Akec Khoc, a medical doctor from the Dinka Bor ethnic group.

CUSTOMS

ACTIVITIES PROHIBITED FOR CHILDREN, MEN OR WOMEN

For small children under 3 years of age

In the Nilotic Culture, children under 3 yrs of age have two main methods of socio-cultural education: customary and protective. As is shown, education plays an important role for the Nilotic population from a very early age. All interviewed persons replied to this question. The indicated percentage of answers shows the priority given to the subject. This does not mean that other people do not have the same point of view. Sometimes more than one priority was given.

1. CUSTOMARY EDUCATION

This is to teach children the traditions of their society. At this age, socio-cultural customary education is initiated. If a child grows without this basic customary education, he may not understand or appreciate traditional norms at a later age. Failure of this education to be effected is felt by the individual concerned but has far reaching ramifications on the whole extended family.

a) Passing urine and/or stools in or around the hut or luak is considered bad. For 32.4% of the studied sample, it was even prohibited.

b) Begging and/or stealing was given by 18.9% of the surveyed population as prohibited.

c) Going to the dance ground without permission of an elder or accompanying person was given by 18.9% of the surveyed population as prohibited for children of this age.

d) Disobeying directives or requests from elders was given by 10.8% as prohibited for these children.

e) Equally so was the idea of eating from the same dish, plate or calabash with older children (8.1%).

f) Some remarks concern: «not to play with dirty things» and «to sleep always inside the tukul».

2. PROTECTIVE EDUCATION

This is the most important type of education at this time. The small child may not appreciate other forms of education. However, he appreciates protection because once he might have had a bad experience about what he is being protected from.

a) Great attention was given to taking care of children. 32.4% indicated that children are not allowed to go far from the tukul and especially by night (8.1%).

b) Walking amongst cattle was prohibited by 21,6% of the sample. The cattle, or tying the sticks used for them, may harm small children. Some cattle are found to be notorious for disliking little children and therefore they frequently harm them.

c) Playing or swimming in deep ponds or rivers was prohibited for children at this age by 13.8%. This is due to the fact that there are many dangerous animals like crocodiles in these ponds or rivers which may or are known to eat people. The Nile or its tributary Sobat are known to contain large numbers of crocodiles that eat people.

d) Playing with or near fire was indicated by 10.8% as prohibited for this age group of children. The reason is that the child may burn himself/herself, with possible further complications.

<u>For older children</u>

At this age, traditional customary education is more vigorous than at any other time.

1. CUSTOMARY EDUCATION

This is the age at which children usually better understand the socio-cultural norms and start to practice them.

a) Begging, stealing and/or insulting elders was prohibited for children by 27.8% of the surveyed population. The Nilotic are a proud people. Therefore, their society does not accept any slight action which may degrade an individual. Such actions are usually lauded (given higher dimensions) by competitors and avoided at all costs by the individuals. Each person therefore teaches his children to live up to his image or even better. Begging was especially prohibited (22.2%).

b) Disobedience: in Nilotic tradition, for 13.9% was prohibited for children. The Nilotic child is usually taught about the cohesiveness of the society. That each and every individual member of the society depends on the others for many things. He/she as a member of this society must fulfil his/her duty towards it. To neglect duties, to drink beer or to work hard was strongly forbidden (8.3%).

c) Sex before puberty: 33.3% of the surveyed population have noted that this is prohibited traditionally. However, the practice is that children are seriously warned against it but they must also learn to play sex at this age (homosexuality is extremely punished, even by death (AK).

d) To keep traditions: to respect age group lines i.e. not to go and sit where elders are sitting alone unless the child is called (13.9%). Especially Shilluk take care of their traditional system.

2. PROTECTIVE EDUCATION

This becomes less important with increasing age because the child is expected to have learned many things either by suggestion or by the hard way of personal experience e.g. burning his/her hand or feet.

a) To stay away from the house area and to walk by night was forbidden (22.2%). At this age curiosity can provoke death if children walk outside the village (lions, hyena, snakes...).

b) Playing with fire was mentioned only by 2.8%. However, this is in a different sense from that of younger children. Here, it is meant not to burn the grass close to a homestead or even the grass in the forest which is intended for building houses or luaks in the dry season.

c) Swimming in deep waters was forbidden for similar reasons to those for younger children.

d) Some remarks (8%) concern the prohibition of drinking beer, eating other's food or cultivating durra. Especially, because of grass « abar » looking similar to young durra «rap» (in Dinka language), children may not recognise durra and remove it with "abar".

For man

There is no great difference between the tribal cultures within the Nilotic community in the South Sudan. However some variations exist in the form of stressing certain norms or having others, specific solely to that ethnicity (tribe). All interviewed replied to this question. Nilotic culture prohibits men from doing :

1. DISGRACEFUL ACTS

Actions which may disgrace the person himself or his entire family. 6O % of the interviewed sample mentioned these as things men are not allowed to do.

a) **Behaving like a woman**: i.e. way of dressing, way of sitting, company, cooking, milking cattle etc.

(i) In the Nilotic tradition as in many other societies, there is a difference between men's and women's clothes. If a man decides to wear women's dresses, then he is considered as disgracing himself and/or his entire lineage (43.2%). Even at times when clothes are not readily available, nobody is expected to wear any clothes he happens to have found.

(ii) In the traditional Nilotic society most people sit on the ground either on animal hides or nets. If a man sits in the same way as a woman, then he would be considered strange. However, if the action is repetitive then it will be taken as disgraceful.

(iii) For any kind of social activity, the society groups itself on the lines of sex and age-groups. If a man decides to be in the company of women (to eat or to walk with a woman) usually, the population will resent such an action and it will be considered disgraceful (16.2%).

(iv) Cooking is considered the duty of the women (up to now) in the Nilotic tradition (56.8%). Certain exceptional cases exist. For example, when the men are alone and far away from the village. If a man decides to cook in the company of women, who are in good health, then this man is considered to dislike or disrespect tradition. Many people therefore will consider this shameful and even disgraceful.

(v) Milking cattle is one of the examples of the differences between the ethnic cultures of the Dinka, Nuer and Shilluk. Whereas the Nuer and Dinka will consider it womanly to milk cattle (24.3%), the Shilluk tradition prohibits women from milking cows, a duty assigned solely to men. For the Dinka and Nuer, if there is no woman or young boy available to milk cattle, the men will have to undertake the duty on condition that they do not drink the milk they have milked. Another person will have to milk that for the other. (If he drinks milk milked by himself, he might become crazy!).

(vi) Not to carry water pot, to make beer or to clean tukuls.

b) **Stealing** has been indicated by 35.1 % as one of the acts prohibited for men. This stems from the fact that stealing is considered disgraceful. Based on his pride, the Nilotic will not want to engage in an activity which may lower his reputation or degrade him. Since stealing is disgraceful, nobody will engage himself with it. Society protects itself against theft by stressing the badness of stealing.

2. CULTURAL ABNORMALITY

About 40% of the surveyed sample has identified certain actions considered deviation from tradition and prohibited for men. Some of these actions include:

a) **Adultery** was for 35.1% of the sample indicated one of the acts prohibited for Nilotic men. There are two forms of adultery: sexual contact with another's legal wife and sex with another's social wife. Social wife means that the husband has paid the deserved dowry but the marriage is not yet consummated. If anybody takes or makes love with such a girl, he is traditionally considered to have committed adultery.

In the first case (18.9%), it is seen as a failure from the side of the man to court girls properly to have sexual relations with them. The woman takes more blame from society which feels that without either invitation or welcoming attitude from the woman, the adultery would not possibly have been committed.

In the second case (16.2%) the story may be quite different. As marriage is sometimes an arrangement between two different groups or families, (different on economic or political grounds) to the exclusion of or disregard for the girl's opinion. If the girl decides either to elope with the young man she loves most or have sex with him with the intention of conceiving a child, it will be difficult for any prior arrangement to take place. Also for the young man to get back all his cattle will be almost impossible. (In the Nilotic tradition a young man has to pay a number of cattle to the future wife's father).

A serious misunderstanding will result between the new husband and the old husband's group; this can lead to a physical confrontation using arms. Also misunderstandings will result between the original husband and the girl's relatives. Therefore it is usually well advised that no young man should engage in a love affair with a married girl or woman. Some young men take pride in having taken the wife of another equally or more important (famous) young man. Therefore the girl may be taken against her wishes.

Sex with very young girls is considered to be bad by all Nilotic traditions where age groups are the rule for any social activities. To have sex with very young girls is considered as an exploitation of them. Therefore, it is advised to protect these young girls.

To have sex with a daughter is strongly forbidden as well as to have sex with a relative or to take some one's fiancé. Homosexuality and masturbation is also mentioned as prohibited.

b) **Insult** to anybody and/or in front of children: 21.6 % of the surveyed sample indicated that to insult one's wife, other women or men (especially a mother or father in law) in front of children was prohibited for Nilotic men. In the extended family system, everybody has to be sympathetic to everybody and to be well regarded by most people. It pays frequently to be gentle with others, children included. Since it is everybody's duty to teach the children or younger people good manners; men or women are not expected to insult others and are prohibited from doing so in front of children.

c) To **disobey** the elderly was strongly underlined as prohibited (10.8%). In the Nilotic society the elderly are always highly respected and their decision is appreciated.

d) **Other remarks**: it's important for each man to have his own tukul and not to sleep outside the hut, not to be drunk and not to beat anyone, especially women. Dignity of a man is highly appreciated.

For woman

In the Nilotic tradition, the woman occupies a central position in the social interactions between families and clans. Much of the tradition is conserved by the woman, therefore any slight variation is considered grave. There are also differences in habits and tradition for women during menstruation, pregnancy or lactation.

From this survey, two main points have been expressed as prohibited by the Nilotic culture for women: disgraceful acts and cultural inconsistency.

A. DISGRACEFUL ACTS meant acts which will bring shame on the individual and/or the whole family. They include:

a) **Adultery**: Whereas 31.5 % of the surveyed population stated that adultery was prohibited for men, 59.5 % emphasized its prohibition for women. Traditionally, many people including women consider that adultery cannot be committed unless the woman is interested in and encourages the man (37.8%). Therefore the emphasis for its prevention is laid on the women. Since the woman is responsible for the education of her daughters, she is expected to be the most decent.

If the adultery results in a conception leading to the birth of a viable baby, that baby frequently suffers socially from this incident. Within the family the baby is considered foreign and unwanted, a sign of traditional breakdown. All people tend to isolate and despise it. This position is easier if the baby is a girl who is expected not to perpetuate the family lineage. The biological father forfeits the child and pays compensation to the husband, as a double punishment. For the Dinka, when this daughter is married later, the biological father is given a minimum share in the dowry: one bull and a calf only. It is also not allowed, for a young girl, to have sex with an old man.

b) **Behaviour like men**: This is for example in the way of dressing, the kind of instruments carried etc. Nilotic women, like women in other societies, have different dress from that of men. Sometimes certain women decide to dress and behave like men (10.8 %). This is seriously objected to by the society. Some women carry clubs, spears (27 % !)... which are absolutely meant for the men. This behaviour is more frequent in the Dinka and Nuer ethnicities than in the Shilluk (if it ever occurred). These two ethnic groups are more liberal with women who can be elected chiefs of villages which is not the practice within the Shilluk kingdom.

Because some women are strong and physically beat their husbands, they order them to do activities of women like, amongst others, going to the forest to collect fire wood for cooking.

c) **Prostitution** is nonexistent in the Nilotic tradition and society. However, with the introduction of western traditions into Nilotic societies, with the evils of the first civil war and the rapid attempts at development which followed, prostitution was introduced into the urban communities of the Nilotic Society. Though only 2.7 % of the surveyed sample stated that prostitution was prohibited, it was highly significant of the change which has occurred as a result of the war and its aftermath. The extended family provides many chances for any single member to get what he/she wants. Therefore, this security does not encourage anybody to employ dignity disgracing actions as a means of getting financial or material benefit.

In the Nilotic tradition, the family's social position is determined by its wealth (cattle or other) which is dependant also on the number of daughters married or marriageable. Therefore every effort is made to protect the daughters from any disadvantage and they are married early and a high dowry is paid, improving or maintaining the family's social position in society. (To better understand the importance of a daughter in the Nilotic families, we questioned if the parents give priority to boys or to girls. The answers obtained were always: «If a boy is protecting the family, a girl is providing dowry which allows brothers to marry and to pay dowry for his wife»).

d) **Other remarks**: It is not advised to eat with men (10.8 %), to be drunk (8.1 %), to build huts or to go to the latrine in front of a man (2.7 %).

B. TRADITIONAL INCONSISTENCY are acts of doing of certain things to which the society objects.

(a) **Theft, begging and lies** were prohibited by 21.6 % of the surveyed sample. These actions depict the family as poor which reflects negatively on the Nilotic culture.

(b) **Insulting** husband and/or children: In 24.3 % insulting another person (especially mother in law) was stated as prohibited.

(c) **Milking** or walking amongst cattle: 2.7 % of the surveyed sample recorded that Nilotic women were prohibited from doing these activities. However, this is one of the examples of the variation in custom between the different ethnic groups within the Nilotic. The Dinka and Nuer do not prohibit their women from milking cattle; actually it is their duty along with very young boys. On the contrary, men are not allowed to milk cattle in the Dinka or Nuer custom, therefore they should naturally walk amongst them. This is why the total percentage is low.

(d) **«Playing sex»** : For the Nilotic women «playing sex» is prohibited after one or more of her daughters is married (indicated by 5.4% of the studied sample) as well as for elderly mothers. Experience has shown that it is not the way the society looks at the woman (if her daughter is married) which discourages her from doing so, rather it is her own will which dissuades her. As a matter of practice we think (AK) that this percentage is particularly high (exaggerated) for the way the Nilotic view this obligation. In the distant past, this was seriously regarded. However at the present time, hardly anyone regards it as a social stigma.

(e) **Other remarks**: It is forbidden for women to sleep outside huts or to travel without permission (32.4 %). The presence of the woman in the family is of great importance. First of all because of the care she has assured to her children, to be present for her husband, and to take care of the whole family (cooking).

In Shilluk society «child's care and feeding is regarded as holy, when it contradicts norms of the society the mother may be condemned even if she is not wrong».

For women during menstruation

In the Nilotic tradition, certain activities which interfere with the cleanliness or the well being of the women during menses are prohibited for her.

A. CLEANLINESS

(a) **Playing sex** during menses: 83.8 % of the studied sample gave this as an activity prohibited for the menstruating women. This is one of the highest single responses to one question. This high percentage also shows how strong the tradition is against having sex during menstruating. However, this result from the fact that sex during menses is considered very dirty by most Nilotic. «We do not know of any Nilotic who considers it otherwise. Again, whereas most Nilotic (married) play sex with the aim of having a baby, they do not consider the time when the woman is bleeding as the most appropriate time for conceiving, so they also deliberately abstain during this time» (AK)

(b) **Visiting sick people** by a menstruating woman was considered as wrong by 2.7 % of the respondents. Probably it is on the basis that a menstruating woman may be considered dirty or vice versa. It might be one of the differences between the Nilotic Ethnicities and may not be a Dinka tradition as well (only mentioned by a Shilluk respondent). The rationale behind this is not quite clear to Dr Akec Khoc having spent most of his time in town. He could have simply not obtained the reason or forgotten it.

B. PROTECTIVE:

Because a menstruating woman loses a lot of blood, she becomes weak. The Nilotic tend to be more protective when they either know or assume that the woman is having her periods. Working hard during periods was stated by 8.1 % of the surveyed sample as prohibited. Many relatives or neighbours come to her aid as soon as they know about it. They go to the river or well to fetch water or grind and sieving pound the family daily food quantity (photo 21 and 22). They collect firewood from the forest for her. They assist in many other domestic daily activities.

C. CULTURAL and/or TRADITIONAL ABNORMALITY

(a) **Drinking cow's milk without traditional ceremony** was stated as prohibited for women during menstruation by 64.8 % of the surveyed sample. This is a very strong tradition among the Dinka and Nuer but not among the Shilluk ethnicity since the females are obliged not to drink milk at all as soon as they reached menstruation.

For the Dinka and Nuer, the bleeding is considered as a cleansing by God and so if a woman drinks cow's milk while bleeding, that cow is expected to become ill of the disease being cleansed from the woman. If certain rituals have been done to the woman who drinks milk, then milk becomes safe. This is usually done for about two or three cattle to guarantee that one of them shall be able to be milked while the woman will be having her period. The woman during this period cannot even drink goat's or sheep's milk.

(b) **Other remarks**: It was also mentioned that women during menstruation may not look after cattle or to go to the luak (5.4%), to cook (5.4 %) or to work hard (2.7 %).

For lactating women

The main objective is to protect the child and mother from:

(a) **Engaging in exhaustive functions** eg. fighting or wrestling (52.8 %), prolonged dancing, drinking beer (8.3 %) and/or practising sex during advanced pregnancy (33.3 %) has been noted by 94.4 % of the surveyed sample. Nearly everybody questioned, whether male or female, adult or adolescent, gave this as one of the activities prohibited for women during pregnancy.

One person indicated: «If pregnant just up to 3 or 4 months, she should not play sex again because the foetus may be spoiled, which has been accepted by God»; Shilluk believes that «if any breast feeding woman plays sex with man she may have the baby sick especially by diarrhoea».

All these activities demand a lot of energy being wasted and some of them, like wrestling may lead to severe physical injury or exhaustion which may interfere with the foetal growth immediately or later. However, sex during advanced pregnancy is considered undesirable because it is believed to lead on the one hand, to premature birth, the result of which is death to the premature child, (the conditions for extra-uterine foetal development are not usually met when coupled with certain deficiencies during the intra-uterine phase - AK). On the other hand, since the woman is already pregnant, there is a lot of scepticism about the reasons for playing sex during that time.

For enjoyment, if a man cannot suspend it until the child is born and has reached a reasonable age, he is advised to marry more wives (polygamy is allowed!).

(b) **Visiting sick people** is prohibited for pregnant women only by 2.7 % of the surveyed population. The reasons behind its prohibition are not very clear.

(c) **Hard work** was in 22.2 % not advised for pregnant women as well as carrying heavy things (25 %).

(d) **Other remarks**: Not to go to luak or to walk among cattle as well as not to sleep on the stomach. «When she gets up in the morning she should sit up properly and rest».

A. PROTECTIVE TO CHILD

86.1 % of the population mentioned facts which are eventually protective to the child as prohibited for a lactating woman.

a) **Going far away from her child** is strongly prohibited (63.9%), as well as to sleep outside the tukul or to travel without permission (22.2%).

b**) Breast feeding** the child as soon as the mother arrives home after a walk in the tropic heat, is prohibited (8.3%). She is advised to rest for at least a few minutes or wash the breast with cool water. «When she is coming from hot sun, she should not suckle her child before washing breast with cool water in order to cool milk».

c) **To be near fire** during breast feeding a child is not advised (8.3%).

d) **Drinking alcohol** (11.1 %) is generally considered to lead the mother not to attend properly to her child's needs. She herself may not be eating enough food or the quality food which will allow her to have more breast milk for the child. For these and other reasons, alcohol intake while lactating is sternly prohibited.

All these measures are aimed at reducing suffering to the child. If a lactating woman leaves her child for long periods, the child may not be able to feed or be fed, may develop an emotional dislike for the mother which is feared and which may continue till adulthood. As there are many dangers which may await the child, the Nilotic do not wish to add a preventable danger or complication.

B. SEX DURING LACTATION

52.7 % of the surveyed group mentioned that sex was prohibited during lactation. Especially it is not advised to play sex at the moment of breastfeeding (5.6%). The Nilotic strongly believe that if a child suckles breast-milk from a pregnant mother, he develops intractable diarrhoea which may lead to death. This idea explains why a child to be weaned has to be taken far from mother during the first month to condition him to bottle milk and food. If the child has to stay close to the mother, she must paint her breast with a foul smelling plant or irritating substance (like pepper) so that the child dislikes and forgets the breast.

It is a tradition that lactating women do not play sex. Before they start to play she decides with her husband the time to start to play sex. It depends on the development of their child. Both of them observe the child and, if they are assured that their child can stay alone and, by himself, find a way of getting food, they can decide to have sex. It means that they have experience that playing sex automatically stops breast-feeding and can have an impact on their child's development and even life. This custom - tradition is very strong amongst the Nilotic.

One person indicated that «lactating woman is not allowed to play sex till the baby is able to walk because the baby will become sick with diarrhea». (In a village, during our survey, a lactating woman asked me to save her child who was extremely malnourished. She had already consulted a magician and offered a cow to save her child but without effect. A clinical examination showed that the breast was very small and there was no more breast milk production since three months. The reason was: her husband started to play sex since a few months and... she became pregnant. Because there was no milk available (no cows !) and the one and half year old child didn't get food, it was too late to save the starving child - ZLO).

C. REMARKS

It is prohibited to walk among cows, to sleep during day time, to fight or wrestle. It is advised not to make children cry.

It is interesting to mention that there is NO difference in breast feeding boys or girls (even twins). It means that the mother gives the same chance to boys as to girls (ZLO).

4. SOCIAL ACTIVITIES

To better understand the life of the Nilotic it was necessary to obtain data concerning their social activities. The subjects we chose to study are cattle, fishing hunting, talking, sex life, marriage, religions and others.

THE VALUE OF CATTLE

With the background that most Nilotic are more nomad than agro-pastoralists, we can therefore imagine the value of the cattle in a traditional society where rains are sometimes unpredictable, leading to crop failure and therefore total dependence on cattle wealth.

MARIAGE AND SOCIAL PRESTIGE

100 % of the surveyed population stated that one of the important values of cattle to Nilotic was their use in marriage for paying dowry. Though they do provide milk for food (rarely meat), especially for children, the primary value of cattle is their use in marriage. For example a dowry varying from 8-10 on cows to more than a hundred, depends on the social status of the bride. Her education and relationship with other members of her family, play an important role in the determination of dowry.

This is because one can eat any kind of food but cannot pay anything else for marriage other than cows. 14.3 % of these same samples indicated cattle as a means for social prestige. This is because the more cattle a Nilotic has, the more prestigious he becomes. The more they have materially (cattle) or financially, the more dominant they become politically, socially and even physically. Then, the people around the wealthy Nilotic work hard to see that one becomes wealthier, and so the vicious circle continues. However, the prestigious individual not only owns the cattle, but also many relatives, friends or other well-wishers support him. The poor usually benefit from the milk of the wealthy man's cattle. These people look after the cattle, protecting them from wild animals, death or loss; these people providing also the traditional veterinary services they require and making the camps comfortable for the cattle.

FOOD AND CASH

Up to 60 % of the surveyed community indicated the value of cattle as food or in cash. All of the 60 % mentioned to eat meat, 51.4 % to drink milk, 2.8 % to produce butter and 57.1 % to sell cows (37.1 % for cash).

As the Nilotic depends mainly on what he owns or can grow around the village for his food. Milk or its products and/or meat provide the best addition to that mainly cereal based food. They like to improve the quality and taste of the food when eaten in company. It is the most readily available food for the Nilotic guest who might not be made to wait for any other food to be prepared. This food is of course also available for a Nilotic who has to go on an urgent journey; especially in cases when some other ethnicity raids and steals the community's cattle. It also acts as a reminder of the value of cattle and therefore the necessity to get them back or protect them.

The cattle are used as commodities for bartering or evaluating other items. This applies to a time when a Nilotic needs grain and the owner may not wish to sell his grain for cash. The same applies to butter (fat) or certain beads worn by young men or girls as a mark for their age groups etc. When the market is available, the cattle among others, provide the best means for acquiring any needed cash.

MEANS OF PROTECTION

The values of a cow for the Nilotics are very important. This consists in different ways:

a) **Compensation**: If anybody has disabled another person, compensation is given by offering a certain number of cattle depending on the degree and severity of the disability. Sometimes when somebody has been killed, the rule is to pay compensation in the form of cattle. Depending on the particular ethnicity, the value of the compensation is assessed and the sex of the deceased individual as also taken into consideration. Many customary law drafters have frequently reviewed the effectiveness of the punishment in stopping or reducing the rate of killing. However, there is a great divergence in the opinions of the proponents and opponents.

b) **Sacrifice**: When a member of a family is ill, whether medical services are available or not, some traditionalists believe in first making a sacrifice to the ancestors or gods to remove the illness. This is usually a goat, sheep, cow or cock depending on the seriousness of the illness and the material conditions of the family.

Another application is when there is an outbreak of epidemic in cattle. Each person makes a sacrifice to God in order to protect his animal wealth or reduce the losses. It remains to be seen the cures that may be effected are resulting from modern medicine (human or veterinary), or from the traditional protective methods.

However, the dual use of the traditional protective methods tends to compound the misunderstanding of their value. Sometimes such sacrifices are done even when there is no threat of an epidemic, there might be some ulterior motives overshadowed by protection.

THE VALUE OF COWS PRODUCTS

a) **Hides** are mostly used for sleeping on (51.4 %) and/or protection from rain or cold in camps where huts or luaks are not available. They are also used for preparing ropes for tying down the cattle so that their offspring do not suckle the milk or that they do not wander away, to be killed at night by wild animals. More important is their use for making drums, either for dancing, or as a signal for an impending or existent danger.

b) **Horns** are used for carving traditional spoons or whistles for young men during dance. Recently, the traditional spoons are fading away and slowly being replaced by metal spoons.

c) **Cow dung** is used as a decoration for the body, houses or for cleaning hands. After being burnt into ashes it is used as tooth-paste. The ashes together with urine are used for hair conditioning and coloration. Ashes are also used for body decoration.

d) **Urine** is used as a decoration for the body, houses or for cleaning hands. The urine together with ashes is used for hair conditioning and coloration. Urine also is providing for body decoration. Urine is also used for body washing (warm and clean).

51.4 % of those surveyed mentioned the sacrificial of cow products. Though these are taken for granted or downplayed by society. There is nothing in a cow which is useless. «The Nilotic take care of the cow and the cow takes care of the Nilotic», is a common Nilotic saying (AK).

THE VALUE OF FISHING

Most Nilotic live along the Nile and/or one of its tributaries or move to its banks during the dry season. Each year, at the beginning of the rainy season, water in the lowlands near the Nile and that which flow throughout the Nile, mix together. Fish from the Nile find a very good opportunity to move to more shallow waters. Some return to the Nile while the water level is receding and others remain in the swamps or are cut off by the water. In the deep waters, fishing-nets or hooks are used. In the swamps or marshes, either nets, hooks or the very traditional «fishing-spears» are used.

Those who live close to rivers get and eat fish throughout the whole year; whereas those who are farther away may get fish only in the dry season. Therefore, the food value of fish is appreciated by most Nilotic. Some of the tribes choose to live near the river in order to fish throughout the year.

Fish is eaten either alone (cooked or grilled) or may be in mixed combinations with cereals like «Kisra» (pancake), «Akello-Akop» or «Kuin», (a delicious roasted sorghum powder paste).

FOOD AND CASH

The cash value of fishing is important, especially for those living close to the river because of the constant supply of fish (much more than they can eat - AK). There is always a greater demand in the towns than in the villages. For example, for those living close to towns like Malakal, Kodok, Bor, Melut etc. Therefore the surplus, in excess of the amount eaten by a normal family, can be sold. For 80.6 % of surveyed persons the value of fishing is to get food and for 30.6% to get cash.

HOBBY OR JOB

For 13.9 % of the surveyed persons, fishing is a hobby. This is the opinion of those Nilotic living further away from the river (mainly Nuer), because they do not normally practice fishing. However, during the beginning of the dry season (December/January), when the swamps are cut off from the main rivers and the water level is rapidly diminishing, many people in these areas go fishing. At this time of the year, there is still enough grain (sorghum) from the second harvest and since there is enough grass to graze the cattle, there is enough milk. Therefore people do not appreciate fish at this particular time. They then consider fishing just as a game to while away that time. It is interesting to note that some young men, including Dinka, refuse to go fishing. Shilluk never consider fishing as just a game or a hobby.

Another 5.6 % mentioned fishing as a job and duty. This is the opinion forwarded by two respondents who happened to be Shilluk. As mentioned earlier, because of the proximity of the Shilluk villages to the Nile or Sobat rivers, most fish throughout the year. Therefore fishing becomes a job to some of them just as cultivation of sorghum is to most of Nilotic.

Moreover, some Dinka consider it as a job or a necessity when they take their cattle camps to the marshes «toich» where fish is abundant. During the dry season, the quantity of milk produced by each cow decreases and therefore food has to be supplemented by fish. Every individual member of the family goes fishing to increase the chance of more fish being caught. In these cases, fishing is done using fishing spears. Therefore, fishing is considered as a dry season, part-time, duty.

For 16.7 % of surveyed persons, fishing has no value. The respondents said that they were not interested in fishing. It was therefore concluded that they considered it to have no value. However, these could have two different meanings: they could appreciate its value but at the same time not be interested in fishing. But mostly, they happened to be far from rivers and they rarely catch or consume fish. They might have grown up without appreciating the value of fishing. Another explanation is that young men usually tend not to take many things seriously and therefore this could be a falsely high figure.

THE VALUE OF HUNTING

For the Nilotic, hunting is the most traditional activity. It has different values.

As food

For 74.3 % of those surveyed indicated food as one of the values of hunting. However, it appeared that hunting was understood as game alone but did not includ river animals (some people explained that «hunting is practiced by those far from the river to get meat for food». But even those near the river also hunt game to get meat for food or for a change of diet.

As trade

Part of those surveyed mentioned that hunting provided meat for sale. It is frequent to find meat being either bartered for sorghum or sold for cash (very rare). Traders travelling a long distance from other parts of Sudan (particularly in the north) come to purchase kids in these areas. Therefore this trade is reason enough for hunting, even if the hunters do not need the meat for food.

As domestic utility

For 77.1 % hunting means to get skins. Many Nilotic prefer to sleep, sit or lie on hides - whether of cows or game animals. The older people particularly rest on chairs made of wood and hides. The hides are also transformed into bags for storing or transporting things: grain, tobacco etc. One or all of these reasons were mentioned by the Nilotic hunters.

As horns

The horns in particularly are turned into beautiful traditional spoons. This practice is historic and still respected and perpetuated up to now in the nilotis community. The horns are also transformed into trumpets for music during the dance. For these reasons as well, the Nilotic hunt animals. This has been indicated by about 8% of those questioned.

As a game or hobby

24% indicated that they hunt as a game or as a hobby (5.7 %). Spears are the weapons used are the spears. One hunter can carry between ten to fifteen spears. Some are designed to be thin and sharp. Others are thick and heavy. In this case a hunter can carry only up to three. Depending on the animal being hunted, the hunter carries a particularly adapted spear. For example hunting antelopes or other small animals requires thin and sharp spears. Hunting giraffes and/or elephants requires thick and long spears. Crocodiles are hunted using a specially adapted short spear with multiple curved ends. (Shilluk use mostly 3 thick, long and heavy spears, including «fishing spear», while Dinka and Nuer use many thin, short and light spears - ZLO).

Young men usually go hunting as a game for training in running and aiming. Often women are also present during hunting, especially in helping the hunter to approach the animals.

THE VALUE OF TALKING

Communication

For Nilotic talking means communication. For 77.8 %, talking, means understanding ourselves. Some of them said «that it's why God gave voice». For 11.1 % «God create man to talk» and for 13.9 % talking means to have power. Another 8.3 % indicated even «if a person does not talk he can die». It is very interesting to underline that in this population oral expression is a way of thinking: 30.6 % said «talking bring thinking».

Since times past, for Nilotic have expressed and communicated facts oraly. From the very beginning of life, infants and children get education and knowledge about life by oral explanation from the parents. (In the South-Sudan, there are very few schools). Very often boys, during long evening hours, listen to elders talking about events of the day, whilst sitting around the fire.

Culture and history

43.2% (16/37) stated that talking was used for passing history and culture from one generation to the other. This is a very important way of passing oral history to children, as the population is mainly illiterate.

Concerning the knowledge of the family, a child is taught to know his great grandparents both from the paternal and maternal side and their contributions to the society. The child is therefore advised or educated to be like them, or a particular individual, according to the kind of contribution he/she may desire. At the community level, each clan is proud of certain historical events associated with it. Therefore when young men are being initiated into manhood, they are frequently reminded of these important historical events so that even if they do not do more important acts, they should do similar acts. When such an attitude of competition between families or clans is established then the society progresses very well by discarding the bad practices and retaining, with improvement, the good ones.

Correction of society

Talking was used also as a means for correcting the society. This is very true for all the Nilotic. When a Nilotic realise that there is something wrong in the society, and he/she cannot correct it by suggestion alone, he/she therefore composes a song to expose that thing or individual. Most traditional songs which do not concentrate around cattle, talk about certain good or bad actions done by members of the society. Especially the Dinka find it as one of the best means correcting their societies (During long evenings, sitting among the elderly around a fire could observe children sitting behind us. They understood each word and sentence but lost interest in listening to elders talking about the most important event of the day, which was usually concerning the behaviour of a cow ! - ZLO).

THE MEANING OF SEX

Pleasure and means of expressing love

77.8 % of the surveyed population mentioned pleasure as «to satisfy our lust for women» or «that which make us love women» as the meaning of sex. Generally, this is the opinion or understanding of the middle aged people and the adolescents. They gave this response as the most immediate meaning for sex. Sexes is practiced for the sake of pleasure alone for 75 % of the sample interviewed Many young people have had the chance to travel away from home either to seek employment or to escape death in the villages (1964-1972). These people therefore interacted with other societies and, coming back, their attitude to sex was more liberal. This applies to women and men, girls or boys. The same population, through the means of story-telling have influenced others who did not have the chance of temporary refuge or migration (AK).

Reproduction was mentioned only by 33.3 % as a reason for sex. For 5.6 % «sex may attract marriage through love of God».

THE MEANING OF MARRIAGE

Reproduction

100 % of those surveyed gave reproduction and/or establishment of a home as the meaning of marriage to them. For 88.9% it means «to have children», for 8.3 % «to create a nation and for 2.7 % «establishment of a home».

In any traditional society, everything is explained in relationship to God. For 5.6 % «God planned these things». This is true for the Nilotic Society as well. (Recently, most Nilotic believes that sex or marriage means the production of children designated by God - AK).

They also understand it as the establishment of Society which will lead to a nation (8.3 %). (This is all in fulfilment of God's wish as He created human beings and animals to live together and reproduce in order to continue the species. They therefore feel that any marriage which does not result in children is not approved by God - A.K.).

The older people 16.7% (6/36) stressed the meaning of marriage as the formation of a home. Probably in their days, as we have been hearing, it was difficult for an unmarried young man or girl to have sex. This was just the way the society felt about it. Therefore, unless one was married, one could not practice sex and sex was synonymous with marriage and the establishment of a home. (These traditions are becoming more lax now due to exposure to other traditions which are quite liberal about sex Movement from or into the Nilotic land has made this change - AK)

Pleasure as «lust» was mentioned by 38.9 % as marriage and in 8.3% as expression of love.

5. COMPORTMENT OF NILOTICS

THE EXISTENCE OF MAGIC AND MAGICIANS

Magic is a common third world belief and so the Nilotic generally believe in the existence of magic and its power.

From the surveyed sample, 75% responded positively to the existence of magic, about 8.3% negatively and 16.7% did not know.

The form in which magic exists

The form was said to be human beings by 47.2% of the studied sample, idol 47.2% and 5.6% did not indicate the form, thought they said it existed. It will be worth mentioning here that most people choose one or two forms of this existence.

As to whom the magician actually is, 43.4% mentioned certain names like «Duop Deang», «Manyang Daw», «Obany Adwok», «Nyay Deng», «Nyang Lual», «Ajwogo» etc. The majority (32%), mentioned idols like some stones, green grass, pieces of wood, pieces of bones etc, as the real magical item (only idols belonging to certain individuals, could have power to do magic). 30.6% also reported that they did not know who the magician was in their village or community. As for the previous question, there was more than one answer per respondent.

As to what the magician does

There were a variety of answers according to how the people felt or probably might have heard others talk about this. They included mainly destruction of either property or the individual or his kin when unhappy with that individual (72.2%). A great number mentioned that the magician can kill people, mostly children (47.2%) or cows (25%). About 58.3 % also mentioned helping people when pleased with them. This means making people becoming well when sick, protecting them or their wealth from any kind of perils like epidemics and/or making a lot of crops grow in their fields. 13.9% did not believe what the magician could do or did not know what exactly the magician did or did not do.

BEHAVIOUR

To better understand the comportment of the Nilotic people, it was necessary to try to get information about each interviewed person's way of life and/or their relation to the society (different cultural groups).

This part of questioner was answered only partially. For example, a man without a wife or children did not respond to questions concerning women or children, a young person did not describe elderly behaviour etc. They described their existence as to the importance of the person or subject they are living. The percentage was calculated only up to the number of answers.

Man lives because of: Herd (48%), cultivation (40%), children (16%), wife (12%), fishing, body decoration or game (4%). For men the society means people with whom they are living or from whom they originated (55%). For young people, the company of girls (29.6%) or other boys (11.1%). Two persons answered they are magicians, so there is nothing else important for them.

A Woman's life depends on: Her husband (68.4%), to bring up her children (15.8%) or upon parents help (15.8%) because still young. For women the society means «people of her husband» (36.8%) or «women in the village and their neighbours» (31.6%). For young people, the company of boys and girls (21%) is important. For two old women, society means the happiness of their children.

Children's lives depend on: their parents (66%) or only their father (33%). Mother alone never has been mentioned!

Whether the persons believe in what they do: 68.6% responded positively that they believed in what they did; 22.9% were not sure whether or not they actually believed in what they did (scarifying, praying...), while 8.6% stated that they did not believe in what they did. The same questioned persons if asked differently revealed similar responses.

Whether the persons do it because others do it: 30.6% answered because other people are doing it (one person said that «he believes in the old way of his father's beliefs»), 61.1% answered negatively and 8.3% don't know.

DREAMS

Like magic, dreams are commonly believed and seriously adhered to by the Nilotic as any other African Community.

Whether they do what they dream about: 65.7% of the sample responded negatively, 31.4% positively and one person (2.9%) dreamed sometimes. These percentages in our opinion are contrary to real Nilotic practice because most Nilotic consult GODS to explain what they have dreamed about and probably acted on them (AK). Maybe the recent influence of Christianity could interfere with their responses (ZLO).

The frequency of dreaming: 68.6% stated that they did not dream very often, 31.4% agreed they dreamed.

As to the content of dreams, almost all (94.3%) mentioned a combination of sex, animals, children, war and 34.3% dreamed also about others: games (2.8%) and frightening (8.6%). Only one person (2.8%) abstained from answering the question. This is not the same individual as in the first or second case.

Whether dreams are sometimes true or not: From the way the question was set; most people were expected to accept that assertion and 97.2% responded approvingly: half of them said that dreams are sometimes true and only one person (2.8%) did not believe so. For 20% the dreams are lies and for 2.9% nonsense. Some made the following remarks: «a true dream comes from God», «because of night evils», «tell you what next will happen to you», «they are what you usually think», «to frighten you»...

DEATH

To better understand the value of life, it was decided to question about the meaning of death.

Whether Nilotic worry about death or not, two thirds claimed not and 1/3 worry about it («I'm worried about death itself»). It would have been expected that the reverse would have been true with more worrying about death and few not worrying about it because many people in this society die either young or when fully grown up. The answers suggest that they do not wish to see themselves or another die (AK). The fact they do not worry can be explained by their traditional way of life: hunting, danger of wild animals, diseases and no health care... (ZLO).

On the existence of life after death or not, 75% stated that it exists, 22.2% said it did not and 2.8% did not know.

In what form can a person exist after death, between those who stated it exist, 50% answered «according to GOD's wish», 42.9% stated that a person will continue to exist as a human being, about 3.6% stated that the human form will change into another creature for example snake. Another 3.6% did not know the form of existence of a person after death.

LIFE

Relationships

As for the meaning of relationship between an individual with his/her children, there were more than one answer in most cases and about 68.6% mentioned blood relationship («child belongs to me»), 34.3% parental emotional love and 28.6% their care (some mentioned support for them for example providing food, security etc).

a) **Education** was indicated in a similar way, as to what people do to their children. For 71.1% the most important was school education for boys. For 11.4%, girls must stay at home (One woman said: «...leave girls at home, if husband allows, because it is a waste to educate girls»).

Most Nilotic are not inclined to send their daughters to school because some of them had bad experience with the first girls. They do not like to let them go to school with children from various tribes; i.e. some of them were not properly married and the relatives did not benefit from their domestic managerial services, as they stayed in towns most of the time (AK).

b) **Culture** was expressed by 60% as education in the traditional way. Between those: 48.6% expressed as «to love nature», 20% «to love the nation» (for 22.9% to be proud to be a Nuer or a Shilluk) and for 8.6% «to be human».

Freedom

Due to the fact that most of the people who answered the questionnaire had either no education or very little, the opinions expressed are quite representative of that of most rural populations of Southern Sudan including the Nilotic community. Freedom for 60 % of the sample means to speak (47.9%) and to think (17.1%). For Nilotic oral expression is very important: «to give a speech means thinking». By this they mean that any Nilotic can think and speak as they wish within their society and age group. Songs are also oral expressions of thinking. Close to them are pictorial expressions: painting their body and/or face, painting on calabashes or on walls inside the tukuls (ZLO). Dance was mentioned by 11.1%.

Very interesting are the additional expressions like «to decide» (34.4%) and «to be a free Nuer» (22.9%) which contrast with a very philosophical expression «no one is free unless he is dead» (20%).

For the Nilotic, freedom to walk is also important (28.6%) and to choose the kind of work they wish to do (28.6%). This is definitely in the village within the community but not in town (AK).

Some persons (3%) stated that they believe in GOD as his/her freedom, to vote for or against community proposals or to take care of his/her family. Other expressions of freedom were: «to breath», «to live as I like», «to help my nation», «to eat» and even «to sleep»! Another 20% stated that they had no freedom at all. They do not fully explain why or who has taken away their freedom.

Life's obligation

The «life's obligations» were summarized under five categories. There were more than one response from a great number of respondents.

a) **Obligations relating to self and family** care was mentioned by 77.8% of the sample studied. This included feeding self (13.9%) or children (19.4%), attending to the family like : looking after family (27.8%) and cattle (16.7%).

b) **Obligations related to duty** mentioned by 36.1% of sample included cultivation (11.1%) and gathering other wealth for the family and work (13.9%), to finish any duty you have already started (2.8%). Marriage (5.6%) is mentioned also as one of the duties. One person added «people who fall under the denomination of marriage always have life different from lives of others who are not concern with reproduction and life whole abilities».

c) **Obligations related to Nation** mentioned by 38.9% of the sample was «Love the country and protect its people», «To be responsible for my people» (8.3%), «To have spears for protection against enemies» (8.3%), «To be respected by the society (Shilluk)», «To determine what my life shall be next year», «To be a man of my own world» or «To be a man like others».

d) **Obligations relating to society** were mentioned by 61.1% of the sample are the following: dance (27.8%), decorating the body (22.2%) and to paint the face (11.1%). These obligations were expressed as: «I am obliged to dance, paint my face carefully so that I shall be observed by girls. I have to show people my talents to be without blame what so ever» or «I am obliged to know dancing, I am obliged to paint my face carefully because I shall be noticed by boys. I am also obliged to decorate my body in time of dancing».

Ego

To determine the impact of «Ego» in the expression of the Nilotic, we noted if a person started to answer with «I» or in any other way, without using «I».

Almost all those who answered this questioner used «I» at the beginning of their answers. This was stated by 88.6% of the sample. 11.4% started a sentence without using «I».

SEXUALITY, LIBIDO or SEXUAL DESIRES

Most Nilotics are usually shy to discuss in public anything related to sex. However, we think that the interviewer must have devised a very good way of putting the subject to the respondents leading to this high level of answers. There were various responses to the questions.

Desire

Whether they feel the desire or not, 83.3% of the sample answered affirmatively. 16.7% responded negatively, that they did not feel it. It is worth mentioning here that these were mainly (almost exclusively) the very old men and menopausal women or very young girls.

How they felt it ?

On how they felt it, 67.7% mentioned «good» and 25.8% even appreciated it as «very good». Four old women and a young girl didn't reply. Between those who replied only 3.2% did not know how it felt. Whether this was the expected answer or that the answer has been dictated by the way the question was put may be seen in a follow up study.

Are they happy about it ?

Whether they were happy about it or not, between the 31 replies 96.8% affirmed (two mentioned they have been even «very happy» and only 3.2% stated they did not know, simply because they no longer felt the desire (lactating woman).

Reasons not to practice sex

What were the reasons not to practice sex? 3O.6% of the interviewed didn't answer, 16.7% said they are too old to practice sex and 2.8% were very young girls.

Between the remaining 50%, many different responses have been given: because of relatives (from relatives of both sides of the family) (77.2%), bleeding (menses) (44.4%), girls too young (38.9%), sisters (16.7%) or sickness of husband (2.9%).

The duration of sex life

On whether they accept sex over a long-time or during a lifetime, 70.6% disapproved and could not accept it while 29.4% approved it. These were mainly those at the extremes of age, the very old (majority) and the very young. Two persons didn't answer.

The difficulties of having sex

As to whether they can't have sex, what could they do? 87.5% of those who disapproved stated that they will definitely look for a partner (mostly wives and/or girls). 8.3% fear their husband and 4.2% did not know what to do (young girl). Between those who disapproved are old women and men (Shilluk mostly) or girls too young «for a sexual life». It is interesting to mention two explanations: «woman cannot refuse me if I wanted her» or «Make my wife love me so that she accepts me».

DISEASES AND LONELINESS

Like death, most Nilotic worries about disease and loneliness. The following answers were given in response to the following questions:

On whether they are worried or not when alone (isolated)? 75% affirmed and 25% were not.

As to what they worry about ? Between those who worry many reasons have been given: 74% were worried about loneliness (1/4 was afraid). But they were worrying as well «about something going wrong in the village» (29.6%), about animals (22.2%), snakes (7.4%) or about killed cows (11.1%), about death (22.2%) or an «independent danger» (18.5%). Some mentioned to worry about children, diseases, «rain who can kill» and magic.

Between those who do not worry still 44% stated simply that loneliness alone worries them.

As to why they worry about it ? All 34 interviewed, except two persons stated following reasons: death (41.2), loneliness (35.3), «no people and cows in the village» (35.3%), «animals who can kill» (11.8%) or «death of cows» (2.9%). Only one person worried without reason and another one simply didn't worry. All those worried stated that they wanted protection or assistance which was usually provided or assured by the presence of another person or other people (AK).

As to whether they are worrying with or without reason, a judgment left to the interviewer, 69.4% of all the sample were stated to be worried with reason while 25% of the whole sample were said to be worried without reason (they often mentioned «imaginative fear») and only 5.6% stated not worrying at all.

COLLECTIVITY

A society/community which is basically rural and not exposed to the advantages or disadvantages of development, like the Nilotic one, usually exhibits many forms of collective behaviour and resents individualism with vigour.

On whether people like dancing, 97% affirmed they liked to dance and only a single person (3%) said he doesn't. Some Nilotic take something as bad (or don't like) when they might have had a bad experience in that place or about that particular thing. If the respondent might either have been harmed or vice versa in a dance, he/she would always take dancing as bad. Others just wish to be different from the majority and whether he believed what he said or not, to be different from the rest.

On their opinions about trouble-shooting, 92 % disapproved of trouble-shooting while the other 8% approved it.

On their opinions about being peace-loving, 92% affirmed the peace-loving nature of the Nilotic (and the Southern Sudanese people in general - AK) whereas 8% claimed not to be peaceful.

On whether they liked or disliked to work, 97 % affirmed to like to work and mentioned some of its advantages while the other 3% did not like to work (one old woman). Probably they like to work while active and young. It will be most unlikely that they did not like hard labour since they worked when young (AK).

6. SUMMARY

The aim to carry out a socio-psychological study in the South-Sudan was the fact, that:

- little scientific knowledge was available about the population living still in a very traditional way,
- this population was submitted to rapid change due to the construction of the Jonglei Canal,
- it is important to collect data about the traditions and the importance of different items.

Because of three main ethnic groups living in this area (Shilluk, Dinka and Nuer), using their own language and of the intimate character of many questioned items it was important to carry out this study by an intelligent local person. Such a person was Mr James Gatluak, from a Nuer tribe, with an excellent knowledge of the three tribal languages as well as English and Arabic. This person had the capacity to adapt himself to local situation, to listen and observe for many hours the questioned persons and to direct the conversation. He was well accepted by the whole population. He even touched many sacred subjects.

It was also important for the questionnaires to be studied by an objective, intelligent, southern Sudanese. Dr Akec Khoc, a medical doctor from a Dinka tribe, agreed to explore the questionnaires and to comment on the answers. Because of the specificity of the population under study, their expressions have been kept unchanged.

It is certain, that this population have a long tradition and an old culture, transmitted orally since generations. The main members of the society who carry this responsibility are men (father or elderly in the village).

The main subjects forbidden in this society have been grouped by age and sex.

For the first three years of life, the main attention was given to customary education such as hygiene («not to pass urine and/or stools in/or around the tukul or luak»), stealing/begging, not to eat from the same dish with older children and obeying elders. Another aspect was to protect the child against accidents (fire, water, wild animals and even cattle («not to walk among the cattle»).

For older children traditional customary education is more vigorous because children at this age understand the message they get. Before puberty, sex is prohibited traditionally but at the same time they must learn to play sex at this age, probably to insure the procreation. Due to the high mortality rate, existence of the society in their meaning is due to high birth rate.

Begging and stealing is not acceptable by the Nilotic society. In their traditional way of life, all people are sharing food and dormitories with others in need. Of course, differences in richness exist. Because of the traditional respect of elders, it is not acceptable to insult elders or disobey them.

A great attention is given to protect life. Because of the most common accidents, playing with fire and swimming in deep water is forbidden.

There are less differences between the three tribal cultures, but some variations of norms exist. Men are considered differently than women, and women are also considered differently especially during menstruation, pregnancy or lactation.

Nilotic culture prohibits men from doing disgraceful acts. Behaviour like a woman is one of the most inacceptable («using women clothes, milking cattle, cooking...»).

Certain actions, considered as deviation from tradition, are prohibited for men, especially adultery and insulting in front of children.

In the Nilotic tradition, women occupy a central position in the social interactions between families and clans. Therefore any slight variation is considered grave for women. Disgraceful acts as adultery, prostitution, and behaviour like man («carry spears...») are not accepted by society.

Other acts like stealing, begging or insulting husband or children are considered as traditional abnormality. Also playing sex, after one or more daughters are married, is prohibited.

For women during menstruation it is absolutely prohibited to play sex, to drink cow's milk (without traditional ceremony) and even to visit sick people. On the other hand these women are protected by relatives and neighbours who help them in daily activities, because of their weakness.

For pregnant women it is prohibited to engage in exhaustive activities like dancing, sex or wrestling, which can interfere with the foetal growth.

The lactating woman is subject to special customs because of the wellbeing of her child. She may not leave a child alone for a long time, cannot breast feed after drinking alcohol and, especially, cannot have.

To better understand the life of the Nilotic, it was necessary to obtain data concerning their social activities. The value of cattle is primordial in marriage for paying dowry and as a means of social prestige. Hunting and fishing was considered as a support of supplementary food, skin or horns.

The value of talking is considered as passing history to the next generation (lack of schools) and correction of society. The existence of magic and magicians, the belief in dreams and life after death, the relationship between an individual and his child, the importance of marriage, sexual desires and libido, the meaning of freedom, life's obligation and EGO are as important as what people are worrying about, who they are (peaceful) and what is their community life (dance, body painting...).

These results, even if the number of studied responses did not reach the aim to obtain at least 100 answers from each ethnic group, gives a scientific approach concerning the traditions in the Nilotic population: Shilluk, Nuer and Dinka.

To add histories and even genealogical trees make such a study more rich and allow better understanding of a population since mankind began in Africa, the «berceau d'humanité», the cradle of humanity.

It is important to mention, that a study to be carry out in this area of the South Sudan, where people still lived in a very traditional way, was very difficult. The environmental conditions, the co-operation of the local population and the acceptance by the local people, was basically due to the existence, since 4 years, of a Southern Sudanese A.D.E. team who lived with these people and gained their confidence.

REFERENCES

1. Fawzi WW, Herrera MG, Spiegelman DL, El Amin A, Nestel P, Mohamed KA, A prospect study of malnutrition in relation to child mortality in the Sudan, American Journal of Clinical Nutrition, 1997, 65(4):1062-1069.

2. Onis de M, Monteiro C, Akre J, Clugston G., The world-wide magnitude of protein-energy malnutrition: an overview from the WHO global database on child growth, Bulletin World Health Organisation, 1993, 71:703-712.

3. Third Report of the World Nutrition Situation, ACC/SCN WHO, 1997: 11-42.

4. World Health Organization, (1985), Prevention and control of vitamin A deficiency, Xerophthalmia and nutritional blindness: Summary of a proposal for a ten-years Programme of support to countries, WHO, Geneva, 1985.

5. Rowland MGM, Rowland SGJ, Cole TJ, Impact of infection on the growth of children from 0 to 2 years in an urban Waest African community, American Journal of Clinical Nutrition, 1988, 47:134-138.

6. Shears P, Berry AM, Murphy R, Nabil MA, Epidemiological assessment of the health and nutrition of Ethiopian refugees in emergency camps in Sudan, 1985, Br Med J, 1987, 295:314-318.

7. Coulter JBS, Suliman GI, Omer MIA, MacFarlane SBJ, Moody JB, Hendrickse RG, Protein-energy malnutrition in northern Sudan: clinical studies, Europ. J. Clin. Nutr., 1988, 42:787-796.

8. Pagezy H, Hauspie R, Growth in weight of African babies, aged 0-24 months, living in a rural area at the lake Tumba, Zaire, Ann Trop Paed, 1985, 5:41-47.

9. Cornu A, Delpeuch F, Chevalier Ph, Etat nutritionnel et croissance au cours des deux premières années de la vie chez des enfants de Yaoundé, Arch Fr Pediatr, 1980, 37:125-129.

10. Roberts DF, A demographic study of a Dinka village, 1956, Hum Biol, 1989, 61(5-6):731-757.

11. Herrera MG, Nestel P, El Amin A, Fawzi WW, Muhammad KA, Weld L., Vitamin A supplementation and child survival, Lancet, 1992, 340:267-271.
12. Broeck JVD, Eeckels R, Vuylsteke J.,Influence of nutritional status on child mortality in rural Zaire, Lancet, 1993, (341):1491-1495.

13. Rush D, Sloan NL, Leighton J, Alvir JM, Horvitz DG, Seaver WB, Garbowski GC,Johnson SS, Kulka RA, Holt M, Devore JW, Lynch JT, Woodside MB, Shanklin DS, Longitudinal study of pregnant women, American Journal of Clinical Nutrition, 1988, 48:439-483.

14. Kunijwok Kwawang, Text and context of genocide, An analysis of the Sudanese Conflict, Document, 18 mai 1993.

15. Josse M.-Ch., Chronologie, *in* Ostrowski Z.L., Soudan, Combats autour des richesses, Ed. L'Harmattan, Paris, 2010

16. Ostrowski Z.L., Soudan, Coulisses d'une guerre oubliée, Ed. L'Harmattan, Paris, 2001

17. WHO, 1986, 64(6):929-941.

18. Payne W.J.A. and El Amin F.M., An interim report on the Dinka livestock industry in the Jonlei Area, UNDP Economic and Social Research Council, Technical Report N° 5, Khartoum, 1977.

19. Makec JW., The customary law of the Dinka people of Sudan, Afroworld Publishing Co, London, 1988.

20. Kigotho AW., Southern Sudan hit by epidemic of sleeping sickness, Lancet, 1997, 350(9076):502.

21. Ostrowski Z.L., Heidrecheid N., Some aspects of nutritional status in the South of the Sudan, J.Trop. Pediatrics, 1982, 28:153-158.

22. Ostrowski Z.L, Josse M.-Ch., L'état nutritionnel des enfants de 0 à 3 ans dans 4 pays européens, A.D.E. Paris, 1990.

23 Josse M.-Ch., Recueil et traitement des informations de l'étude prospective, Exposé d'une methodologie de constitution et d'exploitation des donnees, in: Nutrition and Developpement, Ostrowski ZL, A.D.E. Paris, 1982, 39-72.

24. Ostrowski Z.L, Josse M.-Ch., Longitudinal nutritional study in pregnant women and early childhood in the Jonglei Canal Area; Nutrition and Development - Proceedings, A.D.E., Paris, 1982, 23-38

25. Ilardi S., Staeling N., CDC Anthropometry software package (C.A.S.P.), CDC, Atlanta.

26. Young DS, Implementation of SI Units for clinical laboratory data, Annals Internal Medecine, 1987, 106(1):135-158.

27. Fawzi WW, Herrera MG, Willett WC, Nestel P, Elamin A, Mohammed KA., Dietary vitamin A intake and the incidence of diarrhoea and respiratory infection among Sudanese children, Journal of Nutrition, 1995, 125(5):1211-1221.

28. Roth EA, Kurup KB, Child mortality levels and survival patterns from southern Sudan, J Biosoc Sci, 1990, 22(3):365-372.

29. Ibrahim SA, Babiker AG, Amin IK, Omer MI, Rushwan H, Factors associated with high risk of perinatal and neonatal mortality: an interim report on a prospective community-based study in rural Sudan, Paediatr Perinat Epidemiol, 1994, 8(2):193-204.

30. Taha T. el-T, Gray RH, Malaria and perinatal mortality in central Sudan, Am J Epidemiol, 1993, 138(8):563-568.

31. Kitange HM, Machibya H, Black J, Mtasiwa DM, Masuki G, Whiting D, Unwin N, Moshiro C, Klima PM, Lewanga M, Alberti KG, McLarty DG, Outlook for survivors of childhood in sub-Saharan Africa: adult mortality in Tanzania. Adult morbidity and mortality project, BMJ 1996, 312(7025):216-220.

32. Seaman J, Mercer AJ, Sondorp E, The epidemic of visceral leishmaniasis in western Upper Nile, southern Sudan: course and impact from 1984 to 1994, Int J Epidemiol, 1996, 25(4):862-871.

33. Bergsjo P, African intermezzo. Home birth, Masai style, Acta Obstet Gynecol Scand, 1993, 72(8):597-598.

34. Taylor CB, Ho KJ, Studies on the Masai, Am J Clin Nutr, 1971, 24(11):1291-1293.

35. Maynard EP, The Masai, a pastoral people, N Engl J Med, 1971, 284(13):724-725.

36. Ali BH, Roese PM, Childhood and youth in a population of the Shendi area (Sudan), Arztl Jugendkd, 1989, 80(3):135-139.

37. Dibley MJ, Stachling N, Nieburg P, Trowbridge FL, Interpretation of Z-score anthropometric indicators derived from the international growth reference, Am J Clin Nutr, 1987, 46:749-762.

38. Jelliffe DB, The assessment of the nutritional status of the community, WHO, Monography Series No 5, 1966, 53.

39. Ostrowski ZL, La mesure du pli cutané: la technique et les normes, Arch Fr Ped, 1976, 33:885-893.

40. WHO, A growth chart for international use in maternal and child health care, WHO, Geneve, 1978.

41. World Health Organisation, Development of indicators for monitoring progress towards Health for All by the year 2000, Series N°4, WHO, Geneve, 1981.

42. Hytten FE, Leitch I, The physiology of human pregnancy, Blackwell Scientific publications, Oxford, 1971.

43. Jansen AAJ, Kusin JA, Thiuri B, Lakhani SA, Mannetje WE, Anthro pometric results in pregnancy and lactation. In maternal and child health in rural Kenya, an epidemiological study, Ed JK van Ginneken and AS Muller, Croom Helm, London, 1984, 143-152.

44. Lawrence M, Coward WA, Lawrence F, Cole TJ, Whitehead RG, Fat gain during pregnancy in rural African women: the effect of season and dietary status, A, J Cin Nutr, 45:1442-1450, 1987.

45. Frisancho AR, New norms of upper limb fats and muscle area for assessment of nutritional status, AmJClinNutr, 1981, 34:2540-5).

46. NCHS growth curves for children birth - 18 years. United States, Rockville, MD: National Center for Health Statistics, Vital and health statistics, series 11, no.165 (DHEW publication no.(PHS) 78-1650,1977.

47. Jenss RM., Bayley N, A mathematical method for studying the growth of a child, Human Biology, 1937, 9:556-563.

48. Martin-Prevel Y, Analyse longitudinale de données de croissance d'enfants 0-30 mois au Sud-Soudan. Mémoire de D.E.A. de statistique et Santé, Université de Paris-Sud. UER Médicale de Kremlin-Bicètre, 1988.

49. Wolff MC, Perez L, Gibson JG, Lopez LS, Peniston B, Wolff MM, Nutritional status of children in the health district of Cusco, Peru, Am J Clin Nutr, 1985, 42:531-541.

50. Brown KH, Black RE,Becker S, Seasonal changes in nutritional status and the prevalence of malnutrition in a longitudinal study of young children in rural Bangladesh, Am J Cin Nutr, 1982, 36:303-313.

51. Chali D, Anthropometric measurements of the Nilotic tribes in a refugee camp, Ethiop. Med. J., 33(4):211-217, 1995.

52. Briend A, Wojtyniak B, Rowland MGM., Arm circumference and other factors in children at high risk of death in rural Bangladesh, Lancet, 1987, 2:725-727.

53. Chen LC, Chowdury AKMA, Huffman SL, Anthropometric assessement of energy protein ,alnutrition and subsequent risk of mortality among preschool aged children, Am J Clin nutr, 33:1836-1845, 1980.

54. Stolzfus RJ, Albonico M, Tielsch JM, Chaya HM, Savioli L., Linear growth retardation in Zanzibari school children, J Nutr, 1997, 127(6):1099-1105.

55. Beaton GH, Small but healthy? Are we asking the right question?, European J. Clin. Nutr., 1994, 43:863-875.

56. International Classification of Diseases, Vol 1&2, WHO Geneva, 1978

57. Datry, Parasitologie, Nutrition and Development, Proceeding, A.D.E., Paris, 1982, 146-148.

58. DeMayer EM , Adiels-Tegman M, The prevalence of anaemia in the world. World Health Statistical Quarterly, 38:302-316, 1985.

59. Haggaz AD, Radi EA, Adam I, Anaemia and low birth weight in western Sudan, Trans R Soc Trop Med Hyg, 2010 Mar;104(3):234-6.

60. Snow RW, Bastos de Azevedo I, Lowe BS, Kabiru EW, Nevill CG, Mwankusye S, Kassiga G, Marsh K, Teuscher T, Severe childhood malaria in two areas of markedly different falciparum transmission in east Africa, Acta Trop, 1994, 57(4):289-300.

61. Premji Z, Hamisi Y, Shiff C, Minjas J, Lubega P, Makwaya C., Anaemia and plasmodium falciparum infections among young children in an holoendemic area, Bagamoyo, Tanzania, Acta Tropica 1995, 59(1):55-64.

62. Abdalla SI, Malik EM, Ali KM, The burden of malaria in Sudan incidence, mortality and disability-adjusted life-years, Malaria J. 2007 Jul 28;6:97.

63. Giha HA, Elghazali G, A-Elgadir TM, A-Elbasit IE, Elbahir EM, Baraka OZ, Khier MM, Adam I, Troye-Blomberg M, Theander TG, Elbashir MI, Clinical pattern of severe Plasmodium falciparum malaria in Sudan in an area characterized by seasonal and unstable malaria transmission. Trans R Soc Trop Med Hyg, 2005 Apr,99(4):243-51.

64. Adam I, Ali DM, Elbashir MI, Manifestations of falciparum malaria in pregnant women of Eastern Sudan, Saudi Med J. 2004, Dec;25(12):1947-50.

65. Snow RW, Bastos de Azevedo I, Forster D, Mwankusye S, Bomu G, Kassiga G, Nyamawi C, Teuscher T, Marsh K, Maternal recall of symptoms associated with childhood death in rural east Africa, Int J Epidemiol 1993, 22(4):677-683.

66. Taha T.el-T,Gray RH, Mohamedani AA, Malaria and low birth in central Sudan, Am J Epidemiol, 1993, 138(5):318-325.

67. Elzubier AG, Ansari EH, El Nour MH, Bella H, Knowledge and misconception about malaria among secondary school students and teachers in Kassala, eastern Sudan, J.R.Soc.Health, 1007, 117(6):381-385.

68. Greenwood BM, David PH, Otooferbes LN, Allen SJ, Alonso PL, Schellenberg JRA, Byass P, Hurwitz M, Menon A., Mortality and morbidity from malaria after stopping malaria chemoprophylaxis Transactions of the Royal Society of Tropical Medecine & Hygiene, 1995, 89(6):629-633.

69. Kasongo Project Team. Anthropometric assessment of young children's nutritional status as an indicator of subsequent risk of dying, J Trop Pediatr, 1983, 29:69-75.

70. Dikassa L et al., Maternal behavioural risk factors for severe childhood diarrhoel disease in Kinshasa, Zaire, Int J Epidemiol 1993, 22(2):327-333.

71. Rozov AA, Makhlina VS, Makarovskaia NV, Child mortality in the developing countries of Africa, Sov Zdravookhr. 1989;(3):58-63.

72. Bayoumi RA, Flatz SD, Kuhnau W, Flatz G, Beja and Nilotes: nomadic pastoralist groups in the Sudan with opposite distributions of the adult lactase phenotypes, Am J Phys Anthropol, 1982, 58(2):173-178.

73. Daouda H, Galan P, Prual A, Sekou H, Hercberg S, Iron status in Nigerien mothers and their newborns, Internat J Vit Nutr Res, 61:46-50, 1991.

74. Heese v dc H., (1988), Serum vitamin C, vitamin A and carotene values in infants in SWA/NAMIBIA, SAMJ, 1988, (73):600-602.

75. Underwood BA, Arthur P., The contribution of vitamin A to public health, FASZB J. 1996, (1O):1040-1048.

76. Ostrowski ZL, Suliman GI, Haematology, Nutrition and Development, Proceeding, A.D.E., Paris, 1982, 119-120.

77. Feldmann D, Jardel A, Morgant G, Pressac M, Aymard P, Bilan biologique chez les femmes enceintes, Nutrition and Development, Proceeding, A.D.E., Paris, 1982, 121-126.

78. Bayoumi RA, Trace elements in sera of pregnant women, Nutrition and Development, Proceeding, A.D.E., Paris, 1982, 127-130.

79. Bayoumi RA, Assessment of vitamin B1, B2 and B6 status of pregnant women, Nutrition and Development, Proceeding, A.D.E., Paris, 1982, 131-133.

80. Bayoumi RA, Rosalki SB, Evaluation of methods of coenzyme activation of erythrocyte enzymes for detection of deficiency of vitamins B1, B2 and B6, Clinical Chemistry, 1976, 22:327-335.

81. Thurnham DI, Vitamin assays on erythrocytes, Nutrition and Development, Proceeding, A.D.E., Paris, 1982, 134-139.

82. Thurnham DI, Red cell enzyme tests of vitamin status: do marginal deficiencies have any physiological significance, Proc. Nutr. Soc., 1981, 40:155-163.

83. Bender DA, Niacin status in pregnant women, Nutrition and Development, Proceeding, A.D.E., Paris, 1982, 140-142.

84. Bender DA, Biochem. Pharmacol., 1980, 29:2099-2104.

85. Carpenter HJ, Kodicek E, Biochem. J., 1950, 46:421-426.

86. Holman WIM, Biochem. Pharmacol., 1980, 56:513-520.

87. Watt BK, Merrill AL, Composition of Foods, Agric. Handbk, No 8, US Dept Agric., 1963 Washington.

88. Amino Acid Content of Foods. Food & Agric Org, 1968, Rome, (Microbiological Assay).

89. Dodge JA, Study of plasma and erythrocyte fatty acid content in pregnant women, Nutrition and Development, Proceeding, A.D.E., Paris, 1982, 144.

90. Bertier MC, Apfelbaum M, Serum cholesterol in pregnant women, Nutrition and Development, Proceeding, A.D.E., Paris, 1982, 143.

91. Kamoun P., Parvy P., Rabier D., Indications et interprétation de la chromatographie des acides aminés pour le diagnostic des maladies métaboliques dans: Maladie métaboliques, JM Saudubray, Progrès en pédiatrie 8, Doin, 1991.

92. Cynober L., Giboudeau J., Recueil et traitement des échantillons sanguins destinés aux dosages des acides aminés, Ann.Biol.clin., 1990, 48,713-716.

93. Mourant AE, Kopec A, Domaniewska-Sobczak K, The distribution of the human blood groups and other biochemical polymorphysms, 2nd Edition Oxford University Press, 1976.

94. Dramaix M, Brasseur D, Donnen P, Bawhere P, Porignon D, Tonglet R, Hennart P., Prognostic indices for mortality of hospitalized children in Central Africa, Am J Epid, 1996, 143(12):1235-1243.

95. N'Diaye M, Rougereau A, Gore J, Coulee MD, Etude des protéines sériques au cours des anémies nutritionnelles de la femme enceinte au Senegal, Med et Nut, 6:417-421, 1980.

96. Mann GV, Shaffer RD, Cholesteremia in pregnant Masai women, JAMA, 1966, 197(13):1071-1073.

97. Biss K, Taylor CB, Lewis LA, Mikkelson B, Ho KJ, Atherosclerosis and lipid metabolism in the Masai of East Africa, Afr J Med Sci, 1971, 2(3):249-257.

98. Noseda G, Hypolipidemias, Schweiz Med Wochenschrift 1975,105(39): 1233-1237.

99. Walker ARP, Labadarios D., Haem iron intake in young children - Other health promotion activities would have higher priority in Africa, British Medical Journal, 1996, 313(7051):228-229.

100. Luby SP, Kazembe PN, Redd SC, Ziba C, Nwanyanwu OC, Hightower AW, Franco C, Chitsulo L, Wirima JJ., Using clinical signs to diagnose anaemia in african children, Bulletin of the World Health Organisation, 1995, 73(4):477-482.

101. Hag el Al, Karrar ZA, Nutritional vitamin D deficiency rickets in Sudanese children, Ann Trop Paediatr. 1995;15(1), 69-76.

102. Gordeuk VR, Boyd RD, Brittenham GM., Dietary iron overload persists in rural sub-Saharan Africa, Lancet, 1986, 1:1310.

103. Moyo VM, Gangaidzo IT, Gomo ZAR, Khumalo H, Saungweme T, Kiire CF, Rouault T, Gordeuk VR., Traditional beer consumption and the iron status of spouse pairs from a rural community in Zimbabwe, Blood, 1997, 89(6):2159-2166.

104. Weatherall DJ, The anaemia of malaria. In: Malaria: Principales and practice of Malariology, WH Wernsforder and I McGregor (Eds), Churchill Livingstone, New York, 1988.

105. Suharno D, Muhilal, Vitamin A and nutritional anaemia, Food and Nutrition Bulletin, 1996, 17(1):7-10.

106. Rougereau A, Gore J, N'Diaye M, Coulee MD, Person O, Ferritin and iron status in Senegalese women, Am J Clin Nut, 6:314-318, 1982.

107. N'Diaye M, Rougereau A, Gore J, Coulee MD, Déficience en vitamine A et anémie nutritionnelle en zone sahélienne, Med et Nut, 6:411- 415, 1980.

108. N'Diaye M, Rougereau A, Gore J, Coulee MD, Besnard J, Picaper G, Fer et ferritine sérique au cours des anaemies nutritionnelles chez la femme senegalaise, Med et Nut, 6:401-410, 1980.

109. Bushra M, Elhassan EM, Ali Ni, Osman E, Bakheit KH, Adam Il, Anaemia, zinc and cooper deficiencies among pregnant women in central Sudan, Biol Trace Elem Res, 2010 Dec,137(3);255-61.

110. Salih MA, El Bushra HM, Ahmed M, Kamil IA, Attitudes and practices of breast-feeding in Sudanese urban and rural communities, Trop Geogr Med, 1993, 45(4):171-174.

111. Nur O, The physiological effect of infant mortality in reproductive behavior in the Sudan, Int J Gynaecol Obstet, 1985, 23(2):143-147.

112. Victora CG, Smith PG, Vaughan JP, Nobre LC, Lombardi C, Teixerira AM, Fuchs SM, Moreira LB, Gigante LP, Barros FC., Evidence for protection by breast-feeding against infant deaths from infectious Diseases in Brazil, Lancet, 1987, 2:319-321.

113. Vries de MW, Temperament and infant mortality among the Masai of East Africa, Am J Psychiatry, 1984, 141(10):1189-1194.

114. Fawzi WW, Herrera MG, Willett WC, Nestel P, Elamin A, Mohammed KA., Dietary vitamin A intake in relation to child growth, Epidemiology, 1997, 8(4):402-407.

115. Mata L, Wyan RH, Host resistance to infection, Am J Clin Nut, 24:976-986, 1971.

116. Jelliffe DB, Jelliffe EFP, Human milk in the modern world, Oxford University Press, 84-96, 1978.

117. Ostrowski Z.L., Ojaba. E., Food composition Table adapted to the South-Sudan, A.D.E. Paris, 1985.

118. Richtey S.J., Janette Taper L., Maternal and child Nutrition, Harper and Row publ., New York, 1979.

119. Pagezy H, Hauspie RC, Seasonal variation in the growth rate of weight in African babies, aged 0 to 4 years, Food and Nutrition, 1985, 18:29-41.

120. Maletnlema TN, OAU/ADE Workshop on ideas and methods for tackling nutritional problems in early childhood in Africa, XIII International Congress of Nutrition, Seoul, 1985.

121 Robert Cameron Mitchell, African Primal Religions, Argus Communications, Niles USA, 1977

122 Deng Francis Mading, Tradition and Modernization, Yale University Press, 1987

123 Deng Francis Mading, The Dinka of the Sudan, Holt, Rinehart and Winston, New York, 1972

124 Sienkiewicz H., In desert and Wilderness (W pustyni i w puszczy), Polonia Publishers, Warsaw, 1991

125 Evans-Pritchard E.E., Les Nuer, Ed.Galimard, Paris, 1968, translated from: The Nuer, Oxford at the Clarendan Press, 1937

126 Ostrowski Z.L., Dynastree, Computer Programme for genealogy and genetics, Ed. Dr Ostrowski, Paris, 1989

ANNEXES

1. DATA INPUT AND DATA PROCESSING by M.-Ch. Josse

A.D.E.
PARIS

LONGITUDINAL STUDY ON NUTRITION AND GROWTH IN THE JONGLEI CANAL AREA (SUDAN)

STUDY N° 1 : PREGNANT WOMEN'S SURVEY

TABLE 1: TIME SCHEDULE (this survey covers 6 months)

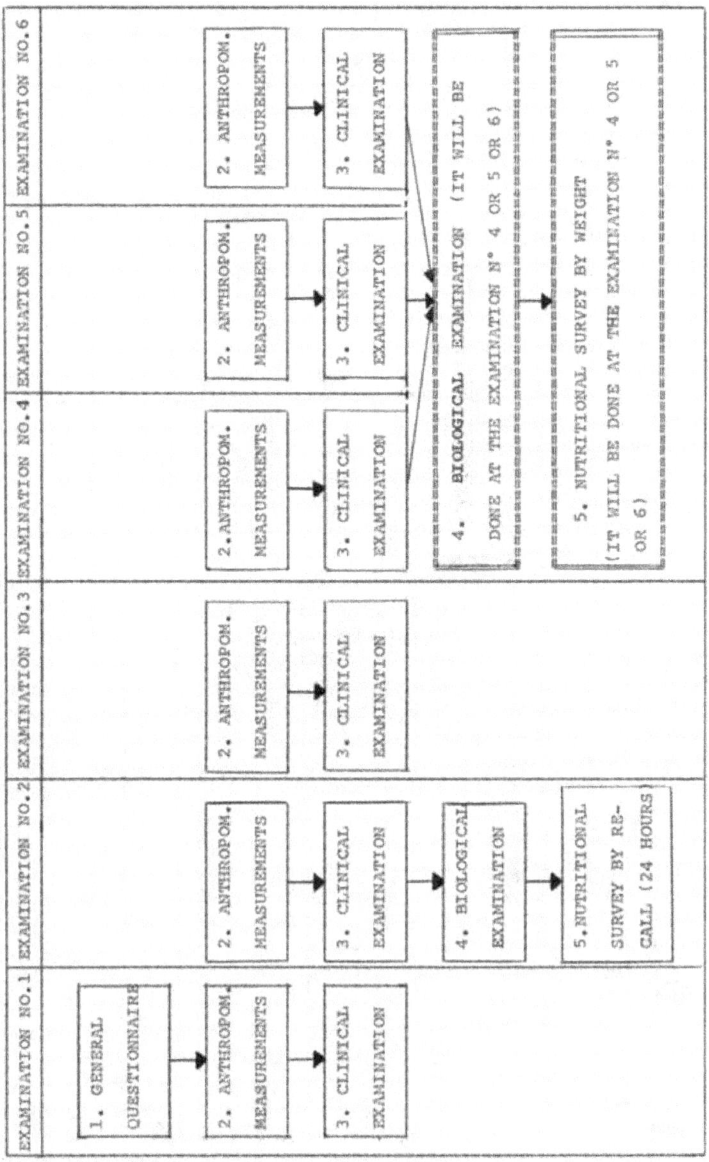

FIGURE 2 : EXTRAIT DU QUESTIONNAIRE GENERAL DE L'ETUDE " PREGNANT WOMEN "

A.D.E. PARIS

Pregnant woman's code: 1 1 1

PREGNANT WOMAN'S SURVEY
1. GENERAL QUESTIONNAIRE

STUDY PW1

1. STUDY N°......... 1 [1]
2. TYPE OF EXAMINATION.......... 2 [1]
3. EXAMINATION N°.......... 3 [1]
4. DATE OF SURVEY.......... 4 day / month / year [8]
5. INVESTIGATOR N°.......... 10

A. IDENTIFICATION

6. VILLAGE N°.......... 11
7. VILLAGE NAME..... 13
8. HOUSEHOLD N°.......... 27
9. NAME OF HOUSEHOLD HEAD.......... 28
10. PERSON'S STUDY N°.......... 42
11. PERSON'S NAME.... 45
12. CODE : 59 [1 1 1] Village n° / h.h. / Person's n°

FIGURE 3 : EXTRAIT DU QUESTIONNAIRE ANTHROPOMETRIQUE DE L'ETUDE " PREGNANT WOMEN "

A.D.E. PARIS

Pregnant woman's code: 1 2 1

2. ANTHROPOMETRIC MEASUREMENTS

STUDY PW 2

1. STUDY N°......... 1 [1]
2. TYPE OF EXAMINATION.......... 2 [2]
3. EXAMINATION N°.......... 3 [1]
4. DATE OF SURVEY.......... 4 DAY / MONTH / [8]
5. INVESTIGATOR N°.......... 10
6. PERSON'S STUDY N° (between 001 and 300).......... 11
7. PRESENT AT ANTHROPOMETRIC SURVEY : 1 = NO 2 = YES....... 14
8. IF NO, REASONS : 1 = refusal 2 = other.......... 15
9. CODE : 16 [1 2 1]

MASS AND LENGHT

10. WEIGHT (kg).......... 25
11. HEIGHT (cm).......... 29
12. TOTAL ARM LENGTH (cm).......... 33

CIRCUMFERENCES (cm)

13. HEAD.......... 36
14. CHEST.......... 39
15. ARM.......... 43
16. CALF.......... 46
17. THIGH.......... 49

SKINFOLDS (mm)

18. TRICIPITAL.......... 52
19. SUBSCAPULAR.......... 55

A D E
PARIS

FIGURE 4 : EXTRAIT DU QUESTIONNAIRE CLINIQUE DE L'ETUDE " PREGNANT WOMEN "

EXAMINATION

BLOOD PRESSURE :

17. SYSTOLIC (mm) 54

18. DIASTOLIC (mm) 57

19. OEDEMA : 1 = NO 2 = YES 60

20. CONVULSIONS : 1 = NO 2 = YES 61

21. WEIGHT : 0 = normal gain, 1 = unchanged, 2 = abnormal loss, 3 = abnormal gain 62

22. IF 2 OR 3, DIFFERENCES (kg) 63

23. URINARY INFECTION : 1 = NO 2 = YES 67

IF YES, WHICH SIGNS OR SYMPTOMS (write clearly) :

WHO Code.

24. (1) ____________________ 68

25. (2) ____________________ 72

26. (3) ____________________ 76

27. GENITAL HAEMORRHAGE : 1 = NO 2 = YES 80

28. ABDOMINAL PAIN : 1 = NO 2 = YES 81

29. IF YES : 1 = unspecified, 2 = suspicion of urinary infection, 3 = suspicion of contractions, 4 = suspicion of appendicitis, 5 = other 82

30. FOETAL MOVEMENTS : 1 = not perceived, 2 = perceived 83

31. VOMITING OR NAUSEA : 1 = NO, 2 = RARE, 3 = FREQUENT 84

32. CONJUNCTIVAL PALLOR : 1 = NO 2 = YES 85

33. OTHER SYMPTOMS / SYNDROMES / ILLNESS : 1 = NO 2 = YES 86

IF YES, WHICH (write clearly) :

WHO Code.

34. (1) ____________________ 87

35. (2) ____________________ 91

36. (3) ____________________ 95

FIGURE 5 : EXTRAIT DU QUESTIONNAIRE BIOLOGIQUE DE L'ETUDE " PREGNANT WOMEN "

A.D.E.
PARIS

pregnant woman's code

1 4 2

BIOLOGICAL EXAMINATION

STUDY PW4

1. STUDY N° .... 1 [1]

2. TYPE OF EXAMINATION .... 2 [4]

3. EXAMINATION N° .... 3 [?]

4. DATE OF SURVEY .... 4 DAY MONTH 8

5. INVESTIGATOR N° 10

6. PERSON'S STUDY N° (between 001 and 300) 11

7. PRESENT AT BIOLOGICAL SURVEY : 1 = NO 2 = YES 14

8. IF NO, REASONS : 1 = delivery, 2 = dead, 3 = sick, 4 = temporary absent, 5 = permanently left village, 6 = refusal, 7 = other 15

9. IF DEAD, REASONS 16

IF LEFT, WHERE ? ____________________

10. CODE : 30 1 4 2

11. EXAMINATION BY COLLABORATORS

1 : not done 2 : done 30

If done, results :

12. W.B.C. (White blood cell) 40

13. R.B.C. (Red blood cell) 43

14. H.G.B. (Hemoglobin) 46

15. H.C.T. (Haematocrit) 49

16. M.C.V. (Mean cell volume) 52

FIGURE 6 : LES DIFFERENTES IMAGES SE SUCCEDANT A L'ECRAN LORSQUE UN UTILISATEUR DEBUTE UN TRAVAIL

Exemple : l'utilisateur veut avoir accès au questionnaire clinique n° 2 de l'étude " Pregnant women " .

IMAGES N° 1 ET 2 (Elles correspondent au niveau 1 page 64)

En tapant " PROC 55 ", l'utilisateur charge en mémoire centrale le programme " SELECT.DEPART ". Une première image apparait à l'écran: elle donne la possibilité de choisir un certain nombre d'options. Pour accéder à l'étude longitudinale, l'utilisateur tape 1 . Une seconde image s'inscrit alors sur l'écran: à ce stade l'utilisateur a la possibilité de changer d'option en tapant 1 ou de continuer sur son choix en tapant 2.

```
A D E  CROSS SECTIONNAL AND LONGITUDINAL STUDIES
ON GROWTH AND NUTRITION IN THE JONGLEI CANAL AREA
TAPE YOUR SELECTION (1 TO 9)
1:Longitudinal survey
2:Cross sectional survey
3:W.H.O. code (creation,modification,suppression)
4:W.H.O. code (impression)
5:Food code (creation,modification,suppression)
6:Food code (impression)
7:List of Pregnant women      8:List of children
9:List of villages            0:[illegible]
ENTER THE CODE AND PRESS EXECUTE =>
```

```
You have selected THE LONGITUDINAL SURVEY

IS IT CORRECT [illegible] YES =>
```

IMAGES N° 3 ET 4 (Elles correspondent au niveau 2 page 65)

A ce stade, le programme qui se trouve en mémoire centrale(" STUDY. SELECT ") donne à l'utilisateur la possibilité de choisir une des 3 études de l'enquête longitudinale.

```
A D E  LONGITUDINAL STUDY
ON NUTRITION AND GROWTH IN THE JONGLEI CANAL AREA

SELECTION OF THE STUDY
TAPE YOUR SELECTION (1,2,3 OR 4)
1: Pregnant women survey
2: Children's survey
3: Lactating women's survey
4: End of job

ENTER THE CODE AND PRESS EXECUTE =>
```

En choisissant l'option 1 à l'image précédente, l'utilisateur sélectionne donc l'échantillon " Pregnant women ". L'image suivante lui donne la possibilité de revenir sur son choix ou de le confirmer.

```
[illegible] THE PREGNANT WOMEN [illegible]

[illegible] YES [illegible]
```

IMAGES N° 5 ET 6 (Elles correspondent au niveau 3 pages 66-67).

Elles permettent à l'utilisateur de sélectionner le type d'examen souhaité.

```
SELECTION OF THE EXAMINATION
[illegible]
1:General questionnaire
2:Anthropometric measurements
3:Clinical examination
4:Biological examination
[illegible] survey
[illegible]
[illegible] of study
[illegible] of [illegible]
ENTER THE CODE AND PRESS EXECUTE => [3]
```

```
You have selected THE CLINICAL EXAMINATION

IS IT CORRECT ? [illegible] YES => [ ]
```

IMAGES 7 ET 8 (Elles correspondent aux niveaux 4 et 5 page 67)

```
STUDY PW3 : CLINICAL EXAMINATION (NO 1 TO 6)

  GIVE THE EXAMINATION NO : [2]
```

```
CLINICAL EXAMINATION STUDY PW3 , NO [illegible]
[illegible] SELECTION [illegible]
1 : Input data
2 : [illegible]
3 : modification
4 : [illegible]
5 : Impression [illegible] Pregnant women
6 : Selection of questionnaire
7 : [illegible]
ENTER THE CODE AND [illegible] => [1]
```

Le questionnaire clinique n° 2 se trouve en mémoire centrale et l'utilisateur peut choisir de l'entrer(1), de l'imprimer (2)...

FIGURE 7 : EDITION DU FICHIER " VILLAGES "

A.D.E LONGITUDINAL STUDY ON GROWTH AND NUTRITION IN THE JONGLEI CANAL AREA

LIST OF VILLAGES

CODE	VILLAGE'S NAME	CODE	VILLAGE'S' NAME	CODE	VILLAGE'S' NAME
01	PACKWACKER	02	PANYAPAR	03	PAADIANG
04	PAONDANG	05	PAATIL	06	PAJUENY
07	PAGACH	08	PAANYANG	09	PAAJOBOM
10	PAPIETLONG	11	POLICE	12	PAONYADW
13	PAONPANG B	14		15	PABWOY A
16	OBIYO	17	PADOOK	18	PAANYANG(OBAI)
19	NYITO A	20	NYITO B	21	PAAKANY
22	PANYACOL	23	PADAK	24	PATAO
25	AGUKO	26	AWAJANG	27	WIRUR
28	NYITOL	29	KALDAK	30	DHEGO
31	ABUJOBO	32	PABWOY B	33	LYEL A
34	LYEL B	35	APIOW A	36	APIOW B
37	ARIDIANG	38		39	CHANGC A
40	CHANGO B	41	ACHOB	42	PATCHAWI
43	CEN	44	WARNENG A	45	WUNTHAU B
46	ACEMRETH A	47	WIKAL A(DOLEIB)	48	WIKAL B
49	ODONE	50	WUNTHAW A	51	PANYAROT
52	CENTER	53	PAALO A	54	DOLEIB A
55	KOANYON	56	WARWENG B	57	ACEMNETH B
58	WICHYLWAL	59	KORFULUS	60	PATENBWONY
61	PANAM A	62	PAKOI	63	PANDI BOM
64	ACHWIR	65		66	PANAM B
67	PAN DWONG	68	WIKAL A(OGOT)	69	ABATAOO
70	WIBALO	71	PAAKWEYWANG	72	KALTANG
73	THANYAPO	74	GOJAK	75	ODWAP
76	NYIKENG	77	LOGDAW	78	OGOT A
79	WIKAL B (OGOT)	80	YEN	81	DELWIC
82	KIROCHOP	83	LUEL	84	
85		86	WARWENG	87	THANAM

FIGURE 8 : EXTRAIT DE L'EDITION DU FICHIER " MALADIES "

O.R.S.T.O.M. LONGITUDINAL STUDY ON GROWTH AND NUTRITION IN THE JONGLEI CANAL AREA

INTERNATIONAL CLASSIFICATION OF DISEASES (W.H.O.)

W.H.O. CODE	DISEASES AND NATURE OF INJURY
0019	CHOLERA
0020	TYPHOID FEVER
0029	PARATYPHOID FEVER
0039	SALMONELLA INFECTION
0049	SHIGELLOSIS
0059	FOOD POISONING UNSPECIFIED
0060	ACUTE AMOEBIC DYSENTERY (NO MENTION OF ABSCESS)
0061	CHRONIC INTESTINAL AMOEBIASIS(NO ABCESS)
0069	AMOEBIASIS UNSPECIFIED
0070	BALANTIDIASIS
0071	GIARDIASIS
0072	COCCIDIOSIS
0073	INTESTINAL TRICHOMONIASIS
0078	OTHER PROTOZOAL INTESTINAL DISEASES
0085	BACTERIAL ENTERITIS UNSPECIFIED
0088	VIRAL ENTERITIS GASTROENTERITIS
0090	COLITIS ENTERITIS GASTROENTERITIS (INFECT)
0091	COLIT ENTERIT GASTROENTERITIS(PRESUMED INF)
0092	INFECTIOUS DIARRHOEA
0093	DIARRHOEA PRESUMED INFECTIOUS ORIGIN
0109	PRIMARY TUBERCULOUS INFECTION
0110	TUBERCULOSIS OF LUNG INFILTRATIVE
0111	TUBERCULOSIS OF LUNG NODULAR
0112	TUBERCULOSIS OF LUNG WITH CAVITATION
0113	TUBERCULOSIS OF BRONCHUS
0114	TUBERCULOUS FIBROSIS OF LUNG
0115	TUBERCULOUS BRONCHIECTASIS
0116	TUBERCULOUS PNEUMONIA
0117	TUBERCULOUS PNEUMOTHORAX
0118	OTHER PULMONARY TUBERCULOSIS
0119	PULMONARY TUBERCULOSIS
0120	TUBERCULOUS PLEURISY
0121	TUBERCULOSIS INTRATHORACIC LYMP
0123	TUBERCULOUS LARYNGITIS
0128	OTHER RESPIRATORY TUBERCULOSIS
0130	TUBERCULOUS MENINGITIS
0149	TUBERCULOSIS INTEST PERITONEUM MESENTERICGLANDS
0150	POTT'S DISEASE TUBERC. OF VERTEBRAL COLUMN
0159	TUBERCULOSIS OF BONES AND JOINT
0160	TUBERCULOSIS OF KIDNEY
0161	TUBERCULOSIS OF BLADDER + URETER
0162	TUBERCULOSIS OF EPIDIDIMIS
0163	TUBERCULOSIS OF TESTIS -PROSTATE- SEMINAL VESICLE
0164	TUBERCULOUS SALPINGITIS
0169	TUBERCULOSIS GENITOURINARY SYST(UNSPECIFIED)
0170	TUBERCULOUS OF SKIN-SUBCUTANEOUS CELLULAR TISSUE
0171	ERYTHEMA NODOSUM-TUBERCULOSIS INDURATIVA
0172	PERIPHERAL LYMPH NODES -SCROFULA-TUBERC.ADENITIS
0173	TUBERCULOSIS OF EYE
0174	TUBERCULOSIS OF EAR
0175	TUBERCULOSIS OF THYROID GLAND
0176	ADDISON'S DISEASE TUBERCULOUS

FIGURE 9 : EDITION D'UN EXTRAIT DU FICHIER " EMPLOI DU TEMPS : FEMMES ENCEINTES"

A LONGITUDINAL STUDY ON GROWTH AND NUTRITION IN THE JONGLEI CANAL AREA

PREGNANT WOMEN'S SURVEY : TIME SCHEDULE

CODE	PREGNANT WOMEN	HUSBAND'S NAME	VILLAGE No	VILLAGE NAME	Md	O	ANTHROPOMETRY	CLINICAL EXAMIN	DIU	QUICK DELIVERY
[illegible]	[illegible]	CUL DENG	63	PARIANG	1	G	1	1		
[illegible]	[illegible]	JAMES YUOT	84	FAUNBANG	1	G	1	1		
[illegible]	[illegible]	HAU LEUAN	61	PAKLACKER	1	G	12	12		
[illegible]	[illegible]	MAJAK COLL	86	PAGRBANG	3	G	1	1		
[illegible]	[illegible]	NYJOK NYAUR	91	PAKWACKER	2	3	1	1		
[illegible]	[illegible]	MAYIK DDOK	17	PAUWIR	1	3	1234	1234		
[illegible]	[illegible] DOUL	GABRIEL AJANG	48	PAKOI DON	1	3	12	12		
[illegible]	[illegible] ADJIL	ARAN DENT	65	PAKOI DON	2	3	1234	1234		
[illegible]	[illegible]	AJANE KAC	63	PAKOI DON	3	3	123	123		
[illegible]	[illegible]	ONEK AJAK	54	DOLEID A	1	3	[illegible]	1		
[illegible]	[illegible]	PETER PAGAN	81	PAKWACKER	3	3	1	1		
[illegible]	[illegible]	DOL TUAL	83	LWLL	1	3	1	1		
[illegible]	[illegible]	YATH YAR	88	YEN	1	G	1	1		
[illegible]	[illegible]	KUR AYIK	54	DOLEID A	2	G	1	1		
[illegible]	[illegible]	GAND XUR	74	PATAO	1	G	1	1		
[illegible]	[illegible]	DOL DAK	19	NYITO A	1	G	1	1		
[illegible]	[illegible]	NYIKAKE CHOL	19	NYITO A	2	G	1	1		
[illegible]	[illegible]	MAYIK DOOK	9	NYITO A	3	G	12	12		
[illegible]	[illegible]	PAULE DUAO	32	PANYAGOL	1	G	1	1		
[illegible]	[illegible]	ACHAKE UTOL	65	PAATI	1	O	1234	1234		
[illegible]	[illegible]	OLYNE JAENY	65	PAJIERY	1	G	1	1		
[illegible]	[illegible]	OKOTH LWAL	53	PAALO A	1	G	1	1		
[illegible]	[illegible]	JEREMIAH ORIEK	97	WIKAL A(DOLLEIB	1	G	[illegible]	1		
[illegible]	[illegible]	ULLAK AJINO	97	WIKAL A(DOLLEIB	2	G	[illegible]	1		
[illegible]	[illegible]	FREWN OBUR	[illegible]	WARNENG A	1	G	[illegible]	1		
[illegible]	[illegible]	KWLL ABAN	13	PADHOY A	1	O	1	1		
[illegible]	[illegible]	AYUOL OWEN	13	PADHOY A	2	O	1	1		
[illegible]	[illegible]	GOJAC CHOL	58	PAALO A	2	G	1	1		
[illegible]	[illegible]	JOHN AKER	31	PAKWACKER	4	G	1234	1234		
[illegible]	[illegible]	JOHN JUOK	52	CENTRE	1	G	12	12		
[illegible]	[illegible]	JAMES ARA	31	PANYAGOT	1	O	1	1		
[illegible]	[illegible]	OKUMDO NYATHR	31	AJUJOOB	1	O	1	1		
[illegible]	[illegible]	KUL AKE	61	ADUJOPO	2	G	1	1		
[illegible]	[illegible]	KEKETO OWET	53	PAALO A	3	G	1	1		
[illegible]	[illegible]	SAMUEL OUREN	51	PANYARO	2	G	1	1		
[illegible]	[illegible]	MOLINO PAYTO	31	ADUJUKO	3	G	1	1		
[illegible]	[illegible]	OLIA DAK	51	PANYAGOT	3	G	1	[illegible]		
[illegible]	[illegible] UOVAN	JAMES OTHAO	35	APIOW A	1	G	1	[illegible]		
[illegible]	[illegible]	SALMON PAGAN	53	PAALO A	6	G	1	1		
[illegible]	[illegible]	JAMES OTCHO	54	DOLLEID A	3	O	1	1		
[illegible]	[illegible]	JAMES ALANG	19	NYITO A	5	3	13	12		

N.B. :

Lorsqu'un 1 est entré dans la colonne "ANTHROPOMETRY", l'examen anthropométrique n°1 est stocké sur la disquette...

FIGURE 10 : EXEMPLE D'ENTREE DE DOSSIER EN MACHINE

```
A__IDENTIFICATION                                    Page : 1 (continued)

06 -VILLAGE N°...... 59               | Value from 01 to 87
07 -VILLAGE NAME... KORFULUS          |
08 -HOUSEHOLD N°... 9                 | Value from 1 to 9
09 -NAME OF PW..... NYADIANG DAK      | Pregnant Woman's Name(14C)
10 -PW  STUDY N°... 212               | Preg. Woman's N°(001to400)
11 -TYPE OF BIRTH.. 1                 | 0=Stillborn 1=Single Birth
                                      | 2=Twin 1  3=Twin 2  4=more
12 -NAME OF CHILD.. UKN(NYADIANG)     | 14 Charact. GL?E9 (maxi)
13 -CODE........... 21015992121       |

To continue,press'EXC';To modify,enter $;To end * =>

           CHILD.GENERAL      0050,0016,0010,9999      6150    87?

--------------------------------------------------------------------------


B  DELIVERY            Code: 21015992121           Pages : 1 / 2

14  RESPONDENT...... 1                | 1=Mother 2=Father 3=Other
15 -REASONS ABSENT. *                 | 1=Dead 2=Sick 3=Absent
                                      | 4=Left 5=Refus 6=Other
16 -DIRECT CAUSE... ****              | W.H.O. Code

17 -INTERVENING ATC ****              | W.H.O. Code

18 -UNDERLYING ATCD ****              | W.H.O. Code

19 -OTHER CONDITION ****              | W.H.O. Code

To continue,press'EXC';To modify,enter $;To end * =>

           CHILD.GENERAL      0058,0016,0010,9999      6150    890

--------------------------------------------------------------------------


B  DELIVERY (continued)        Code: 21015992121         Page : 2

20 -DATE DELIVERY.  220881      | Day Month Year

21 -TYPE DELIVERY.. 2           | 1=>Normal 2=>Difficult

22 -PRESENTATION... 1           | 1=>Cephal. 2=>Breech  3=>Unknow

23 -STILLBORN?..... 1           | 1=>No  2=>Yes

24 -WHO ATTENDED?.. 2           | 1=>Nurse  2=>Woman  3=>Other

25 -SEX OF CHILD... 1           | 1=>Boy  2=>Girl
To continue,press'EXC';To modify,enter $;To end * =>

           CHILD.GENERAL      0050,0016,0010,9999      6150    890
```

N.B. : Ces 3 images-écran sont extraites du questionnaire général de l'étude "Children".

FIGURE 11 : EXEMPLE D'EDITION D'UN QUESTIONNAIRE ANTHROPOMETRIQUE DE L'ETUDE " PREGNANT WOMEN "

PREGNANT WOMAN'S SURVEY :ANTHROPOMETRIC QUESTIONNAIRE No2

DATE OF SURVEY	:20/06/81		
PW'S STUDY NO	:018	PREGNANT WOMAN	:NYAYUO ATWOK
VILLAGE NO	:63	VILLAGE NAME	:PAKET DOM

1 -STUDY No....... 1	2 -TYPE OF EXAMIN. 2	3 -EXAMINATION No. 2
4 -DATE OF SURVEY. 200681	5 -INVESTIGATOR... 2	6 -PW STUDY'S No.. 018
7 -PRESENT SURVEY. 2	8 -REASON ABSENCE.	9 -IF DEAD REASON.
10 -EDD............ 1226330:0	11 -WEIGHT (KG).. 055.2	12 -CHEST CIRCUMF.. 084.2
13 -ARM CIRCUMF.... 27.2	14 -CALF CIRCUMF... 30.7	15 -THIGH CIRCUMF.. 50.0
16 -TRICIPITAL SKF. 67.4	17 -SUBSCAPUL. SKF. 12.0	

N.B. : Ce questionnaire correspond à celui utilisé à la seconde visite. Il diffère donc légèrement de celui de la page 54.

FIGURE 12 : EXEMPLE DE DENOMBREMENT EFFECTUE POUR 3 ITEMS (EFFECTIF ET POURCENTAGE DES DIFFÉRENTES REPONSES)

[illegible] AGE [illegible]....

AGE [illegible]	CLASS 1 ≤ 17	CLASS 2 18 - 20	CLASS 3 21 - 23	CLASS 4 24 - 26	CLASS 5 27 - 29	CLASS 6 30 - 35	CLASS 7 ≥ 36	UNKNOWN	NR	TOTAL
EFFECTIFS	5	49	69	70	49	39	12	7	0	300
%	1.66	16.3	23	23.3	16.3	13	4	2.33	0	100

[illegible] ETHNICITY ....

ETHNICITY ...	CLASS 1 SHILLUK	CLASS 2 DINKA	CLASS 3 NUER	CLASS 4 AUTRE	UNKNOWN	NOT	TOTAL
EFFECTIFS	265	20	8	2	5	0	300
%	88.3	6.66	2.66	.666	1.66	0	100

ITEMS [illegible] MATRIM STATUS.

MATRIM.STATUS.	CLASS 1 SEULE	CLASS 2 MARIEE	CLASS 3 DIVORCEE	CLASS 4 DOUTEUX	UNKNOWN	NOT	TOTAL
EFFECTIFS	6	286	6	1	1	0	300
%	2	95.3	2	.333	.333	0	100

N.B. : Statistiques réalisées sur 300 femmes enceintes.
Dans la colonne "UNKKOWN" figurent le nombre et le % de réponses inconnues.
Dans la colonne "NOT" figurent le nombre et le % de réponses sans objet.

ANNEXE 1 : ORGANISATION GENERALE DES PROGRAMMES

NIVEAU 1 DE LA PROGRAMMATION

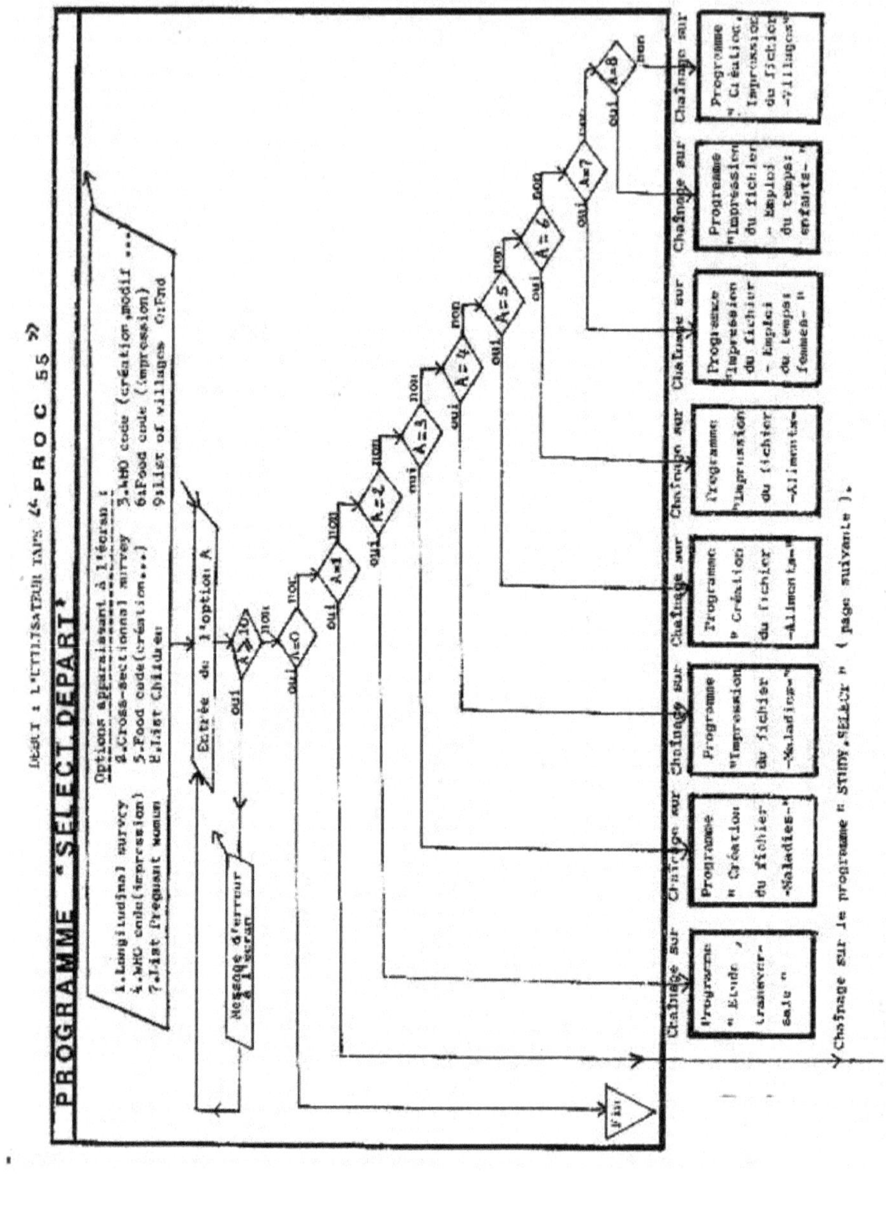

ANNEXE 1 (SUITE)

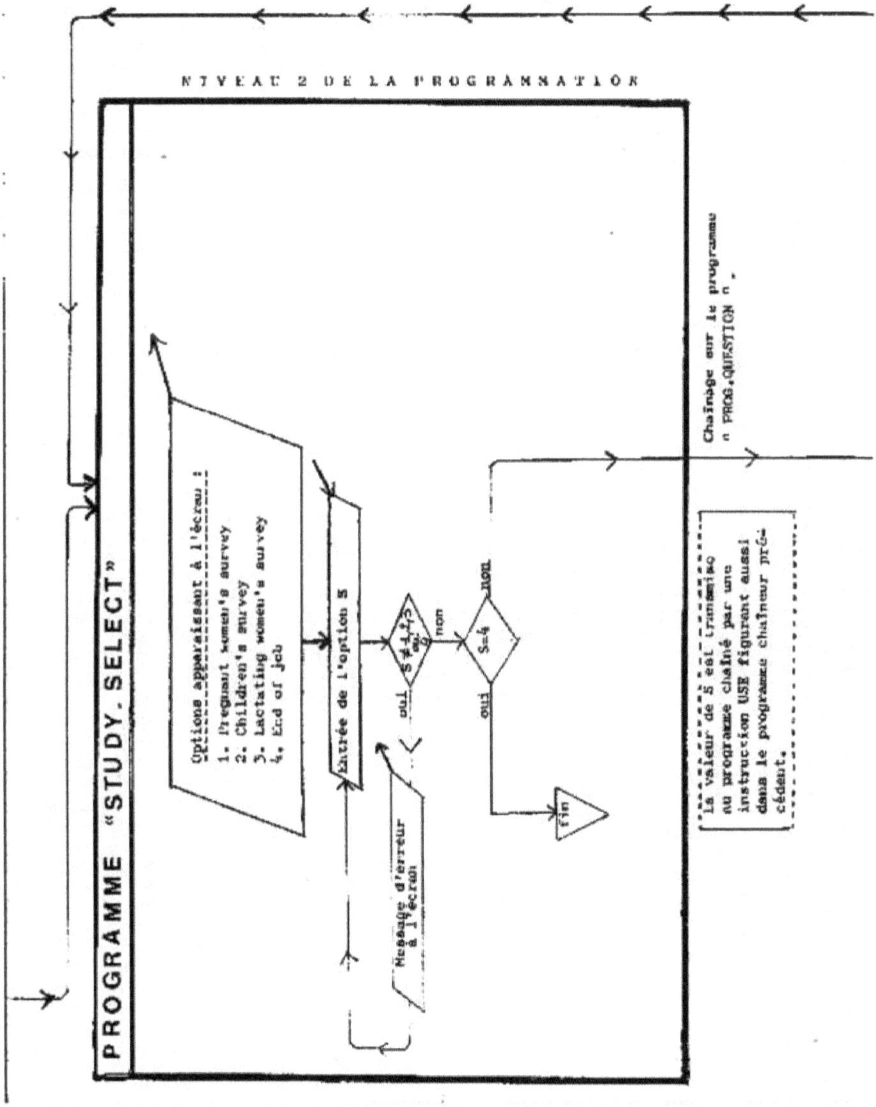

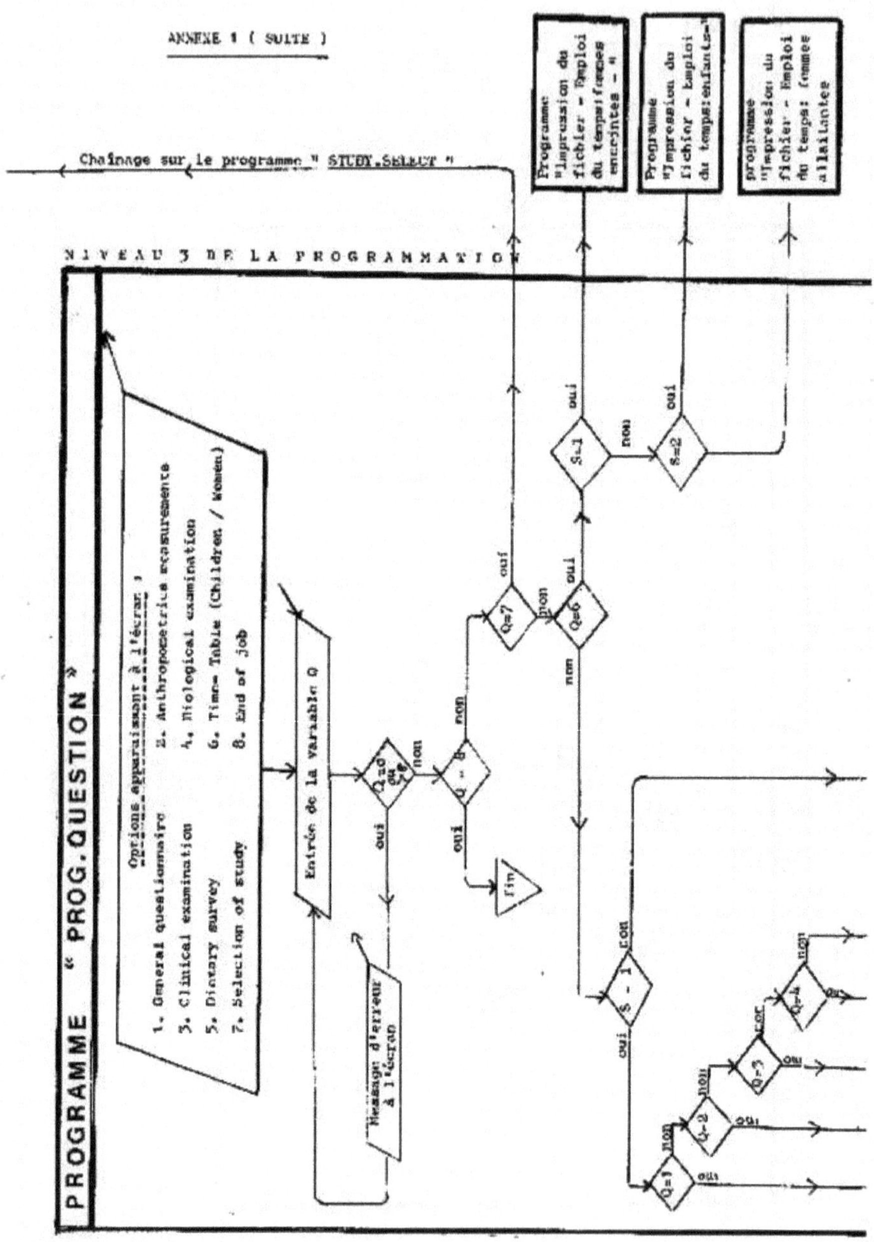
ANNEXE 1 (SUITE)
Chainage sur le programme " STUDY.SELECT "
NIVEAU 3 DE LA PROGRAMMATION
PROGRAMME « PROG.QUESTION »
Options apparaissant à l'écran :
1. General questionnaire
2. Anthropometric measurements
3. Clinical examination
4. Biological examination
5. Dietary survey
6. Time-Table (Children / Women)
7. Selection of study
8. End of job
Entrée de la variable Q
Message d'erreur à l'écran
Fin
oui
non
Programme "Impression du fichier - Emploi du temps:femmes enceintes - "
Programme "Impression du fichier - Emploi du temps:enfants-"
programme "Impression du fichier - Emploi du temps: femmes allaitantes

ANNEXE 1 (SUITE)

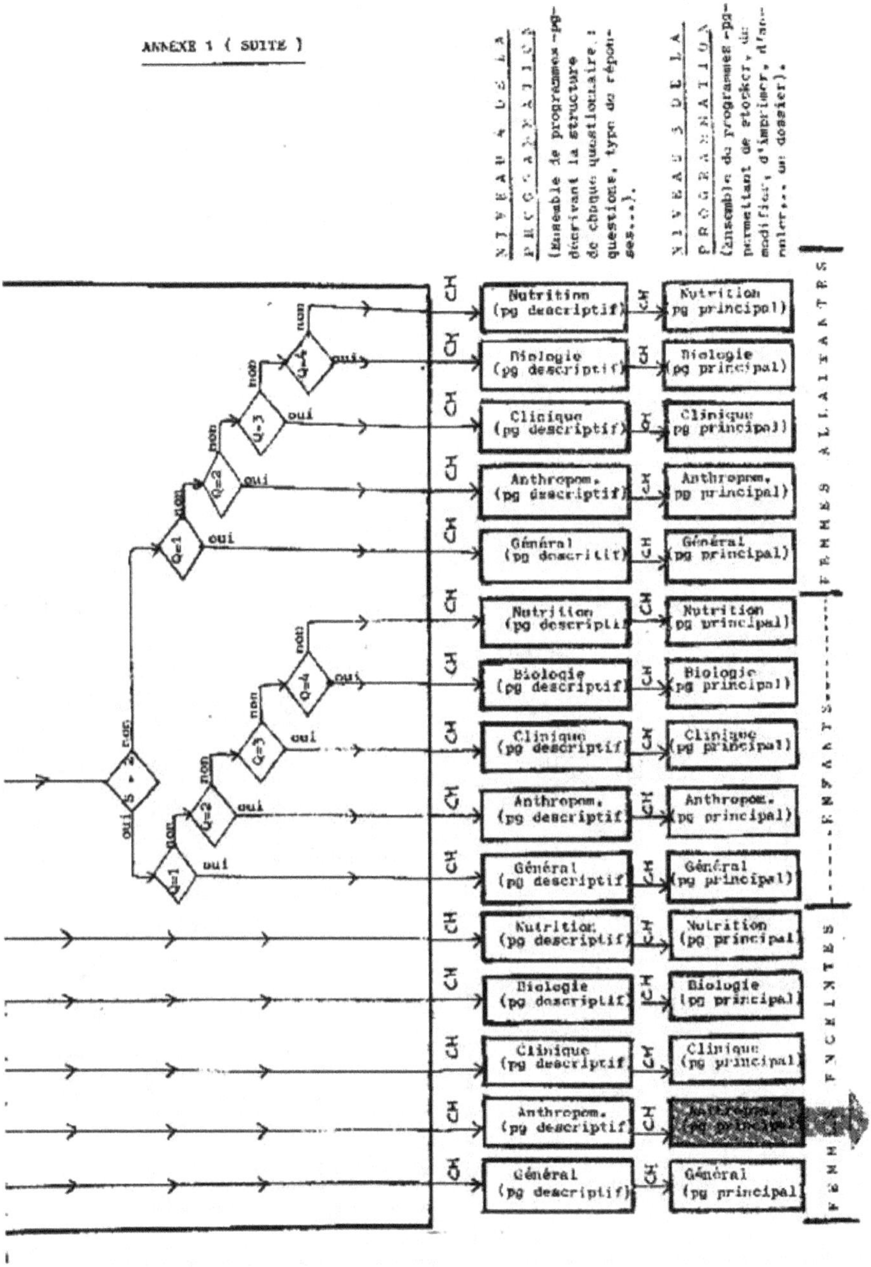

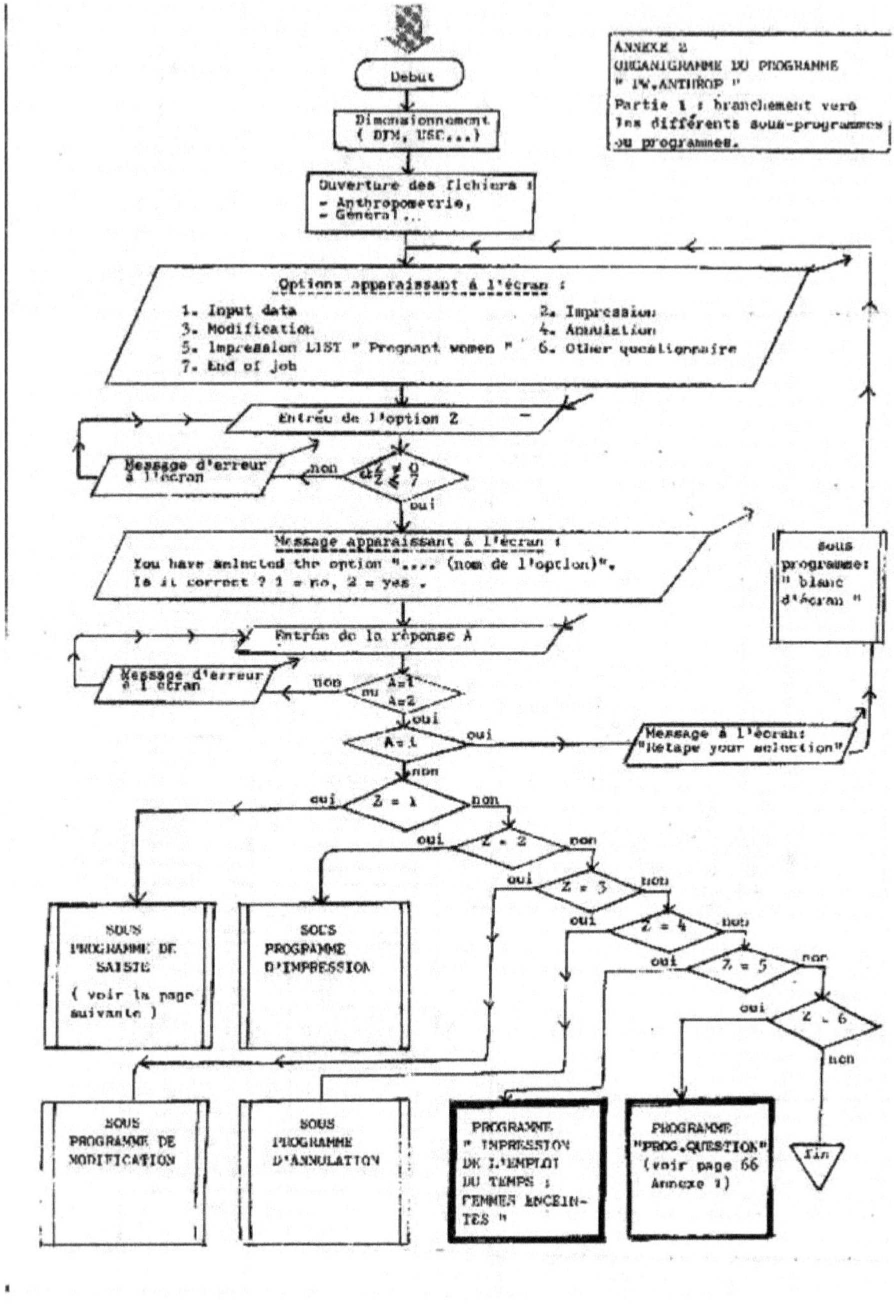

ANNEXE 2
ORGANIGRAMME DU PROGRAMME
" IW.ANTHROP "
Partie 1 : branchement vers les différents sous-programmes ou programmes.
Debut
Dimensionnement (DIM, USE...)
Ouverture des fichiers :
- Anthropometrie,
- Général...
Options apparaissant à l'écran :
1. Input data
2. Impression
3. Modification
4. Annulation
5. Impression LIST " Pregnant women "
6. Other questionnaire
7. End of job
Entrée de l'option Z
Message d'erreur à l'écran
non
oui
Message apparaissant à l'écran :
You have selected the option "…. (nom de l'option)".
Is it correct ? 1 = no, 2 = yes .
Entrée de la réponse A
Message d'erreur à l'écran
A=1 ou A=2
A = 1
Message à l'écran: "Retape your selection"
Sous programme: " blanc d'écran "
Z = 1
Z = 2
Z = 3
Z = 4
Z = 5
Z = 6
SOUS PROGRAMME DE SAISIE (voir la page suivante)
SOUS PROGRAMME D'IMPRESSION
SOUS PROGRAMME DE MODIFICATION
SOUS PROGRAMME D'ANNULATION
PROGRAMME " IMPRESSION DE L'EMPLOI DU TEMPS : FEMMES ENCEINTES "
PROGRAMME "PROG.QUESTION" (voir page 66 Annexe 1)
fin

N.B. : Cet organigramme est à rapprocher de la figure 3

ANNEXE 2 (SUITE)
ORGANIGRAMME DU PROGRAMME " PW.ANTHROP "
Partie 3 : organigramme du sous-programme de saisie (seul, cette partie de "PW. ANTHROP" sera détaillée)

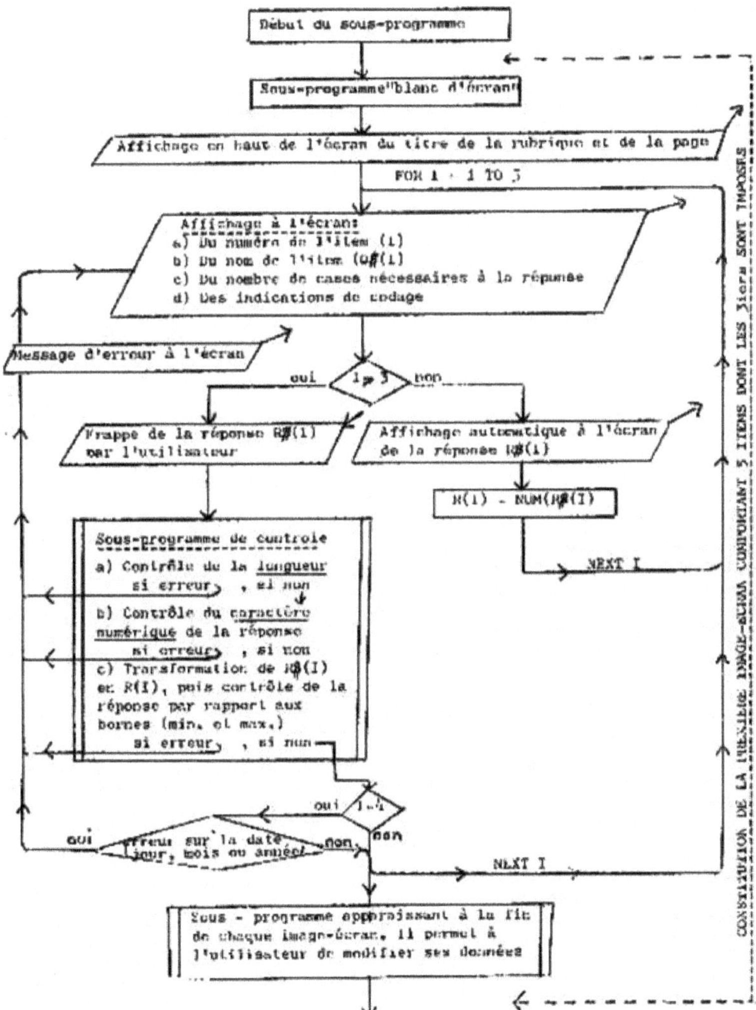

(cf page suivante)

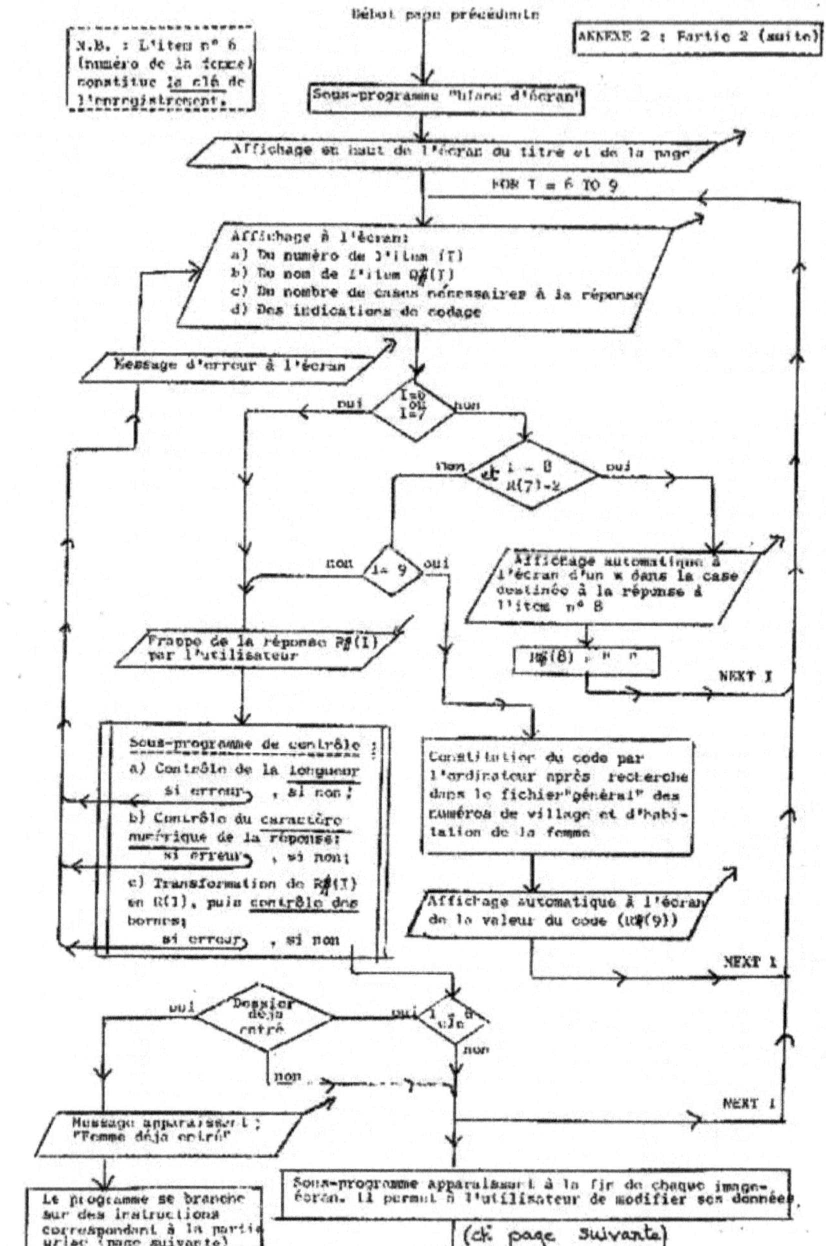
Début page précédente
ANNEXE 2 : Partie 2 (suite)
N.B. : L'item n° 6 (numéro de la femme) constitue la clé de l'enregistrement.
Sous-programme "blanc d'écran"
Affichage en haut de l'écran du titre et de la page
FOR I = 6 TO 9
Affichage à l'écran:
a) Du numéro de l'item (I)
b) Du nom de l'item R$(I)
c) Du nombre de cases nécessaires à la réponse
d) Des indications de codage
Message d'erreur à l'écran
I=6 ou I=7
oui
non
I = 8 et R(7)=2
non
oui
I= 9
non
oui
Affichage automatique à l'écran d'un * dans la case destinée à la réponse à l'item n° 8
R$(8) = " "
NEXT I
Frappe de la réponse R$(I) par l'utilisateur
Sous-programme de contrôle :
a) Contrôle de la longueur
si erreur , si non ;
b) Contrôle du caractère numérique de la réponse:
si erreur , si non;
c) Transformation de R$(I) en R(I), puis contrôle des bornes;
si erreur , si non
Constitution du code par l'ordinateur après recherche dans le fichier "général" des numéros de village et d'habitation de la femme
Affichage automatique à l'écran de la valeur du code (R$(9))
NEXT I
Dossier déjà entré
oui
non
I = 8
oui
non
NEXT I
Message apparaissant : "Femme déjà entrée"
Le programme se branche sur des instructions correspondant à la partie grise (page suivante)
Sous-programme apparaissant à la fin de chaque image-écran. Il permet à l'utilisateur de modifier ses données.
(cf page suivante)

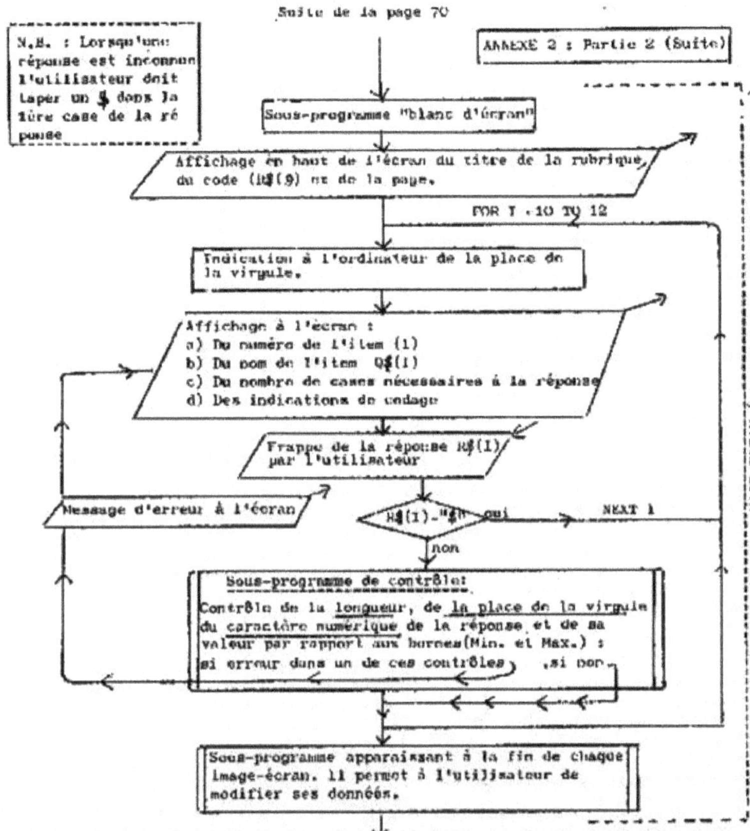

N.B. : PAR LA SUITE, 2 AUTRES IMAGES-ECRAN SE SUCCEDENT :L'UNE CORRESPONDANT AUX ITEMS N° 13 à 17 (CIRCONFERENCES), L'AUTRE CORRESPONDANT AUX ITEMS 18 et 19 (PLIS). LEUR ORGANIGRAMME EST LE MEME ET NE SERA PAS DETAILLE. <u>LORSQUE LE QUESTIONNAIRE EST ENTRE TOTALEMENT, LA SUITE DU TRAVAIL DE L'ORDINATEUR EST:</u>

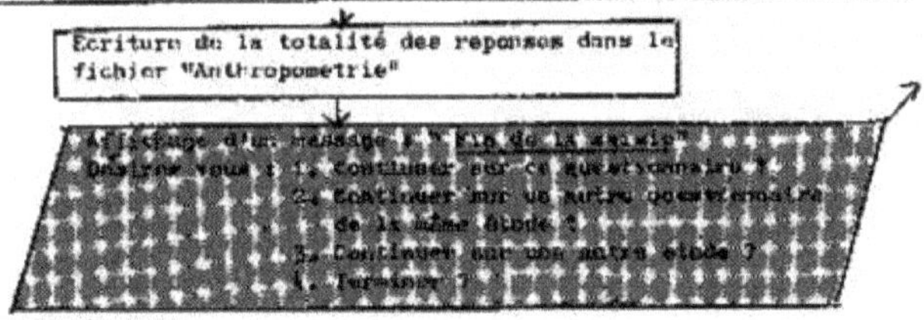

SI L'UTILISATEUR TAPE :
1 - LE MEME PROGRAMME RECOMMENCE,
2 - IL SE BRANCHE SUR LE PROGRAMME " PROG.QUESTION " (voir page 66),
3 - IL SE BRANCHE SUR LE PROGRAMME " STUDY.SELECT " (voir page 65),
4 - IL TERMINE.

BIBLIOGRAPHIE

1) A.D.E. - Conférence sur l'état nutritionnel d'enfants et de femmes enceintes au Sud-Soudan (Région de Jonglei Canal), Compte rendu, Hopital Trousseau, Paris, 23 Octobre 1980.

2) CASTELLANI X. - Méthode générale d'analyse d'une application informatique. Tome 1. Etapes et points fondamentaux de l'analyse fonctionnelle. Masson, Paris, 4ème éd., 1981.

3) CASTELLANI X. - Méthode générale d'analyse d'une application informatique. Tome 2. Etapes et points fondamentaux de l'analyse organique et de la programmation. Masson, Paris, 4ème éd., 1981.

4) DAVIES A.M., TZUR B., PRYWES R., WEISKOPF P. - The Jerusalem Perinatal Study. Methodology manual. Jerusalem, Department of Medical Ecology, Hebrew University-Hadassah Medical School. 1968.

5) DEPARTMENT OF HEALTH AND SOCIAL SECURITY and LONDON SCHOOL OF HYGIENE AND TROPICAL MEDICINE - A survey of growth in the pre-school child in England - 1972 (Fiche d'enquête communiquée personnellement).

6) DEPARTMENT OF HEALTH AND SOCIAL SECURITY and LONDON SCHOOL OF HYGIENE AND TROPICAL MEDICINE - A survey of growth in the pre-school child in England and Wales - 1972 (Fiche d'enquête communiquée personnellement)

7) GREMY F., GOLDBERG R. - Les sciences de l'information dans le domaine de la santé. Rapport fait à l'intention du Bureau Intergouvernemental pour l'Informatique à Rome, 1981.

8) HARLAP S., DAVIES A.M., GROVER N.B., PRYWES R. - The Jerusalem Perinatal Study : the first decade (1964-1973), Isr. J. Med. Sci., 1977. 13, 1073-1091.

9) HEAUME (de) M. - Applications médicales de l'informatique. Les aspects informatiques du traitement des questionnaires . Faculté de Médecine Pitié-Salpêtrière, Paris, 1980.

10) INSTITUT NATIONAL DE LA SANTE ET DE LA RECHERCHE MEDICALE - Enquête médicale sur la grossesse et l'accouchement - 1972 -(Fiche d'enquête communiquée personnellement).

11) LEFEBVRE J., BOITARD M., REY J.F. - Logiciel d'analyses statistiques multidimensionnelles sur micro-ordinateur. 1 vol., Masson, Paris, 1981

12) MUR J.M. - Le dossier médical informatique en milieu hospitalier. Analyse critique des buts, des méthodes et des résultats en France. These de doctorat de médecine, Nancy, 1975.

13) O.M.S. - Classification internationale des maladies. Révision 1975, 2 vol., O.M.S., Genéve, 1977, 1978.

14) O.M.S. - Multipurpose epidemiological surveys Rahad irrigation scheme (Sudan 1974-1975) : Study protocol prepared by IDRIS A.A., LAVOIPIERRE G.J. and SUNDARESAN T. , O.M.S., Genève/Khartoum, July 1974.

15) OSTROWSKI Z.L., FEIDRECHIED K. - Some aspects of nutritional status in the South of the Sudan, J. Trop. Pediatrics, 1982, 28, 153-158.

16) RUMEAU-ROUQUETTE C., BREART G., PADIEU R. - Méthodes en épidemiologie 1 vol., Flammarion, Paris, 2ème éd., 1981.

17) SCHWARTZ D. - Méthodes statistiques à l'usage des médecins et des biologistes. 1 vol., Flammarion, Paris, 1970.

18) SNEDECOR G.W., COCHRAN W.G. - Statistical Methods, 6th ed., Iowa State Univ. Press, Ames

2. SOCIO-CULTURAL QUESTIONNAIRES

Date 10-5-83 Village Ciendol Serial No. 49
The Interviewer James J. Gatluak
The Interogater Bilia Kuer
ETHNICITY; Nuer; Dinka; Shilluk

In Nilotic's Customs what is forbiden =

1. For children under three years ? should not walk about among cows. should not beg big people.

2. For other children ? should not beg other big men who are outside the family

3. For Man. should not cook – should not insult woman [illegible] – should not dress like woman should not covit other people

4. For Woman. should not spend night [illegible] outside the hut without the husbands notice. Should not comit adultery.

(a); Woman under Menstruation should not sleep with man during bleeding period. should not drink cows milk

(b) During Pregnancy. should not comit adultery – should not work hard – should avoid fight.

(c). During breast feeding. should avoid fighting should not sleep outside the hut during night. should not go far from child.

COMMENTARY = ...

SOCIAL ACTIVITIES

What do you do with Herds ? we marry woman with cows
We drink milk - eat meat - sleep in the skins of herds

What do you with fishing ? this is a surplus hobby - we fish to get fish for food.

What do you with Hunting ? we hunt animals for their skins and meat

What do you do with talking ? this is the way of thinking. God gave man a powerful and reasonable voice in order to understand others

What do you do with Sex life ? this is lust which makes man love woman

What do you do with marriage ctivities ? we marry to satisfy freely our lust desires - we marry also to reproduce ourselves freely.

What do you do with religion ? this is ~~a~~ a human fear for death that makes him think there is God who will provide an eternal life

OTHER GENERAL IDEAS ?

COMMENTARY?

DATE .... NAME OF VILLAGE

The Interviewer

The Interogated

the Sect Woman/Man

MAGIC EXISTANCE :-

In which case does Magics Exists ? this happen's indirectly. Idols speak through people and say good or evil as he likes

Who does the Magics in your Area ? many unnumbered person

What does the Magician do to the people in your Area ? the magician kill people when he is angry and save many people from their deseases when they need magical help and should pay the magician.

To Determine (Describe the type of his compartments i.e the way he lives)

(a). MAN .... Himself .... Society

He is a Herds man - His life is composed of cattle cultivation and his children. | people of his village are his society.

WOMAN dependable on her husband only | woman likewise women of his village are her society)

CHILDREN also dependable on their parents.

(a). Does he believe in what he is doing e.g. sacrificing/praying ....
yes he is believing in what he is doing because he has a [illegible] of his own

(b). Does he do it because people do it or does he do it of his own will ?
No - he does things because he brought them over [illegible] with him for 2 days

COMMENTARY ....

DREAMS - If you dream do you usually do it ? Yes/No..................

Is it often ? ......No......................................

About what do you dream ? (Sex; children; wars; animals make you afraide during dreams)

Do you believe dreams are true sometimes ? ....

Sometimes dreams are true and those true dreams are said to have come from God. evil dreams are lies

What is your relationship with your sons ? ... I born them and I bring them up - and they are from my blood - blood relationship is stronger than friendship relationship

What do you do to your children ? Education; Culturising them in what way ?

Send them to School to be Educated and culturised them to Love Nature and people.

DEATH - Do you worry about death Yes/No .

Do you believe there is life after death Yes/No .

If the answer is yes; What do you think you shall be e.g.

Man as you are now; animal; reptile; snakes; birds; fly etc.

Or what do you say ....

God is free to make me any thing

What is your freedom ? I am not free. No man is free unless he is dead. dead men are free men

He answers with I

He answers without "I"

What is your life's obligation ? I am obliged to cultivate more food for the next year - obliged to ~~cook~~ Look after my cattle.

COMMENTARY ....

S E X U A L I T Y = L I B I D O = S E X U A L D E S I R E S =

(a). Do you have it ? Yes/No

How do you feel it ....good..

....

Do you feel happy about it ....Yes....................................

If you do not do it why ? I can not when the woman (is)
I can not do it if the girl is one of my relative
" " " " " " " " " relative to my wife.

D I S E A S E = Do you ever worry when you are alone ? Yes/No .

If yes; then about what are you worry ? I can not
worry about loneliness, but should it
be that cows & the village people are not
there – I can not for sure be puzzling.

Why do you worry about them ? that cows and
village people are not there, this alone
can make one feel- think dead
and I can be worried because I can't like such a state

C O M M E N T A R Y = is he worrying with reasons ? ....

Is he worrying without reasons ? ....

....

COLLECTIVITY = AGRESSIVITY =

Do they like dancing ? Yes/No

Are you troublesome ? Yes/No.

Are you peaceful ? Yes/No.

Do you like work ? Yes/No.

Do you accept living without sexual intercoast ?

Yes/No.

If you cannot what do you do ? I can not
do it if the woman is too old.
if the girl is too young – if the
woman is bleeding.

C O M M E N T A R Y ....

....

....

....

....

....

3. PROCEDURE OF TAKING BLOOD SAMPLES

The blood samples have been taken as a support for diagnosis and treatment (diseases, parasite infections, anaemia,..). Due to the fact that the population under study was a priori illiterate, an oral agreement (for use of their blood samples for research) has been obtained through the translator. The amounts of the blood samples were not always enough to carry out all analyses, proposed by the study protocol. In a number of cases additional biological analyses could be made because of remaining blood volumes.

Venous blood was collected in vacutainers tubes in early morning in the field (after clinical examinations). The tubes with the blood samples were stored in cool boxes (+4°C) and transported within 1 to 3 hours to the A.D.E. field laboratory in Sobat (photo 28). In this laboratory (+15°C) all samples were submitted to a similar treatment before analysis. A blood drop was taken for malaria and parasitological research (thick and thin blood film). 47 μl was taken for a haematogram (Coulter Counter). The remaining blood was centrifuged at 3000 x g for 8 minutes. Serum was removed to different special tubes (2 ml, 1 ml and O,5 ml) depending of the analysis and the amount of the available blood sample. The erythrocytes were divided in 2 tubes. All samples, well codified, were stored in a deep freezer (-80°C) (only red cells samples at -20°C).

Every 1 to 2 weeks the samples were send in cool boxes (-20°C) by plane to different laboratories in Khartoum (a), Paris (b,c,d) and London (e,f,g). The blood samples arrived frozen (<-10°C) at place and were immediately stored in deep-freezers (-80°C) for specific analysis.

Because of priorities given to diagnostic reasons, only a few samples were available for such analysis like amino-acids, zinc, copper, magnesium, etc... and vitamin A or E.

The following micro-methods have been used:

- Enzymatic: uric acid, cholesterol, triglycerides, phosphor-lipids, glucose, Alkaline phosphatise.
- Colorimetric: phosphor, iron, creatinin, proteins.
- Immuno-turbidimetry: IgG
- Immononephelometric: transferrin.
- Immunoenzymatic: ferritin.
- High performance liquid chromatography: vitamin A and vitamin E.
- Spectometry by atomic absorption: zinc.
- Coulter Counter S5: Haematology - Hb, RBC, WBC, MCV, MCH, MCHC, Haematocrit.

Some values have been suppressed from the study because blood has been contaminated, when blood samples have been taken or, accidentally during transport in the field. Two blood samples (from the Dinka population), because of wrong storage, have not been taken into consideration for statistical analyses.

Some analyses have been done by micromethods in A.D.E. laboratories (Coulter Counter and Kemo Mat) (photo 29 and 30) at the local A.D.E. Research Center in Sobat (photo 28), others, at the departments of biochemistry in Khartoum, Paris, London and Cardiff.

* * *

The biological data are drawn from two different studies carried out in the Jonglei Canal area: from two cross-sectional studies in the Shilluk and Nuer area as well as from the longitudinal study of pregnant women and their children until age three years, in the Shilluk area.

Data were compared with usual reference values used in the university Hôpital Armand Trousseau in Paris, based on Hitachi 911 references (25) and SI conversion factors for values in clinical chemistry (26).

4. FOOD TABLES ADAPTED TO SOUTHERN SUDANESE

by Z. L. Ostrowski and E. Ojaba

INTRODUCTION

This edition was intended for use in evaluation dietary data based on records of food consumption as a part of the A.D.E. Longitudinal Study on Growth and Nutrition carried out in the South Sudan in 1979-1984 with the agreement of the Ministry of Health of the Democratic Republic of the Sudan and the National Research Council. This edition was prepared in the response to the need for evaluating the diet and nutrition status of the population who have a similar cooking and feeding habits as those under study.

Even if the data in these tables are only indicative, they can be used for nutritional investigations in the South Sudan as well as similar regions in Africa. More precise data could be obtained only by chemical analysis of all food items. But still seasonal variations, food habits and way of preparation could interfere in nutritional values.

For certain food items only few analytical results were available. For other food items, representative values given by other authors have been adopted in the present tables. Some of the foods values have been taken from tables published by the Food Agriculture Organization (F.A.O. 1953, 1954) and, for certain European types of food, from food tables published by Ostrowski and Josse (1978). These data have been compiled with data from other food tables (see references). In some cases only a mean value was used. Certain food items have been analysed by A.D.E. in French laboratories, other has been calculated using local recopies obtained during the study period.

INSTRUCTION

Food items are grouped into nine categories and each item appears in only one group. Food items are arranged in alphabetic order according to the names by which they are most commonly known.

Values for food items are expressed in terms of 100 grammes edible portions. Values for protein, lipids and carbohydrates are expressed in grammes (g). Values for minerals and vitamins are expressed in miligrammes (mg). Values for vitamin A are expressed in International Units (IU). If values have more than 4 figures, they are expressed as «9999» (see list 1). Abbreviations and measurements used in this food tables are indicated in list 2 and 3. References for each food item and/or nutriment are indicated by a letter in list 4.

LIST 1 : VALUES FOR VITAMIN A (instead of «9999»)

Calf liver raw	: 20 000 (P)
Lamb liver raw	: 20 000 (P)
Lamb liver cooked	: 25 000 (C)
Chicken liver cooked	: 25 000 (A)
Oil palm	: 62 167 (F)
Carrot fresh raw	: 11 000 (A)
Carrot fresh cooked	: 10 500 (A)
Juta lvs. fresh raw	: 10 683 (F)
Juta lvs. dry raw	: 30 000 (C)
Palm purée	: 10 250 (F)
Salt	: 38 809 (A)

LIST 2 : ABREVIATIONS

FR	: Fresh
AVG	: Average
YNG	: Young
C	: Calculated values
FAO	: F.A.O. values
WHL	: Whole
COND	: Condensed
DIL	: Diluted
FTF	: Fortified
PRP	: Prepared
M	: Mongo
I	: Groundnut butter added
LVS	: Leaves
VEGE	: Vegetables

LIST 3 : MEASUREMENTS

1 cub of fresh milk	: 160 g
1 cub of dry fish	: 220 g
1 cub of fresh fish	: 240 g
1 cub of sour milk	: 165 g
1 cub of porridge	: 170 g
1 cub of dry rice	: 120 g
1 cub of cooked rice	: 110 g
1 cub of dry rice = 3 cups cooked	
1 tea spoon of sugar	: 7 g
1 table spoon of Apwoto	: 32 g
1 table spoon of Akelo	: 25 g
1 table spoon of boiled fish	: 30 g
1 tarha of kisra	: 115 g
1 hand full of Asida	: 150 g

LIST 4 : REFERENCES

A - Food values of proportions commonly used, by Bowes & Church, 12th Edition, J.B. Lippincott Company, 1937.

C - Calculated values, A.D.E. Research Center, Paris, 1985.

D - Mc Cance and Widdowson, The composition of foods, A.Paul, D.A.T. Southgate, 4th Edition, H.M.S.D., London, 1967.

E - Les principaux aliments : composition, conservation et transformation, Centre International de l'Enfance, Paris, 1984.

F - Food composition tables for use in Africa, F.A.O., U.S. Dept. of Health, Education and Welfare, 1968.

G - Tables scientifiques, Ciba-Geigy S.A., Bâle, 1973.

I - Dosages microbiologiques, Laboratoire vitaminologie, Institut Pasteur, Lyon, 1978, 1979,1980.

L - A.D.E. analyses du Laboratoire du Centre multidisciplinaire d'études et de recherches nutritionnelles, Institut Pasteur, Lyon, 1985.

M - Mean values, calculated based on : Vitamins in medicine, B.M. Baker and DA.Bender,William Henemann Medical Books Ltd, London, 4th Edition 1980

N - Livsmedels tabeller, Energi och vissa näringsämnen, Schmidts Boktryckeri A.B., Helsingborg, 1981.

O - Ostrowski Z.L. and Josse M.-C., Tables nutritives des aliments, A.D.E., Ed. J. Lanore CLT, Paris, 1978.

P - Tables of representatives values of foods commonly used in tropical countries, B.S. Platt, Medical research Council, London, 1962.

R - Randoin L., Tables des compositions des aliments, J.Lanore Ed. Paris, 1947

S - Composition of foods in term of 100 gr edible portion, compiled by U. Zacharias, Ahfad University College for Women, Omdurman, 1978.

W-The Health Aspect of Food and Nutrition, W.H.O. Regional Office for the Western Pacifique, Manila, 1979.

Z - Tables of the values of Zambian foodstuffs, The National Food and Nutrition Commission of Zambia, 1971.

Commission of Zambia, 1971.

FOOD TABLES FOR THE SOUTHERN SUDANESE POPULATION

ALIMENTS (100 gr)	ENG Cal	PRO g	LIP g	GLU g	Ph mg	Mg mg	Ca mg	Fe mg	Na mg	K mg	Asc mg	Try mg	B1 mg	B2 mg	Nia mg	VitA IU	VitE mg	ref
MEAT																		
AVG.MEAT FR RAW	117	20.6	3.8	0.0	141		22	4.6			0.0		0.06	0.17	3.20	0	0.50_{G}	(F)
AVG.MEAT FR COOK	128	23.1	4.0	0.0	158		25	5.1			0.0		0.04	0.17	3.36		0.33_{B}	(C)
AVG.SOUP	8	1.7	0.3	0.0	8		1	0.3			0.0		0.02	0.03	0.53		0.02	(C)
ANTELOPE FR RAW	141	30.4	2.2		102		65	2.1			0.0		0.07	0.28	7.80		0.11_{M}	(F)
ANTELOPE FR COOK	186	41.0	2.5		328		73	2.3			0.0		0.06	0.31	8.74		0.10_{M}	(C)
ANTELOPE DRY RAW	335	81.8	0.9	0.0	577		145	2.2			0.0		0.02	0.29	1.54		0.10_{M}	(C)
ANTELOPE DRY COOK	290	71.2	0.6		416		105	1.8			0.0		0.01	0.20	1.28		0.10_{M}	(C)
CALF FR RAW	111	20.4	3.2	0.0	205	15	13	2.2	96	340	0.0		0.15	0.26	6.40_{F}	0	0.90_{H}	(D)
CALF FR COOK	130	24.5	3.6	0.0	250	18	16	2.6	80	408	0.0		0.12	0.29	6.48_{C}		0.86_{E}	(D)
CALF KIDNEY RAW	128	16.7	6.4	0.8	260		10	11.5	200	290	12.7		0.37	2.48	7.00_{F}	1000_{F}	0.18_{D}	(D)
CALF KIDNEY COOK	130	18.4	6.7	0.9	286		11	12.6	165	319	6.3		0.30	2.59	5.21_{I}	2	0.38_{B}	(D)
CALF LIVER RAW	113	15.9	5.1	1.0	180	25	16	13.8	104	265	5.4		0.55	1.90	13.00_{F}	9999	0.90	(D)
CALF LIVER COOK	132	19.2	4.3	4.1	311	46	4	10.6	84	295	41.0		0.28	2.56	12.10_{C}	416	0.90	(D)
CHICKEN FR RAW	141	20.5	6.5	0.0	206		10	1.1	70_{A}	285_{A}	0.0_{A}	219_{A}	0.08_{A}	0.16_{A}	8.00_{A}	0	0.21_{M}	(A)
CHICKEN FR COOK	169	26.0	7.2	0.0	217		11	1.2	67	362	0.0	278	0.07	0.18	8.40		0.11_{G}	(C)
CHICKEN BREAST COOK	125	29.0	1.0	0.0	269	25	15	1.4	63	335			0.58	0.90	10.00		0.27_{M}	(D)
CHICKEN LEG COOK	161	26.2	6.2	0.0	254	47	13	2.3	78	456	1.6		0.07	0.17	10.00		0.27_{M}	(D)
CHICKEN FRIED	126	18.4	5.8	0.0	180	15	9	1.0	63	254	0.0	197	0.05	0.13	5.76		0.27_{M}	(C)
CHICKEN LIVER COOK	147	24.3	4.9	1.3	254	0	20	8.1	56	239	14.0	440	0.22	2.60	1.56_{A}	9999_{A}		(D)
CHICKEN SOUP	24	2.1	1.7	0.0	21		1	1.0	30	29	0.0	22	0.04	0.04	2.00		0.01	(C)
COW FR RAW	122	20.6	3.8	0.0	141		22	4.6			0.0		0.06	0.17	3.20		0.50_{G}	(F)
COW FR COOK	128	23.1	4.0	0.0	158		25	5.1			0.0		0.04	0.17	3.36		0.33_{B}	(C)
COW DRY RAW	235	55.4	1.5	0.0	269		49	4.9					0.02	0.18	6.30	0	0.10_{M}	(F)
COW DRY COOK	204	48.2	1.2	0.0	234		43	4.2			0.0		0.01	0.14	5.10		0.10_{M}	(C)
COW LIVER RAW	138	19.0	4.7	5.0	360		8	10.0			71.0				5.20	300		(F)

FOOD TABLES FOR THE SOUTHERN SUDANESE POPULATION

ALIMENTS (100 gr)	ENG Cal	PRO g	LIP g	GLU g	Ph mg	Mg mg	Ca mg	Fe mg	Na mg	K mg	Asc mg	Try mg	B1 mg	B2 mg	Nia mg	ViA IU	ViE mg	ref
MEAT																		
COW LIVER COOK	124	20.9	4.5	5.5	396		9	11.0			39.0				5.72	330		(C)
COW TRIPES FR RAW	94	19.1	2.0	0.0	132		69	0.9	46	19	0.0		0.01	0.09	1.60	0	0.08_c	(A)
COW TRIPES FR COOK	101	20.9	1.9	0.0	145		76	1.0	51	21	0.0		0.01	0.10	1.76	0	0.08_w	(C)
COW BLOOD RAW	73	17.8	0.1	0.1	19	5	6	49.0	330	44	0.0		0.09	0.03		3		(D)
COW SOUP	8	1.2	0.3	0.0			1	0.3			0.0		0.02	0.03	0.53		0.02	(C)
DUCK FR RAW	227	18.1	17.2	0.0	187	15	11	2.1	80	292	7.5		0.30	0.20	0.77_w	0_p	0.28_w	(D)
DUCK FR COOK	271	24.4	19.3	0.0	252	20	12	2.8	81	394	3.7		0.26	0.22	0.69	0	0.27	(D)
DUCK ROASTED	304	22.8	23.6	0.0	230		19	3.3								0	0.27_w	(A)
DUCK SOUP	48	1.2	5.1	0.0	13	1	1	0.1	32	20	2.0		0.14	0.04	0.15		0.02	(C)
GOAT FR RAW	159	18.7	9.4	0.0			11	2.2			0.0		0.17	0.32	5.60	0	0.11_w	(A)
GOAT FR COOK	173	20.9	9.9	0.0			12	2.5			0.0		0.12	0.30	6.27		0.10_w	(C)
GOAT DRY RAW	235	50.3	3.7	0.0			25	2.3			0.0		0.06	0.33	11.90		0.10_w	(C)
GOAT DRY COOK	202	43.7	3.0	0.0			21	2.0			0.0		0.04	0.26	8.90		0.10_w	(C)
GOAT SOUP	14	1.0	1.1	0.0			1	0.1			0.0		0.05	0.04	0.71		0.01_w	(C)
GUINEA FOWL COOK	134	27.9	2.2	0.6											11.00_c		0.27_w	(B)
HIPPO FR COOK	305	90.2	2.7	0.0	234			10.2			0.0		0.02	0.09	0.29		0.10_w	(C)
HIPPO DRY RAW	346	80.6	2.6	0.0	209			9.1			0.0		0.04	0.24	4.50	0	0.10_w	(F)
HIPPO DRY COOK	302	70.1	2.4	0.0	182			7.9			0.0		0.03	0.22	4.12		0.10_w	(C)
HIPPO SOUP	25	5.5	0.3	0.0	13			0.6			0.0		0.00	0.01	0.30		0.01	(C)
LAMB FR RAW	280	16.0	24.0	0.0	160	24	10	1.7	90	250	0.0		0.20	0.25	5.00	0	0.11_w	(D)
LAMB FR COOK	293	20.3	26.5	0.0	203	30	11	2.2	86	318	0.0		0.16	0.28_c	0.25_c	0	0.10_w	(D)
LAMB KIDNEY RAW	101	16.8	3.3	0.9	218	13	13	7.5	151	205	15.0		0.51	2.42	7.00_p	1000_p	0.45_s	(B)
LAMB KIDNEY COOK	105	18.5	3.2	0.5	239	14	12	8.2	124	225	7.5		0.36	2.32	8.09_c		0.41_s	(D)
LAMB LIVER RAW	131	21.0	3.9	2.9	349	14	13	10.9	51	170	33.0		0.40	3.28	13.00_p	9999_p	0.46_s	(B)
LAMB LIVER COOK	132	23.1	3.7	1.6	384	15	12	12.0	42	187	16.0		0.29	3.14	0.47	9999	0.41_c	(D)

FOOD TABLES FOR THE SOUTHERN SUDANESE POPULATION

ALIMENTS (100 gr)	ENG Cal	PRO g	LIP g	GLU g	Ph mg	Mg mg	Ca mg	Fe mg	Na mg	K mg	Asc mg	Try mg	B1 mg	B2 mg	Nia mg	VIA IU	VIE mg	ref
MEAT																		
RABBIT FR RAW	154	20.8	7.6	0.6	224	29	14	3.5	47	382	3.0		0.11	0.07	9.00_p	0	0.11_m	(D)
RABBIT FR COOK	189	29.1	8.5	0.0	259	29	15	3.8	41	368	1.5		0.09	0.07	0.30	0_0	0.10_m	(D)
SHEEP FR RAW	260	16.9	21.4	0.0	148	16	10	2.0	84	301	1.0	379	0.17	0.27	5.00_p	0_p	0.12_c	(F)
SHEEP FR COOK	279	19.0	22.5	0.0	166	18	11	2.2	70	337	0.0	424	0.14	0.28	5.80		0.11_0	(C)
SHEEP DRY RAW	255	44.8	8.4	0.0	282	30	22	2.1	160	574	0.5	424	0.11	0.28	0.39	80	0.10	(C)
SHEEP DRY COOK	218	39.0	6.9	0.0	245	26	19	1.8	104	499	0.2	369	0.07	0.22	0.36	9	0.10_m	(C)
SHEEP FRIED	293	50.9	8.8	0.0	315	34	25	2.3	136	642	0.5	475	0.10	0.23	0.43	95	0.10_m	(C)
TERMITES FR RAW	356	20.4	28.0	4.2			12_p	1.0_p										(F)
TERMITES DRY RAW	656	35.7	54.3	3.5	780		142	52.0			0.0		0.03	5.97	0.58			(F)
TERMITES FRIED	534	31.8	42.6	5.8	520		80	17.4			0.0		0.12	3.28	8.30			(F)
TURTLE FR RAW	79	16.0	1.0	2.0			100	1.0			0.0		0.20	0.50	3.00	0	0.11_m	(Z)
TURTLE FR COOK	90	17.9	1.1	2.2			112	1.1			0.0		0.17	0.52	3.12		0.10_m	(C)

ALIMENTS (100 gr)	ENG Cal	PRO g	LIP g	GLU g	Ph mg	Mg mg	Ca mg	Fe mg	Na mg	K mg	Asc mg	Try mg	B1 mg	B2 mg	Nia mg	ViA IU	ViE mg	ref
FISH																		
AVG.FISH FR RAW	113	21.6	3.0	0.0	113		32	1.7			0.0	314_{C}	0.05	0.08	2.80		0.60_{D}	(F)
AVG.FISH FR COOK	110	21.3	2.8	0.0	89		25	1.4			0.0	310	0.04	0.07	0.88		0.74_{M}	(C)
AVG.FISH FR COOK+SAUCE	67	10.9	2.6	0.0														(L)
AVG.FISH DRY RAW	256	47.3	7.4	0.0	749		1018	4.9			0.0	687_{C}	0.07	0.23	6.20	0	0.74_{M}	(F)
AVG.FISH DRY COOK	207	38.7	5.8	0.0	409		664	3.4			0.0	562	0.05	0.22	4.30		0.74_{M}	(C)
AVG.FISH ROASTED	132	25.9	3.2	0.0	126		38	2.0			0.0	600	0.06	0.06	2.02		0.74_{M}	(C)
AVG.FISH SOUP	19	3.5	0.6	0.0	42		11	0.5			0.0	53	0.01	0.02	0.90		0.07	(C)
CATFISH FR RAW	85	17.6	1.6	0.0	97		61	1.2	60_{A}	330_{A}		314	0.05	0.08	2.80		0.80_{M}	(F)
CATFISH FR COOK	83	17.4	1.5	0.0	155		48	1.0	30	277		310	0.04	0.07	2.35		0.74_{M}	(C)
CATFISH DRY RAW	307	62.5	6.3	0.0	440		1370	3.6				687	0.03	0.02	6.00		0.74_{M}	(F)
CATFISH DRY COOK	256	51.1	5.7	0.0	330		894	2.9				562	0.05	0.22	4.30		0.74_{M}	(C)
CATFISH SOUP	14	2.9	0.3	0.0	72		22	0.4	36	187		53	0.01	0.02	0.88		0.07	(C)
LUNGFISH FR RAW	72	16.4	0.2	0.0													0.86_{M}	(F)
LUNGFISH FR COOK	64	15.6	0.2	0.0													0.74_{M}	(F)
LUNGFISH DRY SMOKED	371	82.1	2.8	0.0													0.74_{M}	(F)
NILE PERCH FRESH RAW	101	21.9	1.5	0.0	137		89	4.1			0.0	314_{C}	0.05_{C}	0.08_{C}	2.00_{C}		0.80	(F)
NILE PERCH FRESH COOK	99	21.6	1.4	0.0	108		70	3.4			0.0	310	0.04	0.07	2.35		0.74_{M}	(C)
NILE PERCH DRY RAW	401	70.0	13.4	0.0	662		170	8.5_{S}				687_{C}	0.03_{S}	0.02_{S}	6.00_{S}		0.74	(F)
NILE PERCH DRY COOK	323	57.2	10.5	0.0	432		110	5.9			0.0	562	0.05	0.22	4.30		0.74_{M}	(C)
NILE PERCH SOUP	17	3.7	0.3	0.0	50		32	1.3			0.0	53	0.01	0.02	0.88		0.07_{M}	(C)
MUDFISH FR RAW	85	17.6	1.6	0.0	197		61	1.2				314_{C}	0.05_{C}	0.08_{C}	2.80_{C}		0.80_{M}	(F)
MUDFISH FR COOK	83	17.4	1.5	0.0	155		48	1.0	30	277		310	0.04	0.07	2.35		0.74_{M}	(F)
MUDFISH DRY RAW	307	62.5	6.3	0.0	440		1370	3.6				687_{C}	0.03_{S}	0.02_{S}	6.00_{S}		0.74_{M}	(F)
MUDFISH DRY COOK	256	51.1	5.7	0.0	330		894	2.9				562	0.05	0.22	4.30		0.74_{M}	(C)
SARDINES CANNED	227	24.1	13.9	1.3	430	23	330	2.7	505	397	0.0	237_{A}	0.04	0.30	5.33_{A}	220_{A}	0.30_{D}	(D)

FOOD TABLES FOR THE SOUTHERN SUDANESE POPULATION

ALIMENTS (100 gr)	ENG Cal	PRO g	LIP g	GLU g	Ph mg	Mg mg	Ca mg	Fe mg	Na mg	K mg	Asc mg	Try mg	B1 mg	B2 mg	Nia mg	ViA IU	ViE mg	ref
FISH																		
TILAPIA FR RAW	96	19.7	1.9	0.0	344		112	3.2				314_{C}	0.03	0.05	1.50		0.80_{M}	(F)
TILAPIA FR COOK	94	19.5	1.8	0.0	271		88	2.7				310	0.02	0.04	1.30		0.74_{M}	(C)
TILAPIA FR COOK	117	22.0	2.8	0.0	275		90	2.6				251	0.02	0.04	3.70		0.74_{M}	(F)
TILAPIA DRY RAW	319	54.3	11.3	0.0	1766		2406	10.4				750	0.08	0.61	5.80		0.74_{M}	(F)
TILAPIA DRY COOK	257	44.4	8.8	0.0	1152		1570	8.3				613	0.06	0.42	4.60		0.74_{M}	(C)
TILAPIA FRIED	512	39.4	39.4	0.0	688_{C}		224_{C}	6.4_{C}				600_{C}	0.03_{C}	0.07_{C}	3.30_{C}		0.74_{M}	(F)
TILAPIA SOUP	17	3.3	0.4	0.0	126		41	0.9				53	0.01	0.01	0.50		0.07	(C)
TUNA CANNED	283	22.8	20.9	0.0	294	27_{A}	7	1.2	361	343	0.0	290_{A}	0.05	0.06	12.90_{A}	80_{A}	6.30_{D}	(D)

FOOD TABLES FOR THE SOUTHERN SUDANESE POPULATION

ALIMENTS (100 gr)	ENG Cal	PRO g	LIP g	GLU g	Ph mg	Mg mg	Ca mg	Fe mg	Na mg	K mg	Asc mg	Try mg	B1 mg	B2 mg	Nia mg	VitA IU	VitE mg	ref
EGGS AND FATS																		
EGG CHICKEN RAW	136	11.8_{F}	9.6_{F}	0.6_{F}	200	10	45	2.6	123	129	0.0	206	0.10	0.29	0.30_{F}	1188	1.00_{G}	(A)
EGG CHICKEN COOK	158	12.9	11.5	0.8	204	10	54	2.3	123	129	0.0	206	0.08	0.27	0.00	1138	0.50_{G}	(A)
EGG CHICKEN FRIED	208	12.4	17.2	0.8	222	10	60	2.4	338	140	0.0	198	0.10	0.30	0.20	1420	0.80_{G}	(A)
EGG CHICKEN WHITE RAW	49	11.1	0.2	0.7	21	12	11	0.2	170	154	0.3	229_{A}	0.02	0.32	0.11_{A}	0_{A}	0.00	(D)
EGG CHICKEN YOLK RAW	353	16.1	31.9	0.2	590	16	140	7.2	51	138	0.0	165_{A}	0.29	0.40	0.04_{A}	3407_{A}	3.00	(D)
OMELET IN OIL	217	11.6	17.9	2.4	189	11	81	1.6	258	147	0.0	185	0.08	0.27	0.16	1081		(A)
BUTTER	752	0.7	83.0	0.6	15	1	12	1.8	22	12	0.0			0.01	0.00_{F}	3000_{F}	1.50	(D)
OIL AVERAGE	882	0.0	98.0	0.0													25.00	(D)
OIL GROUNDNUT	899	0.0_{E}	99.9_{E}	0.0_{E}	0		0	0.0	0	0	0.0		0.00	0.00	0.00	0	25.00_{G}	(A)
OIL PALM	891	0.0	98.9	0.3	7		6				0.0		0.01	0.02	0.00	9999_{C}	25.00_{G}	(F)
OIL SESAME	899	0.2	99.7	0.1			10	0.1			0.0		0.01	0.07	0.10		25.00_{G}	(W)
SEMIN (GHEE)	702	0.0	77.3	1.5												908	25.00_{G}	(F)

ALIMENTS (100 gr)	ENG Cal	PRO g	LIP g	GLU g	Ph mg	Mg mg	Ca mg	Fe mg	Na mg	K mg	Asc mg	Try mg	B1 mg	B2 mg	Nia mg	VIA IU	VIE mg	ref
MILK AND MILKPRODUCTS																		
AVG. MILK RAW	64	3.3	3.6	4.7	92	13	12	0.1	50	144	1.0	49	0.04	0.14	0.08$_A$	145	0.08	(D)
AVG. MILK SOUR	44	3.8	2.0	2.7	97	14	140	0.1	55	150	0.6	51	0.03	0.11	0.06	115	0.04	(C)
COND.MILK NON SWEETENED	133	6.5	7.6	9.7	189	27	242	0.1	98	322	2.1	112$_C$	0.07	0.37	0.21$_F$	320$_F$	0.17	(D)
COND.MILK SWEETENED	332	8.2	8.8	51.1	236	27	238	0.2	88	360	3.8	113$_A$	0.09	0.39	0.20$_F$	350$_F$	0.42$_D$	(D)
COW MILK WHL.RAW	64	3.3	3.6	4.7	92	13	112	0.1	50	144	1.0	49	0.04	0.14	0.08$_A$	145	0.08	(D)
COW MILK WHL.BOILED	64	3.3	3.6	4.7	92	13	112	0.1	50	144	0.4	49	0.03	0.12	0.04	145	0.08	(C)
COW MILK WHL.BOILED+SUGAR	78	3.2	3.5	8.5	88	12	108	0.1	48	138	0.4	47	0.03	0.12	0.04	139	0.08	(C)
COW MILK RAW DIL.	55	2.8	3.1	4.0	78	11	95	0.0	43	122	0.9	42	0.02	0.12	0.06	123	0.07	(C)
COW MILK BOILED DIL.	55	2.8	3.1	4.0	78	11	95	0.0	43	122	0.4	42	0.03	0.10	0.03	123	0.07	(C)
COW MILK SOUR	44	3.8	2.0	2.7	97	14	140	0.5	55	150	0.0	51	0.03	0.11	0.06	115	0.04	(C)
COW MILK SOUR+SUGAR	108	3.1	1.6	20.2	80	12	115	0.1	45	123	0.0	42	0.02	0.09	0.05	94	0.07	(C)
COW MILK FRESH/SOUR	64	3.3	3.6	4.7	92	13	112	0.1	50	144	0.6	49	0.03	0.11	0.06	145	0.07	(C)
DRY SKIMMED MILK	357	35.0	1.0	51.9	1020	143$_A$	1290	0.8	557	1580	2.0	500$_A$	0.34	2.18	1.10$_F$	40$_F$	0.03$_B$	(D)
GOAT MILK WHL.RAW	96	3.4	4.9	7.0	106$_A$	17$_A$	129$_A$	0.1$_A$	34$_A$	180$_A$	1.0$_A$	38$_A$	0.04$_A$	0.11$_A$	0.30	160	0.52$_M$	(F)
GOAT MILK WHL.BOILED	85	3.4	4.9	7.0	106	17	129	0.1	34	180	0.0	38	0.03	0.09	0.15	160	0.07	(C)
GOAT MILK WHL.BOILED+SGR	89	2.9	4.2	10.0	91	15	111	0.1	29	155	0.0	33	0.02	0.07	0.13	138	0.07	(C)
GOAT MILK RAW DIL.	73	2.9	4.2	6.0	90	14	110	0.9	29	153	0.1	32	0.03	0.10	0.26	136	0.08	(C)
GOAT MILK BOILED DIL.	73	2.9	4.2	6.0	90	14	110	0.9	29	153	0.0	32	0.02	0.08	0.13	136	0.08	(C)
GOAT MILK SOUR	56	3.9	2.7	4.0	111	18	135	0.1	36	190	0.0	40	0.03	0.09	0.24	128	0.07	(C)
GOAT MILK SOUR+SUGAR	118	3.2	2.2	21.2	91	15	111	0.1	30	156	0.0	33	0.02	0.07	0.20	105	0.08	(C)
GOAT MILK FRESH/SOUR	85	3.4	4.9	7.0	106	17	129	0.1	34	180	0.6	38	0.03	0.07	0.18	160	0.04	(C)
HUMAN MILK	69	1.1	3.1	9.1	18	4$_A$	32	0.1$_A$	16$_A$	51$_A$	1.0$_A$	18$_A$	0.01$_A$	0.04$_A$	0.20$_A$	240$_A$	0.70$_B$	(F)
MIXED MILK WHL.RAW	92	4.6	5.3	3.9	90	12	110	0.1	50	144	1.0	49	0.04	0.14	0.10	145	0.08	(C)
MIXED MILK WHL.BOILED	92	4.6	5.3	3.9	90	12	110	0.5	50	144	0.5	49	0.03	0.12	0.09	130	0.08	(C)
POWDER MILK	506	26.4	27.5	38.2	708	98	909	0.5	405	1330	6.0	370	0.29	1.46	0.70	1130	0.90	(A)

ALIMENTS (100 gr)	ENG Cal	PRO g	LIP g	GLU g	Ph mg	Mg mg	Ca mg	Fe mg	Na mg	K mg	Asc mg	Try mg	B1 mg	B2 mg	Nia mg	ViA IU	ViE mg	ref
MILK AND MILKPRODUCTS																		
POWDER MILK FTF.	506	26.4	27.5	38.2	708	98	909	0.5	405	1330	6.0	370	0.29	1.46	0.70	6130	0.70	(C)
POWDER MILK FTF.REC.+SGR	77	2.5	2.6	10.8	71	9	92	0.1	37	116	0.0	37	0.01	0.06	0.02	613	0.04	(C)
POWDER MILK REC.+SUGAR	77	2.5	2.6	10.8	71	9	92	0.1	37	116	0.0	37	0.01	0.06	0.02	113	0.04	(C)
SHEEP MILK WHL.RAW	101	5.9	7.0	3.5	92	13	112	0.1	50	144	1.0	49	0.04	0.14	0.08	145	0.08_{E}	(F)
SHEEP MILK WHL.BOILED	101	5.9	7.0	3.5	92	13	112	0.1	50	144	0.5	49	0.03	0.12	0.04	145	0.08	(C)
SHEEP MILK RAW DIL.	86	5.0	6.0	3.0	78	11	95	0.0	43	122	0.9	42	0.03	0.12	0.06	123	0.07	(C)
SHEEP MILK BOILED DIL.	86	5.0	6.0	3.0	78	11	95	0.0	43	122	0.4	42	0.02	0.10	0.03	123	0.07	(C)
SHEEP MILK SOUR	70	6.8	3.9	2.0	95	14	118	0.1	52	151	0.0	51	0.03	0.11	0.06	116	0.07	(C)
SHEEP MILK FRESH/SOUR	101	5.9	7.0	3.5	92	13	112	0.1	50	144	0.6	49	0.03	0.11	0.06	145	0.08	(C)
WHITE CHEESE	129	16.3	3.5	5.7	180		112	1.4					0.03	0.27	0.40	42	0.52_{M}	(F)
YOGHURT PLAIN	67	4.2	3.4	4.9	87_{A}		111	0.0_{A}	47_{A}	132_{A}	0.8_{A}	33_{A}	0.03	0.16	0.10	139_{A}	0.52_{M}	(S)

FOOD TABLES FOR THE SOUTHERN SUDANESE POPULATION

ALIMENTS (100 gr)	ENG Cal	PRO g	LIP g	GLU g	Ph mg	Mg mg	Ca mg	Fe mg	Na mg	K mg	Asc mg	Try mg	B1 mg	B2 mg	Nia mg	VitA IU	VitE mg	ref
CEREALS AND GRAINS																		
BISCUIT	418	7.0	10.0	75.0			30	2.0					0.02	0.03	1.00		0.19_M	(S)
BREAD MIXED	260	8.0	1.5	53.6	123		29	2.6			0.0		0.22	0.01	1.30		0.19	(S)
BREAD WHITE	256	7.7	2.0	51.7	95		37	1.7			0.0		0.16	0.04	1.00	0	2.00_B	(F)
BREAD WHL.WHEAT	248	7.7	1.6	50.8	151	78_A	43	2.2	526	274_A	0.0_A	126	0.20	0.08	2.10	0_A	1.30_B	(F)
CORNFLOUR	362	7.8	2.6	76.8	164_A		6	1.8			0.0_A		0.20	0.06	1.40	340_A	0.20_M	(S)
CUSTARD FLOUR	360	4.5	0.8	3.1			10	4.0									0.20_M	(S)
CUSTARD+MILK COOK	81	2.5	2.6	11.9	64	9	79	0.2	35	101	0.3	49	0.02	0.08	0.04	100	0.06	(C)
DOUGHNUTS	416	6.3	26.7	37.7	77	20	37	1.7	233	80	0.0	80	0.17	0.17	1.30		0.19_M	(A)
DURRA ASIDA	184	4.1	1.6	38.2	118		23	1.2		175	0.0	40	0.09	0.04	1.36	6	0.10	(C)
DURRA DRY BOILED	118	3.4	0.8	24.2	63		9	1.3		122	0.0	38	0.08	0.04	0.92	5	0.19	(C)
DURRA DRY GRAINS	361	11.1	2.5	73.5	263		23	3.6		351_A	0.0	119	0.37	0.15	3.30	17	0.20_M	(F)
DURRA DRY ROASTED	391	10.3	2.8	78.7	390		8	3.8		375	0.0	128	0.02	0.10	4.00	0	0.19_M	(C)
DURRA FR ROASTED	361	11.1	2.5	73.5	263		23	3.6		351	0.0	119	0.24	0.12	2.64	14	0.19_M	(C)
DURRA KISRA (CREPE)	257	5.7	2.2	53.5	166		32	1.7		245	0.0	56	0.13	0.05	1.90	9	0.13	(C)
DURRA MONGO AKELO	191	5.0	1.6	39.2	142		28	1.4		210	0.0	48	0.11	0.04	1.63	7	0.11	(C)
DURRA M.AKELO+FISH+SAUCE	108	4.2	1.6	19.2														(L)
DURRA MONGO APWOTO	153	3.3	1.9	30.6	95		18	1.0		140		32	0.07	0.03	1.09	4	0.08	(C)
DURRA/MAIZE M.APWOTO	86	2.4	1.0	16.9	92_C		13_C	1.4_C			0.2_C	19_C	0.05_C	0.03_C	0.62_C	4_C	0.08_C	(C)
DURRA MEAL	367	8.2	3.2	76.4	237		46	2.4		350_A		80	0.28	0.09	3.40	14	0.20_M	(F)
DURRA PORRIDGE	36	0.8	0.3	7.6	24		5	0.2		35		8	0.03	0.01	0.30	1	0.02	(C)
DURRA PORRIDGE+SUGAR	60	0.8	0.3	13.4	22_C		5_C	0.2_C		32_C		7_C	0.03_C	0.01_C	0.27_C	1_C	0.02_C	(C)
MACARONI DRY	375	11.8	1.3	77.8	169	48_A	23	1.5	8_A	197_A	0.0_A	149_A	0.09_A	0.06_A	1.73_A	0_A	0.20_M	(F)
MACARONI COOK	151	4.7	0.9	30.9	67	18_A	8	0.6	1_A	61_A	0.0_A	41_A	0.01_A	0.04_A	0.29_A	0_A	0.19_M	(F)
MAIZE ASIDA	183	4.7	1.9	36.7	109		9	2.1			0.7	24	0.10	0.03	0.72	17	0.10	(C)
MAIZE DRY GRAINS	369	8.6	4.3	73.9	182		6	2.8			5.0		0.36	0.08	1.40	33	0.20_M	(F)

FOOD TABLES FOR THE SOUTHERN SUDANESE POPULATION

ALIMENTS (100 gr)	ENG Cal	PRO g	LIP g	GLU g	Ph mg	Mg mg	Ca mg	Fe mg	Na mg	K mg	Asc mg	Try mg	B1 mg	B2 mg	Nia mg	VIA IU	VIE mg	ref
CEREALS AND GRAINS																		
MAIZE DRY ROASTED	392	8.0	4.8	79.2	270		2	3.0				0	0.02	0.09	2.20	0	0.19$_M$	(F)
MAIZE FR RAW	111	3.5	1.0	22.1	111	48	3	0.1	0	280	12.0	21	0.15	0.12	1.76	200	0.28$_M$	(A)
MAIZE FR BOILED	106	3.3	1.0	21.0	89	22	3	0.6	0	196	9.0	20	0.12	0.10	1.40	200	0.19$_M$	(A)
MAIZE FR ROASTED	150	2.7	1.3	29.8	150	65	4	0.1	0	378	8.1	28	0.13	0.13	1.80	200	0.19$_M$	(C)
MAIZE KISRA (CREPE)	256	6.5	2.7	51.4	153		12	2.9			1.2	33	0.14	0.05	1.01	24	0.13	(C)
MAIZE MONGO AKELO	219	5.6	2.2	44.0	131		10	2.5			0.9	28	0.12	0.04	0.86	29	0.11	(C)
MAIZE MONGO APWOTO	146	3.7	1.5	29.4	87		7	1.7			0.6	19	0.08	0.03	0.58	13	0.08	(C)
MAIZE MEAL	365	9.3	3.8	73.4	218		17	4.2			3.0	47$_A$	0.30	0.08	1.80	42	0.20$_M$	(F)
MAIZE PORRIDGE	36	0.9	0.4	7.3	218		2	0.4			0.3	5	0.02	0.01	0.14	3	0.02	(C)
RICE COOK	117	2.4	0.6	25.4	42	8	4	0.3	2	38	0.0		0.02	0.01	1.80$_E$		0.19$_M$	(D)
RICE DRY GRAINS	354	7.6	1.7	77.6	100	28	10	0.8	4	120	0.0		0.06	0.03	2.80$_E$		0.35	(D)
SPAGHETTI COOK	109	3.4	0.4	23.0	50	20	8	0.4	1	61	0.0	41	0.01	0.01	0.30	0	0.19$_M$	(A)
WHEAT MEAL	357	12.4	1.8	72.9	279	113$_A$	54	6.1	3$_A$	370$_A$	0.0$_A$	160$_A$	0.36	0.09	3.80	0	1.00$_B$	(F)

FOOD TABLES FOR THE SOUTHERN SUDANESE POPULATION

ALIMENTS (100 gr)	ENG Cal	PRO g	LIP g	GLU g	Ph mg	Mg mg	Ca mg	Fe mg	Na mg	K mg	Asc mg	Try mg	B1 mg	B2 mg	Nia mg	VitA IU	VitE mg	ref
VEGETABLES AND PULSES																		
BROAD BEAN	354	26.2	1.3	59.4	301		104	6.7			1.6	162	0.38	0.24	2.10	217		(F)
CABBAGE FR RAW	32	1.7	0.1	6.0	40	13_A	47	0.7	20_A	233_A	54.0	10_A	0.04	0.04	0.30	147	0.25_M	(F)
CABBAGE FR COOK	22	1.0	0.2	4.0	17	21	42	0.3	13	151	24.0	3	0.02	0.02	0.10	120	0.20_M	(A)
CARROT FR RAW	44	1.2	0.3	9.0	37	15	39	1.2	56	300	9.0	9	0.06	0.06	0.60_A	9999_A	0.25_M	(D)
CARROT FR COOK	32	0.6	0.3	6.4	26	10	26	0.6	35	200	4.0	7	0.05	0.05	0.50_A	9999_A	0.20_M	(D)
CAULIFLOWER FR RAW	28	2.5	0.3	3.9	54	17	20	0.6	16	328	70.0	25	0.11	0.10	0.70_A	60_A	0.15_B	(D)
CAULIFLOWER FR COOK	24	2.2	0.3	3.1	42	15	16	0.4	10	220	45.0	30	0.10	0.10	0.60_A	60_A	0.10_B	(D)
CHICKPEA DRY RAW	366	19.6	3.7	63.5	127	130_D	252	11.1	26_A	797_A	0.0_M	223	0.48	0.16	1.80	100		(F)
CHICKPEA DRY COOK	373	18.5	3.7	64.3	250_D	130_D	123_D	8.2	20_D	400_D	0.0_D		0.38	0.14	1.80			(F)
CHILI FR RED	48	1.1	0.1	10.7	78		5	1.2			99.9		0.04	0.05	2.00	500	0.25_M	(S)
CHILI DRY RED	364	13.9	9.4	56.0	190	538	130_A	7.8_A	374_A	1203_A	12.0		0.00	0.20	0.50	1768	0.20_M	(W)
COWPEA LVS.FR RAW	55	4.7	0.3	8.3	62		256	5.7			5.6		0.20	0.37	2.10	9999	0.25_M	(F)
COWPEA LVS.FR COOK (1)	108	5.6	6.4	7.1	76		104	5.2									0.20_M	(F)
COWPEA LVS.DRY RAW	338	22.6	3.2	54.6	348		1555	12.0			8.6						0.20_M	(F)
COWPEA SEEDS FR RAW	130	9.0	0.8	21.8	172	92	27	2.3	2	541	29.0	90	0.43	0.13	1.60	370		(A)
COWPEA SEEDS FR COOK	112	8.1	0.8	18.1	146	78_C	24	2.1	1	379	17.5	81	0.03	0.11	1.38	350		(A)
COWPEA SEEDS DRY RAW	352	22.8	1.5	61.7	426	230	74	5.8	35	1024		228	1.05	0.21	2.20	30		(A)
COWPEA SEEDS DRY COOK	78	5.1	0.3	13.8	95	50_C	17	1.3	8	229		51	0.16	0.04	0.40	10		(A)
CUCUMBER RAW	15	0.8	0.1	3.4	30	10_A	13	0.5	6_A	160_A	14.0	4_A	0.02	0.01	0.03	0	0.25_M	(F)
EGGPLANT FR RAW	37	1.0	0.2	7.7	26	16_A	14	1.3	2_A	214_A	0.9	11_A	0.05	0.05	0.50	57	0.25_M	(F)
EGGPLANT FR COOK	28	1.0	0.2_A	5.6	29	16_A	13	0.4	1_A	150_A	0.3_A	9_A	0.05_A	0.04_A	0.50_A	10_A	0.20_M	(A)
EGGPLANT DRY RAW	351	15.7	2.0	67.5													0.20_M	(F)
GARLIC FR RAW	143	5.2	0.1	30.2	195		33	1.7	19_A	529_A	11.0		0.25_A	0.07_A	0.48_A	0_A	0.25_M	(F)
GARLIC FR COOK	105	3.3	0.1	22.6	157		29	1.4	13	370	7.0		0.20	0.05	0.40	0	0.20_M	(C)
GREEN VEGE.LVS.FR RAW	46	5.0	0.7	5.0			250	4.0			100.0		0.10	0.30	1.50	3000	0.25_M	(Z)

ALIMENTS (100 gr) -	ENG Cal	PRO g	LIP g	GLU g	Ph mg	Mg mg	Ca mg	Fe mg	Na mg	K mg	Asc mg	Try mg	B1 mg	B2 mg	Nia mg	ViA IU	ViE mg	ref
VEGETABLES AND PULSES																		
GREEN VEGE.LVS.FR COOK	41	5.0	0.8	2.6			219	4.7			50.0		0.08	0.28	1.40	2000	0.20	(C)
GROUNDNUT BUTTER	597	25.6	47.2	18.0	425	173	61	6.0	120	820	0.0	330	0.12	0.13	16.20	0		(A)
GROUNDNUT DRY RAW	580	23.2	44.8	23.0	409		49	3.8	2	720	0.1	321	0.79	0.14	15.50	25		(F)
GROUNDNUT DRY BOILED	247	16.0	8.3	26.3	260		45	5.1					0.44	0.16	14.00		7.70	(F)
GROUNDNUT DRY ROASTED	634	23.2	56.9	21.7	324		42	3.4	2	740	0.1	335	0.45	0.11	15.30	0	7.70	(F)
JUTE LVS.FR RAW	70	4.5	0.3	12.4	122		360	7.2			80.0		0.15	0.53	1.20	9999	0.25	(F)
JUTE LVS.FR COOK	39	1.5	2.6	2.3	40	51		3.4			6.0						0.20	(F)
JUTE LVS.DRY RAW	291	19.0	1.6	50.1	525		1540	8.0			8.0		0.30	1.00	2.60	9999	0.25	(C)
JUTE LVS./MEAT SAUCE	23	1.9	0.1	3.7	46	18	43	0.7	1	112	5.0	11	0.01	0.04	0.70	111	0.06	(C)
KIDNEY BEAN DRY RAW	344	21.7	1.5	60.9	323	163	120	8.2	10	984	0.1	808	0.27	0.16	2.40	17		(F)
KIDNEY BEAN DRY COOK	147	5.9	5.7	17.9	129		46	1.9	3	340		78	0.11	0.06	0.70	0		(A)
LENTIL DRY SPLIT RAW	325	25.8	1.8	58.8	271		24	10.6	30	790	0.0	222	0.47	0.21	1.30	100		(F)
LENTIL DRY SPLIT COOK	78	5.7	0.4	12.9	60		6	2.3	7	174	0.0	49	0.07	0.04	0.27	22		(C)
LETTUCE	24	1.2	0.2	4.3	40		26	0.7	9	264	10.0	13	0.05	0.08	0.40	1900	0.06	(A)
OKRA FR RAW	46	2.1	0.2	8.2	90	41	84	1.2	3	249	47.0	24	0.04	0.08	0.60	388	0.25	(F)
OKRA FR COOK	35	2.0	0.3	6.0	41		92	0.5	2	174	20.5	29	0.12	0.18	0.90	490	0.20	(A)
OKRA FR/FISH SAUCE	23	3.2	0.6	1.2	42		27	0.5		35	4.0	46	0.04	0.05	0.88	98	0.10	(C)
OKRA FR/MEAT SAUCE	26	4.4	0.4	1.2	30		22	0.7		35	0.0	4	0.05	0.06	1.10	98	0.06	(C)
OKRA DRY COOK	65	2.2	1.6	10.4	68		84	0.8									0.20	(F)
OKRA DRY/FISH SAUCE	24	3.3	0.6	1.4	45		18	0.5			0.0	48	0.01	0.01	0.80		0.08	(C)
OKRA DRY/MEAT SAUCE	50	4.6	0.5	7.0	41		102	4.3			1.0	12	0.05	0.07	1.54	28	0.04	(C)
OKRA DRY POWDER	329	10.7	0.8	69.7	390		968	26.4			10.0	123	0.26	0.43	4.60	283	0.25	(F)
ONION FR RAW	44	1.2	0.1	9.6	45	16	27	0.8	7	180	11.0	18	0.02	0.04	0.20	40	0.26	(F)
ONION FR COOK	32	1.2	0.1	6.5	29	18	24	0.4	7	110	5.5	18	0.03	0.03	0.20	40	0.26	(A)
ONION FRIED	94	1.2	7.0	6.5	29	18	24	0.4	7	110	5.5	18	0.03	0.03	0.20	40		(C)

FOOD TABLES FOR THE SOUTHERN SUDANESE POPULATION

ALIMENTS (100 gr)	ENG Cal	PRO g	LIP g	GLU g	Ph mg	Mg mg	Ca mg	Fe mg	Na mg	K mg	Asc mg	Try mg	B1 mg	B2 mg	Nia mg	VitA IU	VitE mg	ref
VEGETABLES AND PULSES																		
ONION IMMATURED+LVS.RAW	26	1.3	0.1	4.9	24		90	0.6	5	231	1.7	16	0.05	0.04	0.40	0	0.25	(F)
PIGEONPEA DRY RAW	352	19.5	1.3	65.5	285		161	1.5					0.72	0.14	2.90	92		(F)
PUMKIN FR RAW	27	1.0	0.1	5.5	32	12	25	1.4	1	340	8.0	13	0.05	0.02	0.50	5942	0.25	(F)
PUMKIN FR COOK	18	1.0	0.1	3.2	29	9	18	1.3	1	323	4.0	13	0.03	0.01	0.15	4518	0.25	(C)
PURSLANE FR RAW	29	2.4	0.3	4.2	31		104	1.4			58.0		0.03	0.15	0.50	2500	0.25	(F)
PURSLANE FR COOK	19	1.2	0.3	2.8	24		86	1.2			12.0		0.02	0.06	0.40	2100	0.20	(A)
RADISH RAW	21	1.1	0.1	4.0	30	15	42	1.0	18	322	2.6	4	0.03	0.03	0.03	10	0.25	(F)
SPINACH FR RAW	33	3.2	0.3	4.3	51	88	93	3.1	71	470	5.1	51	0.10	0.20	0.60	8100	2.50	(A)
SPINACH FR COOK	29	3.0	0.3	3.6	38	88	93	2.2	50	324	28.0	47	0.07	0.17	0.50	1800	2.50	(A)
SQUASH FR RAW	22	1.1	0.1	4.2	29	16	28	0.4	1	202	2.2	9	0.05	0.09	0.10	410	0.25	(A)
SQUASH FR COOK	17	0.9	0.1	3.1	25		25	0.4	1	141	1.0	7	0.05	0.08	0.80	390	0.20	(A)
SWEETPOTATO PALE RAW	122	1.6	0.2	28.5	38	31	33	2.0	10	243	37.0	29	0.09	0.04	0.70	125	0.25	(F)
SWEETPOTATO YELLOW RAW	122	1.6	0.2	28.5	38	31	33	2.0	10	243	37.0	29	0.09	0.04	0.70	2091	0.25	(F)
SWEETPOTATO COOK	104	1.9	0.2	23.7				0.3									0.20	(F)
SWEETPOTATO FLOUR	344	12.5	0.2	73.1														(F)
TAMIA	431	10.0	31.0	26.3	153		72	6.1										(S)
TOMATO RIPE RAW	25	1.0	0.2	4.8	24	14	10	0.6	3	244	26.0	10	0.06	0.04	0.60	750	0.27	(F)
TOMATO DRY	290	12.1	2.0	55.8	279	155	403	7.3	3934	3518	41.0	104	0.52	0.40	13.50	1310	0.20	(A)
TOMATO KETCHUP	113	2.0	0.4	25.4	50	21	22	0.8	1042	363	1.5		0.09	0.07	1.60	1400		(A)
TOMATO PASTE	92	3.4	0.4	18.6	70	20	27	3.5	38	888	4.9		0.20	0.12	3.10	2300		(A)

FOOD TABLES FOR THE SOUTHERN SUDANESE POPULATION

ALIMENTS (100 gr).	ENG Cal	PRO g	LIP g	GLU g	Ph mg	Mg mg	Ca mg	Fe mg	Na mg	K mg	Asc mg	Try mg	B1 mg	B2 mg	Nia mg	VitA IU	VitE mg	ref
FRUITS																		
APPLE RIPE	55	0.3	0.4	12.6	12	6	7	0.5	3	144	12.0		0.04	0.03	0.10_P	20_P	0.20_D	(D)
BANANA RIPE	89	1.5	0.1	20.6	21	32_A	9	1.4	2_A	370_A	0.9	18_A	0.03	0.03	0.80	200	0.45_D	(F)
DATE FR RIPE	158	1.6	0.6	36.6	350		34	6.0			30.0			0.54	5.40	242	0.48_M	(F)
DATE DRY	327	2.7	0.6	77.6	85	50_B	82	9.4	35_B	650_B	3.3_B	13	0.06	0.15	1.80	50	0.42_M	(F)
GRAPE	73	0.7	0.3	16.8	20	9	18	0.5	2	192	4.2		0.05	0.03	0.30_A	50_P	0.48_M	(D)
GRAPEFRUIT RIPE	44	0.7	0.2	9.8	17	10	20	0.3	2	131	45.0	1	0.05	0.03	0.20_P	42_P	0.25	(D)
GUAVA RIPE	73	1.1	0.4	15.7	31		24	1.2_A	4_A	289_A	326.0	8_A	0.06	0.04	0.30	483	0.48_M	(F)
KARKADEH POWDER	315	21.0	1.3	54.9			1030	16.0									0.42_M	(S)
LIME JUICE+SUGAR	50	0.1	0.1	12.1	5	2	5	0.2		25	11.0	1	0.01	0.01	0.07	2		(C)
LIME RIPE	44	0.6	0.8	8.7	21	9_D	19	0.7	2_A	102_A	45.0	3_A	0.03	0.02	0.30	10_A	0.48_M	(F)
MANGO RIPE	67	0.6	0.2	15.8	22	17_D	24	1.2	6_A	175_A	4.2	1_A	0.03	0.05	0.04	5333	0.48_M	(F)
OLIVE	123	0.9	11.0	5.0	17	22	61	1.5	2400_A	91			0.02	0.06	0.00_P	300_A	0.48_M	(D)
ORANGE JUICE	47	0.6	0.2	10.6	15	12	11	0.2	1	157	54.0		0.04	0.03	0.40_A	200_A		(D)
ORANGE RIPE	54	1.0	0.2	12.0	23	14	42	0.4	1	177	50.0	3	0.08	0.04	0.40_A	200_A	0.24	(D)
ORANGE SYRUP	280	0.0	0.0	70.0	30	10	100	10.0	250	500	27.5		0.07	0.08	1.70_W			(D)
ORANGE SYRUP DIL.	56	0.0	0.0	14.0	6	2	20	2.0	50	100	5.5		0.01	0.01	0.46			(C)
PALM RIPE	583	1.9	58.4	12.5	47		82	4.5			12.0		0.20	0.10	1.40	667	0.48_M	(F)
PALM PUREE	260	0.4	27.6	2.6	110		50	2.4			3.0	2	0.05	0.05	0.80	9999	0.48_M	(F)
PAPAYA RIPE	36	0.4	0.1	8.3	15		21	0.6	2_A	234_A	5.2	12_A	0.03	0.03	0.40	1583	0.48_M	(F)
PINEAPPLE RIPE	52	0.4	0.1	12.4	14	17_D	16	0.4	2_D	173_D	34.0	5_A	0.06	0.03	0.10	150	0.48_M	(F)
PINEAPPLE CANNED	95	0.4	0.2	22.9	7	8	13	0.3	1	75	7.0	4_A	0.07	0.02	0.30	60		(D)
SWEET MELON	31	0.8	0.2	6.5	18	15	18	0.4	19	260	10.0	1_A	0.02	0.05	0.50_P	500_P	0.48_M	(D)
TANGERINE	48	0.7	0.3	10.6	20	11	33	0.3	1	210	30.0		0.06	0.03	0.20_P	383_P	0.48_M	(D)
WATER MELON	25	0.5	0.1	5.5	9	8_A	8	0.3	1_A	100_A	8.0		0.04	0.05	0.10	417	0.10_D	(F)

FOOD TABLES FOR THE SOUTHERN SUDANESE POPULATION

ALIMENTS (100 gr).	ENG Cal	PRO g	LIP g	GLU g	Ph mg	Mg mg	Ca mg	Fe mg	Na mg	K mg	Asc mg	Try mg	B1 mg	B2 mg	Nia mg	VitA IU	VitE mg	ref
SUGARS AND SWEETS																		
CANDY	380	0.8	0.1	9.4	147$_A$		94$_A$	1.4$_A$	33$_A$	269$_A$	0.0$_A$		0.02$_A$	0.14$_A$	0.33$_A$	13$_A$		(0)
HONEY	322	0.4	0.0	80.1	4		11	0.6	5$_A$	51	1.0$_A$		0.00$_A$	0.04$_A$	0.26$_A$	0$_A$		(F)
ICE CREAM	202	3.9	11.7	20.2	117	13$_A$	140	0.1	110	99	2.0$_A$	57$_A$	0.04	0.25	0.17$_A$	520$_A$		(0)
JAM	283	0.5	0.1	7.0	12		12	0.2	12	12	5.0		0.02	0.02	0.18$_A$	11$_A$		(0)
RIVER GRASS STALK	58	0.5	0.0	14.0			25	1.0			0.0$_P$		0.00			0		(C)
SORGHUM STALK	58	0.5	0.0	14.0			25	1.0			0.0$_P$		0.00			0		(Z)
SUGAR	399			99.7			1	0.0										(0)
SUGAR BROWN	344	0.0	0.0	88.8														(0)
SUGAR CANE	69	0.6	0.1	16.5	6		8	1.4			3.0		0.02	0.01	0.10	0$_P$		(F)

ALIMENTS (100 gr)	ENG Cal	PRO g	LIP g	GLU g	Ph mg	Mg mg	Ca mg	Fe mg	Na mg	K mg	Asc mg	Try mg	B1 mg	B2 mg	Nia mg	ViA IU	ViE mg	ref
MISCELLANEOUS																		
ATABOBA LOCAL BEER TH	117	2.6		21.2														(F)
BEER (IMPORTED)	35	0.3	0.0	4.0	11	5	8	0.1	3	40	0.0		0.00	0.02	0.21 A	0 A		(G)
COCA COLA	44	0.0	0.0	11.0	15		4		6	1	0.0		0.00	0.00		0		(G)
MERISSA LOCAL BEER CL	31	0.5		3.6	7		1	0.6					0.04	0.05	0.40			(F)
MERISSA+SUGAR	83	0.4		5.1	6		1	0.5					0.03	0.04	0.34			(C)
TEA LVS.DRY	320		0.0	80.1			11	1.6		4526				0.95	3.90			(A)
TEA+MILK FR+SUGAR	66	1.4	1.5	11.6	38	6	47	0.1	200	60	0.2	21	0.01	0.06	0.04	61		(C)
TEA+MILK POWDER+SUGAR	87	1.6	1.6	16.6	42	6	54	0.0	24	80	0.2	22	0.02	0.09	0.04	68		(C)
TEA+SUGAR	86			21.5			0	0.1	90					0.20	0.18			(C)
PEPPER (BLACK)	347	12.0	7.0	59.0	130	45	120	10.0	7	42			0.04	0.20	1.00			(G)
SALT	0	0.0	0.0	0.0			253	0.1	9999	4	0.0		0.00	0.00	0.00	9999		(A)
VINEGAR	0	0.0	0.0	0.0	20	16	15	0.4	20	90								(G)

5. SOME LIGHTS ON THE DAILY ACTIVITIES OF A.D.E. TEAM
by Z. L. Ostrowski and G. Habib

The A.D.E. Research Centre was established at the Sobat-Nile Mouth, about 25 km southern of Malakal (see map 6). The camp was surrounding by the Nile and Sobat River.

The A.D.E. team was composed by two medical doctors (one of them French, another Sudanese), two nutritionists (one of them Dutch), two medical assistants, a laboratory technician, a social worker, a translator and a driver/translator). The team was supervised by two paediatricians (one, French and one Sudanese) and a French medical Doctor (nutritionist and statistician).

The team worked every day in the field, except Wednesday which was allocated for special consultation in the A.D.E. Dispensary in Obang (for pregnant women and children).

The work started early in the morning by preparing the questionnaires, files, drugs and equipment. The whole team (composed by a medical doctor, a nutritionist, a laboratory technician, a translator and a driver/translator) moved always by car or by boat to the study area. Every 6 – 8 weeks two supplementary French doctors reinforced the team during a period of 2-3 weeks.

Because the climate in the study area is a typical tropical one (with dry and rainy seasons), during the rainy season, the unique mean of transport was the speed boat. To reach the villages under study the team needed to walk in high grass or through water, which reaches sometimes the knees. The water was muddy and the soil sticky. The heavy gum boots make the walking really hard because they stiff in the mud.

In the dry season a 4-wheels drive Landcrusier «Toyota» was used. To reach the villages it took about 30 minutes up to 3 hours. On arrival in the villages, all children laughing and happy shouted «*Kawajat*» (*). They run and helped the team by carrying their bags and equipment.

When the team tried to identify the case under study, nobody can imagine how difficult it was! In the villages all huts (tukuls) are hazardless scattered. All tukuls looks similar for a stranger. With the help of well done lists, drawings and registers it was possible to identify the cases because each pregnant women and

* .«*Kawajat*» *mean white people*

the child had his own number and the date of examination noted. The Sudanese nutritionist (Elisabeth Ojaba, from a Madi tribe) helped very much in the identification of the cases. She was permanent in the study area since 4 years, so she knows all cases and without her help sometimes it was impossible to find the mother and/or the child, especially if the person was not in his own hut.

The nutritionist as well as the translator (Luciano, a Shilluk native from this area) was a great help because he also worked with the team from the beginning of the study. But, when he sometimes disappeared, the team faced often a lot of troubles.

After the identification of the case under study, a place for examination was found mostly under a tree or inside a hut. Sometimes even the team worked inside a luak (special hut for animals). The mate on which we sat was made of leafs of fine branches of palm trees. *One day, we have been invited to a new constructed hut, not yet used. Sitting on the ground covered with a piece of tissue, the medical doctor examined the babies putting them on his knees. After an hour of examinations, one of the baby urinated on the knees. When the doctor stands up and the mother removed the tissue we discovered that the doctor sat on 7 scorpions!*

Each member of the team has its own role. The cooperation between them was very important especially to fill the files for each child and each examination. Usually the medical doctor begins the work by codification the case on a well prepared questionnaire. Then he asked whether the child received any treatment at the last examination. If any, he asked after how many days he got cured. The following questions concerned the diseases the child had got since the last examination. Then the child was examined with special attention for: pallor, eye infection, oedema, heart sounds, femoral pulse, umbilical infection, splenomegalia hepatomegalia skin rash, etc...

The general status of the child and the diagnosis as well as any treatment been given was codified. The nature of any investigation was noted. Then the nutritionist begins the food recall during the last 24 hours. At the end anthropometric measurements have been taken: weight, length, skin folds, head, arm and calf circumferences, number of teeth and size of fontanel. There were a lot of difficulties for taking these anthropometric measurements from the children who were scared and fighting, especially at age two years. The investigation has been taken at the end of examination. Some of them have been done at place (for ex. uristix), others like blood samples have been analysed in the A.D.E. Laboratory in Sobat or send to the University Laboratory in

Khartoum, Paris or London. At the end of the survey, if necessary, treatment was given and special advises have been explained to the mother. Any treatment and food supply was registered.

Also, all ill people from the villages who came seeking medical advice were examined and treatment was given immediately. Sometimes also food supply was given (gived from EEC). If these people needed some investigation and/or a follow up, they have been asked to come to A.D.E. Centre in Sobat where a good number of investigation could be done : e.g. urine, stool, complete haemogramme (by Coulter Counter S5), serum chemistry (by Kem-O-mat). Urgent cases have been taken by the team to the A.D.E. Centre or have been sending to the hospital in Malakal.

Beside the treatment of ill people, health and nutrition education was given when needed. Some of the traditional believes were a great obstacle to the investigation, like fear from giving a blood sample.

The weather in the study area is hot, and during the dry season, very dusty with a temperature between 35°C to 40°C. The team worked sweating all the time, which obliges them to change the whole wears and under wears every day and use showers at least twice a day.

Often, the team came back to the camp after 5 - 8 hours of hard work in the field. After few minutes of rest, they began to analyse the blood samples which could not be done at side. The results were codified, some investigations which could not be done in the A.D.E. Laboratory were prepared in micro tubes, well preserved in a cool chain, and sent (every week, if necessary) to Khartoum, Paris and London for further analysis.

Still remained an important work to be compiled: the administration. The medical doctor had to check all the code numbers which identify the child and his mother (submitted to the longitudinal study) : the household number and the number in the village, the code number of the village, number of examination, type of examination... After this work compiled, all symptoms and diagnosis were codified according to WHO codes (56). Then, the medical doctor had to arrange the examination files in each village envelope and in chronically order in respect the other examination for each child. But, the end of the working day was still far, because it was usual that the villagers come in the night awaking the doctor for urgent medical problems.

This description shows one usual day of the A.D.E. team during the longitudinal study. But there were many unusual things that could be happened. One day, for example, the team took the speed boat to a place called Godjak, 3 hours far away from A.D.E. Center. When we just arrived some of the people, who sympathised our team, advised us to go back quickly because there was some armed people of a political movement. The team returned immediately. A trip of six hours by boat under strong sun rays for nothing!

Sometimes, we arrived to a village and we found nobody, except one or two old women who told us that all people left the village because of «tribal fights». When another tribe attacked the village, all young people run away to form a bigger agglomeration in other place. Another time, we found only one small child alone with a small sister or a brother. We tried to recall about its health problem, but usually no enough data were given by the small sister. Once, in the beginning of the rainy season, the Landcrusier stuck in mud and the team had to walk many hours on feet for a long distance (> 20 km) to arrive to the camp extremely tired. Sometimes, the team had a chance to return to the camp in a CCI lorry which carried material for the construction of the Jonglei Canal who might change the life of this people (!).

But nothing could stop the team to follow this study, which might provide data to better resolve the adaptation of these people submitted to the extreme rapid change of their traditional life since thousands of years...

6. THE GENEALOGY OF THE SOUTH-SUDANESE

By Z. L. Ostrowski

An extended family system still exists on the whole African continent. The traditional great family was a must to continue the existence of the different ethnicities. Due to high mortality and morbidity rate, a family needed to produce at least 7 to 10 and more children per wife. Moreover, to increase the place of the family in the tribe it was important to have a great family size. Polygamy allowed developing the family size up to a few hundred members over only three generations.

In the South-Sudan we observed that in the Dinka and Nuer societies the knowledge of the family is mostly horizontal. The smallest genealogical unity, described by Evans-Pritchard (11) as «thok dwiel» (for the Nuer) can reach up to three or five generations. A clan, as a group of people having the same ancestor, is therefore a genealogical structure and have their own rules (no intermarriage or sexual rapports). An example of a typical extended Dinka family could be described thanks to data obtained from Dr Akec Khoc and his wife Anti (see Genealogical tree 1).

Contrary in the Shilluk society, due to the political system (kingdom) the knowledge of the family could be determined up to ten, twenty and even more generations. The example of the traditional oral transmission of data since a hundred years could be described thanks to data obtained from Dr Lam Akol, a member of the Shilluk royal family (see Genealogical tree 2).

With the help of a logistic support «Dynastree» (computer programme for genealogy and genetics (Ostrowski - 12) it was possible to draw the family trees and to calculate some hereditary traits.

In the tradition of the South-Sudanese, the knowledge even by name, of the members of their family is of great importance. This is why it was possible to develop the two following families.

The family of Akec Khoc is a well known Dinka Bor family. The family is more developed from the maternal branch. The maternal grandfather had three wives, 17 children and 109 grand children. The paternal grandfather had one wife, 5 children and 15 grand children. The known number of members in Akec generation was 114 persons (3 died), in the generation of his parents 21 persons (2 died) and in the grandparents generation 4 persons. Only 35 great grand children have been registered (from 11 grand children's families). The total number of Akec family, known to him by names is 174 (8 died).

The family of Anti Ajok (wife of Akec) is also a well known Dinka Bor family. The family is more developed from the paternal branch because of frequent polygamy. The maternal grandfather had one wife, 3 children and 13 great children (included Anti). The paternal grandfather had also one wife, 11 children and 33 grand children (included Anti), because Anti's father had 8 wives and 29 children. The known number of members in Anti generation was 47 persons (11 died), in the generation of her parents 24 persons (5 died) and in the grandparents generation 11 persons. Only 40 great grand children have been registered (from 6 grand children's families) and 4 great great grand children. Anti's family (known to her by names) count 164 (23 died) plus 23 great uncles and aunts. Up to the present, Dr Akec's and Ajok's three generations family count 448 members (34 died).

The family of Dr Lam Akol is a well known Shilluk royal family. The family is first of all developed from the paternal branch the family has existed since the 13th century. The earliest known date of birth being 1298 (21st generation). In this family we found mostly monogamy, only in 3 cases polygamy (2 to 3 wives). The number in the paternal family (included Lam) reached 49 persons, but only 3 persons from the maternal family (until the 2nd generation).

The family of Rebecca (wife of Lam) is also a Shilluk family but the members are known only until the 2nd generation. The number of known members in her family reached only 7. The total family of Lam and Rebecca, until 20 generations family, count 61 members, including their two children.

The royal family tree of the Reth of Shilluk was developed following the indications obtained from Dr Lam Akol and Oriji Kwongo, son of the Reth.

GENEALOGICAL TREE OF THE RETH OF SHILLUK

Generation		First Name	Surname	Birth – Death	
0		Oriji	Kwongo Dak	1987	
1	Reth	Kwongo	Dak Padiat	1946	
2		Dak	Padiat Kwathker	1912	1956
3		Padiat	Kwathker Akwot	1889	1948
4		Kwathker	Akwot Yor	1860	1932
5		Akwot	Yor Kondit	1821	1905
6		Yor	Kondit Kudit	1779	1862
7		Kondit	Kudit Okon	1740	1819
8		Kudit	Okon Tugo	1682	1765
9		Okon Nyaba	Tugo Dhokoth	1643	1708
10		Tugo	Dhokoth Bwoc	1618	1697
11		Dhokoth	Bwoc Diwaad	1595	1669
12		Bwoc	Diwaad Ocolo	1572	1637
13		Diwaad	Ocolo Daag	1554	1618
14		Ocolo	Daag Nyikango	1530	1590
15		Daag	Nyikango Okwa	1511	1565
16		Nyikango	Okwa Mol	1480	1556
17		Okwa	Mol Kolo	1442	1517
18		Mol	Kolo Omaro	1409	1488
19		Kolo	Omaro Nyadhyang	1377	1461
20		Omaro	Nyadhyang	1343	1414
21		Nyadhyang	Nyadhyang	1298	1376

Indications from Dr Lam Akol and Oriji Kwongo

@ Dr Zygmunt L. Ostrowski, Paris, 2012

GENEALOGICAL TREE 1

A Genealogical Tree of a typical extended Dinka family of Dr Akec Khoc

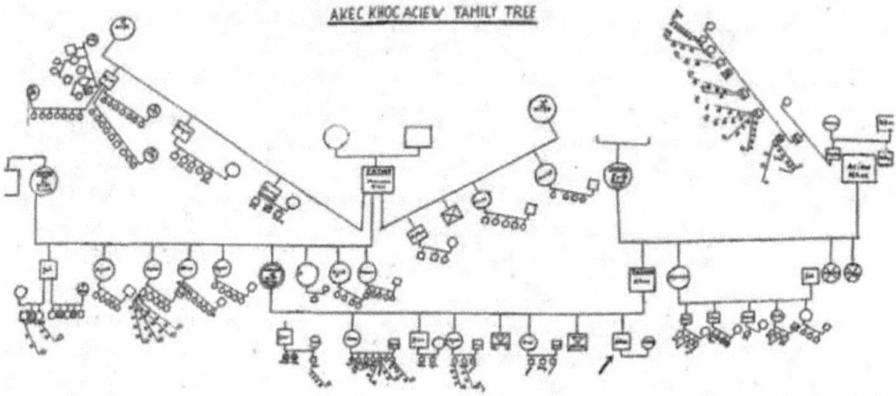

A Genealogical Tree of a typical extended Dinka family of Dr Akec Khoc wife Anti Simon

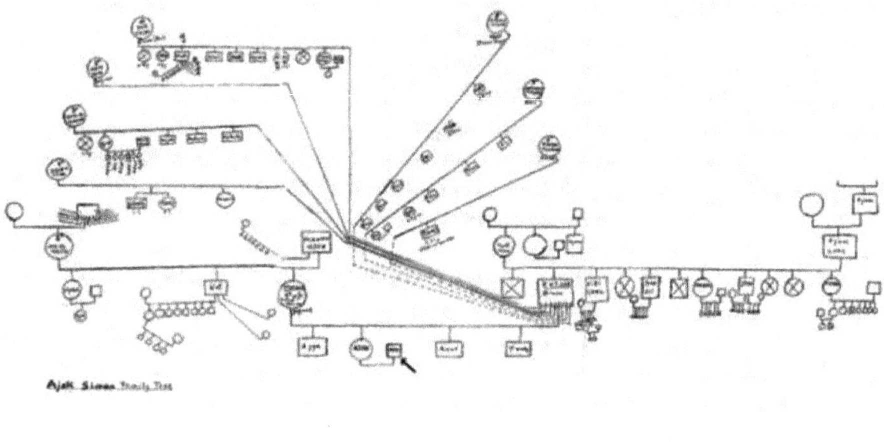

GENEALOGICAL TREE 2

A Genealogical Tree of the Shilluk royal family obtained from Dr Lam Akol

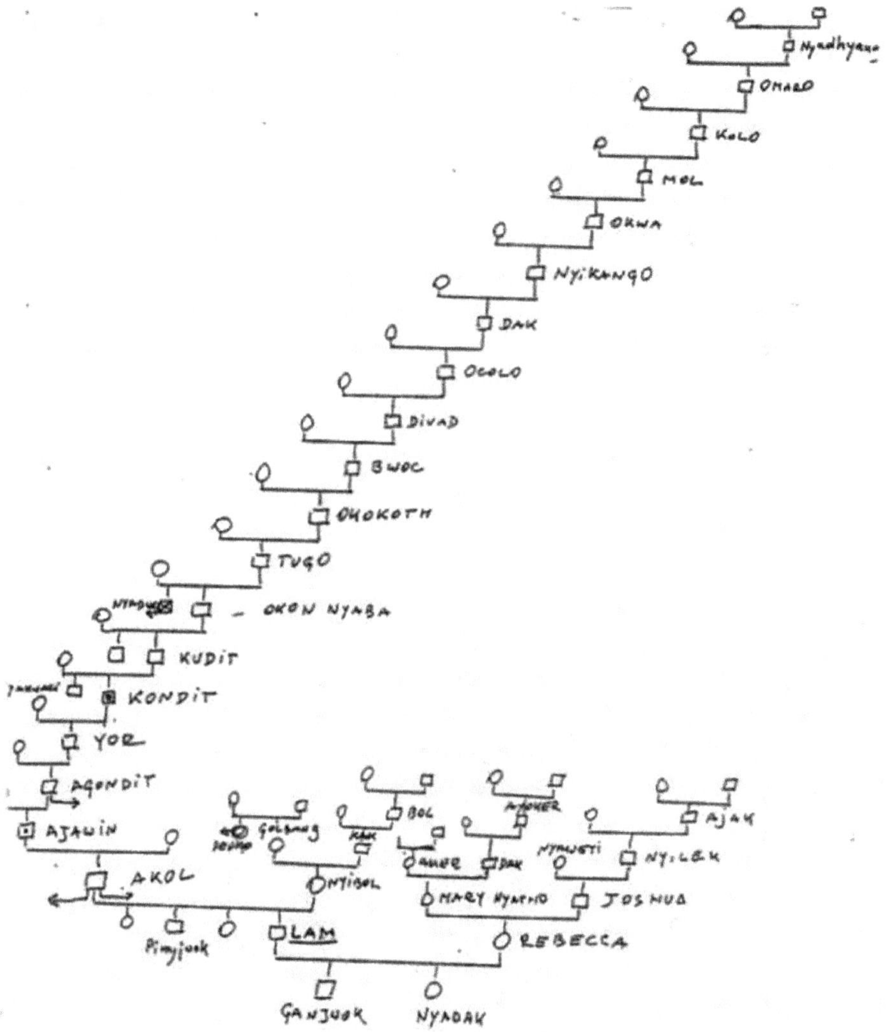

Development of the Genealogical Tree of the Shilluk royal family

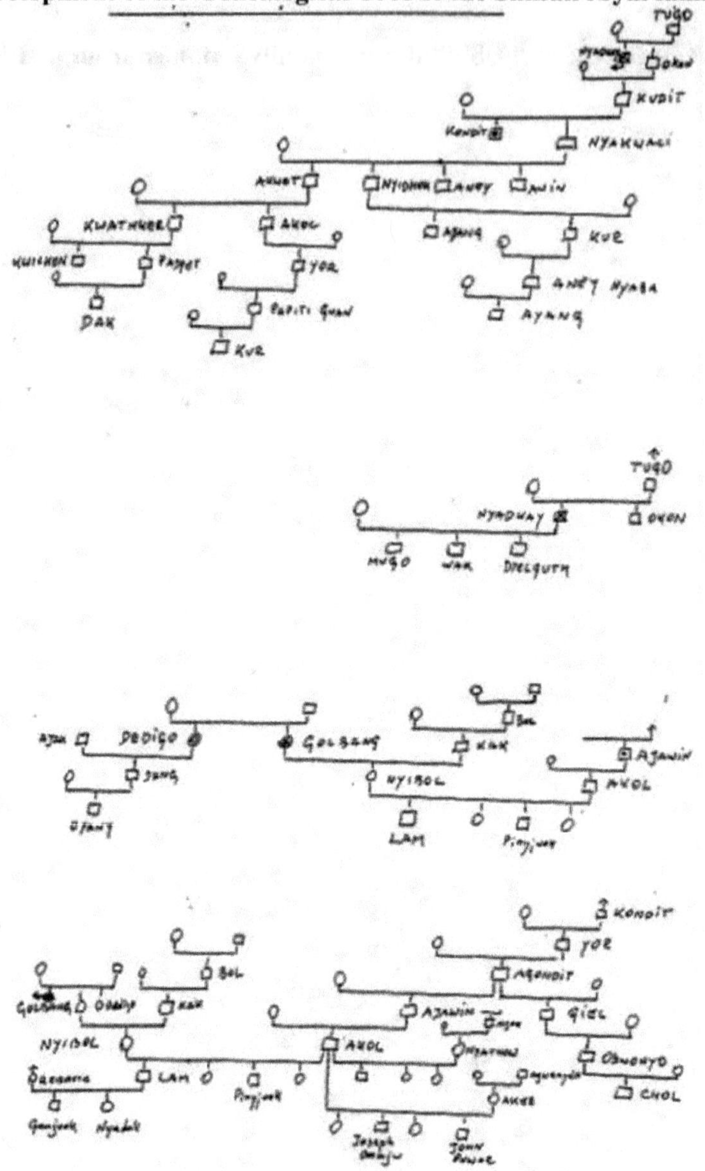

Development of the Genealogical Tree of the Shilluk royal family
Descendant lineage of Dak Nyikango Okwa

```
*Ocolo                DAK NYIKANGO
**Dewad                OCOLO DAK
***Bwoc                 DIWAD OCHOLO
****Dhokoth              BWOC DIWAD
*****Tugo                 DHOKOTH BWOC
******Okon Nyaba           TUGO DHOKOTH
*******Kudit                OKON TUGO
********Kondit               KUDIT OKON
*********Yor                  KONDIT KUDIT
**********Agongdit Lwal        YOR KONDIT
***********Ajawin               AGONDIT YOR
************Akol                 AJAWIN AGONDIT
*************Lam                  AKOL AJAWIN
**************Ganjwok              AKOL AJAWIN
**************Nyadak               AKOL AJAWIN
**************Dominica             AKOL AJAWIN
*************Christine            AKOL AJAWIN
*************Pinyjwok             AKOL AJAWIN
*************Vivianne             AKOL AJAWIN
*************Joseph Omujwok       AJAWIN AGONDIT
*************                     AJAWIN AGONDIT
*************John Onwar           AJAWIN AGONDIT
*************                     AJAWIN AGONDIT
*************                     AJAWIN AGONDIT
*************                     AJAWIN AGONDIT
*************                     AJAWIN AGONDIT
***********Giel                 YOR KONDIT
************Obwonyo              YOR KONDIT
*************Chol                 YOR KONDIT
*******Nyakwaci              KUDIT OKON
********Akwot                 NYAKWACI KUDIT
*********Kwathker              AKWOT NYAKWACI
**********Kwickon               KWATHKER AKWOT
**********                       KWATHKER AKWOT
**********Padyet                KWATHKER AKWOT
***********Dak                   PADYET KWATHKER
************Kwongo                PADYET KWATHKER
*********Akoc                  AKWOT NYAKWACI
**********Yor                   AKOC AKWOT
***********Papiti Gwang          YOR AKOC
************Kur                   PAPITI YOR
********Nyidhok               NYAKWACI KUDIT
********                       NYIDHOK NYAKWACI
*********Kur                   NYIDHOK NYAKWACI
**********Aney Nyaba            KUR NYIDHOK
***********Ayang                 ANEY KUR
*********Ajang                 NYIDHOK NYAKWACI
********Aney                  NYAKWACI KUDIT
********Awin                  NYAKWACI KUDIT
*****Nyadway Fachoda TUGO DHOKOTH
******Mugo                 TUGO DHOKOTH
******Dyelguth Nyutho TUGO DHOKOTH
******Wak                  TUGO DHOKOTH
***Labudo              BWOC DIWAD
```

Development of the Genealogical Tree of the Shilluk royal family
Descendant lineage of Omaro Nyadhyang

```
*Kolo                OMARO NYADHYANG
**Mol                 KOLO OMARO
***Okwa                MOL KOLO
****Nyikango            OKWA MOL
*****Chol                NYIKANGO OKWA
*****Dak                 NYIKANGO OKWA
******Ocolo               DAK NYIKANGO
*******Dewad               OCOLO DAK
********Bwoc                DIWAD OCHOLO
*********Dhokoth             BWOC DIWAD
**********Tugo                DHOKOTH BWOC
***********Okon Nyaba          TUGO DHOKOTH
************Kudit               OKON TUGO
*************Kondit              KUDIT OKON
**************Yor                 KONDIT KUDIT
***************Agongdit Lwal       YOR KONDIT
****************Ajawin              AGONDIT YOR
*****************Akol                AJAWIN AGONDIT
******************Lam                 AKOL AJAWIN
*******************Ganjwok             AKOL AJAWIN
*******************Nyadak              AKOL AJAWIN
*******************Dominica            AKOL AJAWIN
******************Christine           AKOL AJAWIN
******************Pinyjwok            AKOL AJAWIN
******************Vivianne            AKOL AJAWIN
******************Joseph Omujwok      AJAWIN AGONDIT
******************                    AJAWIN AGONDIT
******************John Onwar          AJAWIN AGONDIT
******************                    AJAWIN AGONDIT
******************                    AJAWIN AGONDIT
******************                    AJAWIN AGONDIT
******************                    AJAWIN AGONDIT
****************Giel                YOR KONDIT
*****************Obwonyo             YOR KONDIT
******************Chol                YOR KONDIT
*************Nyakwaci            KUDIT OKON
**************Akwot               NYAKWACI KUDIT
***************Kwathker            AKWOT NYAKWACI
****************Kwickon             KWATHKER AKWOT
*****************                    KWATHKER AKWOT
****************Padyet              KWATHKER AKWOT
*****************Dak                 PADYET KWATHKER
******************Kwongo              PADYET KWATHKER
***************Akoc                AKWOT NYAKWACI
****************Yor                 AKOC AKWOT
*****************Papiti Gwang        YOR AKOC
******************Kur                 PAPITI YOR
**************Nyidhok             NYAKWACI KUDIT
***************                    NYIDHOK NYAKWACI
***************Kur                 NYIDHOK NYAKWACI
****************Aney Nyaba          KUR NYIDHOK
*****************Ayang               ANEY KUR
***************Ajang               NYIDHOK NYAKWACI
**************Aney                NYAKWACI KUDIT
**************Awin                NYAKWACI KUDIT
***********Nyadway Fachoda TUGO DHOKOTH
************Mugo               TUGO DHOKOTH
************Dyelguth Nyutho TUGO DHOKOTH
************Wak                TUGO DHOKOTH
*********Labudo             BWOC DIWAD
*****Nyidoro            NYIKANGO OKWA
```

The paternal lineage of the family Akol Ajawin

Generation	First Name	Surname	Birth - Death	
-1	Ganjwok	Akol Ajawin	1993	
0	Lam	Akol Ajawin	1950	
1	Akol	Ajawin Agongdit	1902	1981
2	Ajawin	Agongdit Yor	1858	1942
3	Agongdit Lwal	Yor Kondit	1821	1904
4	Yor	Kondit Kudit	1779	1862
5	Kondit	Kudit Okon	1740	1819
6	Kudit	Okon Tugo	1682	1765
7	Okon Nyaba	Tugo Dhokoth	1643	1708
8	Tugo	Dhokoth Bwojd	1618	1697
9	Dhokoth	Bwoj Diwaad	1595	1669
10	Bwoc	Diwaad Ocolo	1572	1637
11	Diwaad	Ocolo Daag	1554	1618
12	Ocolo	Daag Nyikango	1530	1590
13	Daag	Nyikango Okwa	1511	1565
14	Nyikango	Okwa Mol	1480	1556
15	Okwa	Mol Kolo	1442	1517
16	Mol	Kolo Omaro	1409	1488
17	Kolo	Omaro Nyadhyang	1377	1461
18	Omaro	Nyadhyang	1343	1414
19	Nyadhyang	Nyadhyang	1298	1376

The maternal lineage of the family Akol Ajawin

Generation	First Name	Surname	Birth – Death
-1	Ganjwok	Akol Ajawin	1993
0	Rebecca	Joshua Okwaci	1960
1	Mary Nyathow	Dak	1931
2	Aker	Aker	1895

7. THE HISTORY OF GOJAK VILLAGE
By James Gatluak

Gojak is a village near the Sobat River (map 7). The meaning of GOJAK was explained to James J. Gatluak by Nyong Koal in the presence of Nyago Korial (chief Thanyapore), Aban Waajan (chief), Ayul Ayiang Dak and Nyul Nyawale.

«Gojak» is a Dinka word. It derives from two words: «gok» means "durra which is still growing", «jak» means "white durra which is ripe".

There is no data when Gojak was established. There are tales saying that people have lived since five generations before the English ruled. Gojak was a Dinka village. It was taken by the Shilluk through terrible wars. The Shilluk belongs to a section called «oputhiwan». They were first in Ogot but a quarrel arose between them which were terrible and their grandfather brought them to Abejogo. The grandfather «Akuot» bought land in the village Panyiduaw, but the enemy was stiil near. One of their grandfathers, Akol Wu Kuath Ker, went further to Thanyapore village where quarrels with Dinka followed thousands of times and where they have been helped by the Nuer from the other side. Dinka became tired of wars and they fled to the Dinka land. Some have remained up to the present days, living together with the Shilluk, near the Gojak forest. During the English rule, Akol Wa Kuath Kiir, who reigned over the Shilluk land as a king, was killed by the English people.

The people of Gojak claim to be relatives to the actually ruling king. Othow Nyanyireth, the present chief, explained the relationship by the fact that «Nyireth» indicates that any person who bears this name is a relative to the royal family.

Regarding the Court or Law, the English changed some of the kings rights (the king have no written documents). Before, the king could kill a person without any redress. But though they are guarded by law, their conservativeness makes them still law abiding and obedient to the king's rule.

There are differences between the old generations and the new one. Now, the people started to understand the meaning of money as a support of life. They can get cash selling vegetables, okra, lemons, tomatoes etc. When there is rain they grow durra for food and vegetables for cash. Also fishing and making nets increase their cash. The Shilluk started doing something to get money and this is unlike the old Shilluk who depended only upon the mercy of nature for food.

The chief of the village explained how the Shilluk accepted the Dinka and how they are living together. The Dinka became friendly people and are Shilluk speaking because most of them adapted part of Shilluk customs. «The Dinka are clever men anywhere. Now all together we are guarded by the same Sudanese law and we abide within that law, only we are different by blood».

The second village's name, close to Gojak, but far from the Sobat River is an old name. It does not represent anything. Following belief, a mad man who used blow a horn of an animal brought the name Thanyapore.

Gojak is a group of 12 villages with a number of huts and luaks lying along the Sobat River. The huts were constructed in mud mixed with cow dung and grass, mostly in a circle around a big tree. Each group of huts had a place for idols.

In the surveyed Gajak and Thanyapore village, 34 families have been visited. The total number of people living in 69 tukuls was 230 (58 men, 54 women and 118 children). The mortality between children was important: 188 children died. The families had 12 luaks with 200 cows (40 bulls, 62 calves, 42 heifers, 67 pregnant cows and 49 milking cows), 178 goats and 83 sheep. There were as well twelve pirogues and 22 fishing nets.

8. THE HISTORY OF POTTERY

By James Gatluak

Many thousands of years ago, people knew nothing about pottery. Once, a herding boy started the use of the calabash. The calabash is a big bulk fruit which was the only bitter fruit that could not be eaten. The boy cut this fruit one day into two halves and played with it while he was looking after his father's cows. After he finished playing he threw the fruit into the river.

Two days later he returned to the same place carrying other calabashes to play with. While looking into the river he saw his two halves of the calabash floating on the water. They were very clean inside because the water had taken away the dirty unwanted flesh away. The boy took the two clean halves and dried them in the sun. In the evening he took them home and he milked his cows into one. Other boys copied or imitated the same idea. Every one of the village boys cut himself two halves of the calabash. So the halves of calabash spread rapidly in the Nuer land.

Women saw the calabash and found that it was good and they asked their sons to cut more of this fruit. This calabash was used for drinking water and for milking cows. One day a cow broke Deng's calabash. So the boy made a mud calabash. But the milk destroyed the mud calabash rapidly. Another day the boy left the mud calabash on the fire and it roasted. He found that the calabash made of mud became strong and was not destroyed by milk. Women also imitated the boy's calabash of mud and roasted their mud calabash and used them in the same way as the boy. Later women made lids and have since used pottery calabashes as containers.

In summary:

1) Pottery is now done by women. It is no longer done by boys as years ago.
2) It is mostly successful only during the rainy season because it cracks rapidly during the dry season.
3) It has become a traditional vessel for cooking purposes, for drinking water and for brewing beer with "holy food".
4) It is used in funeral ceremonies for brewing holy beer and cooking "holy food".
5) In some areas, people leave a pot with a dead woman who was a maker of pots.
6) It is not traditional to colour all pots, but its some women own wish to colour pots.
7) The colour is not painted, but they collect some special stones known to them and roasted them and grind them till soft. With this colour they decorate the

pot before it is roasted. Later, when roasted, the colours appear especially when they put the strings round the pot.

8) It is up to the woman concerned to make any shape she likes either cylindrical, round or returning to the very old, boy's calabash shape.
9) There is nothing holy about the pot itself, only when a holy beer or holy cow oil is contained in it.
10) It is useful for holding water, beer making and brewing, milking cows, keeping holy oil, cooling water and cooking...

PHOTOS

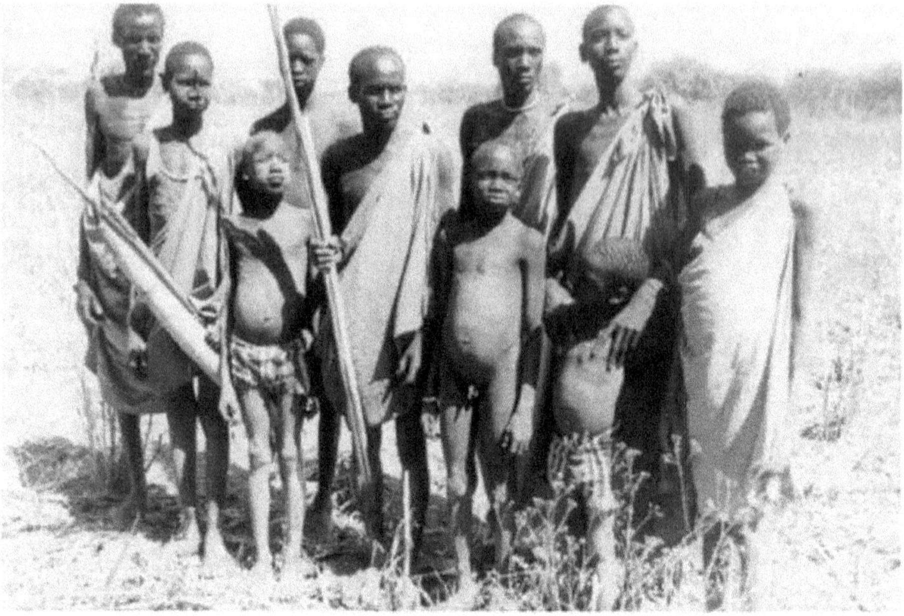

Photo 1. Children

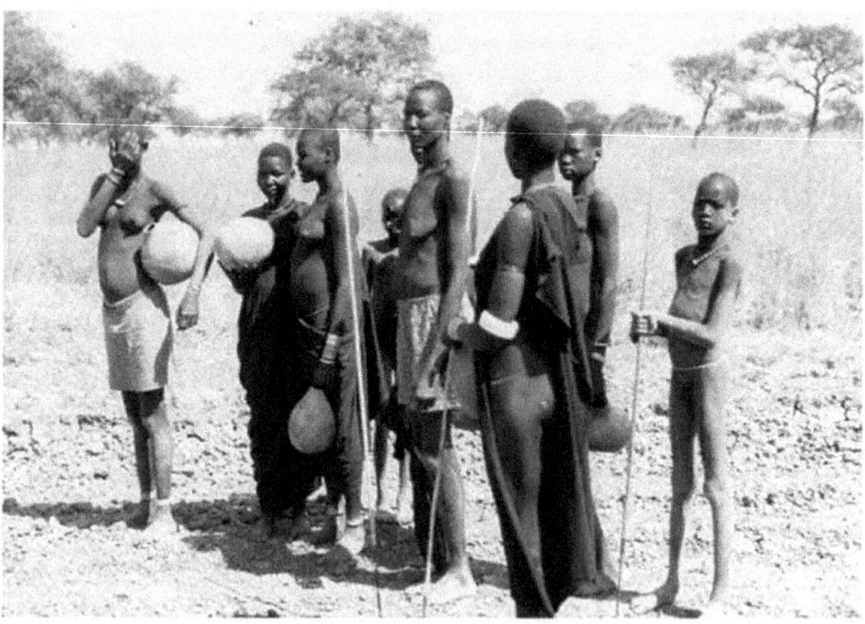

Photo 2. Women

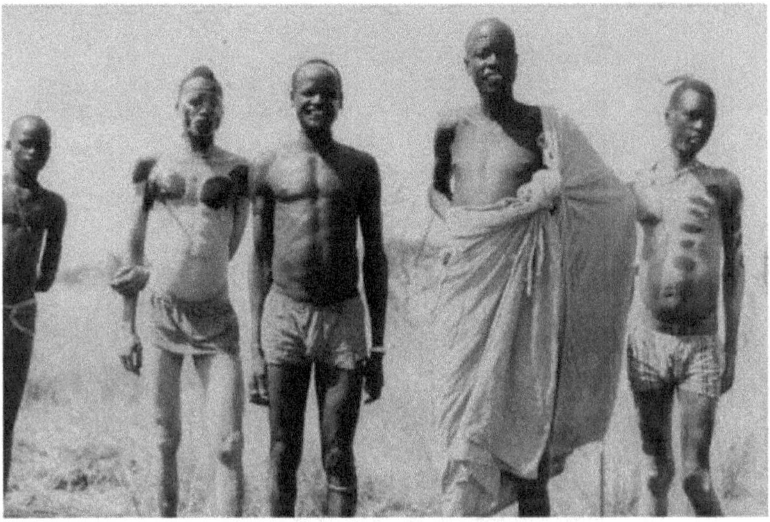

Photo 3. Men

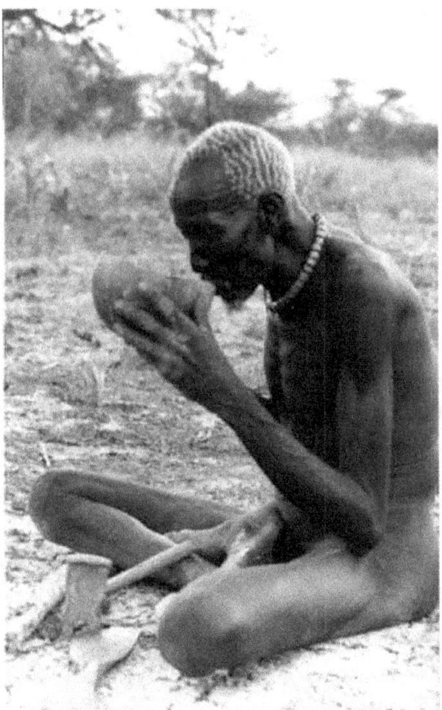

Photo 4. Traditional way of life

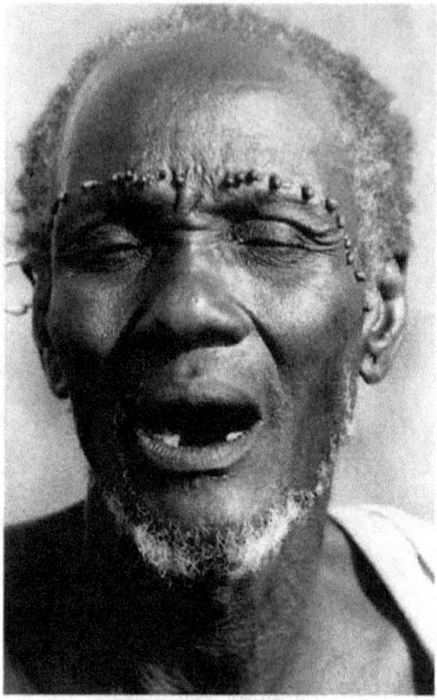
Photo 5. Shilluk

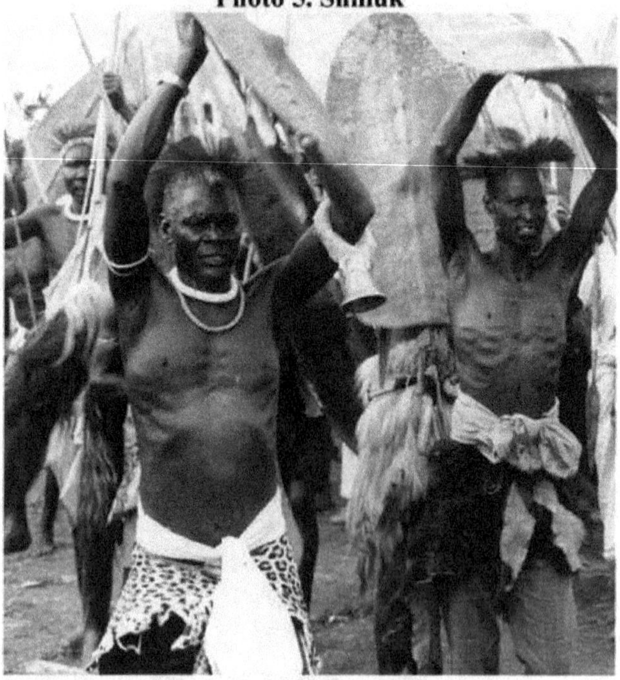
Photo 6. Shilluk worriors

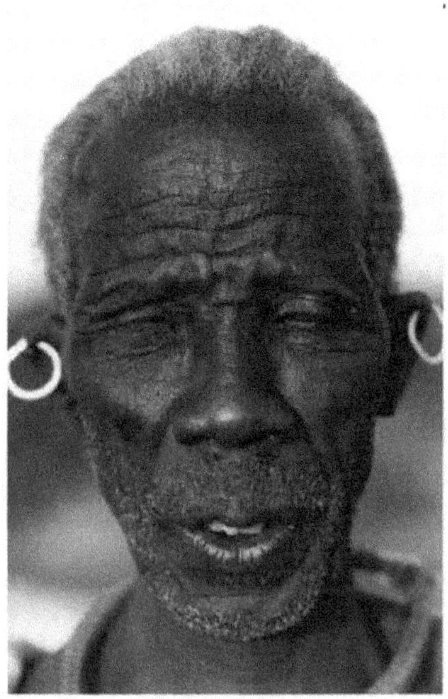

Photo 7. Dinka

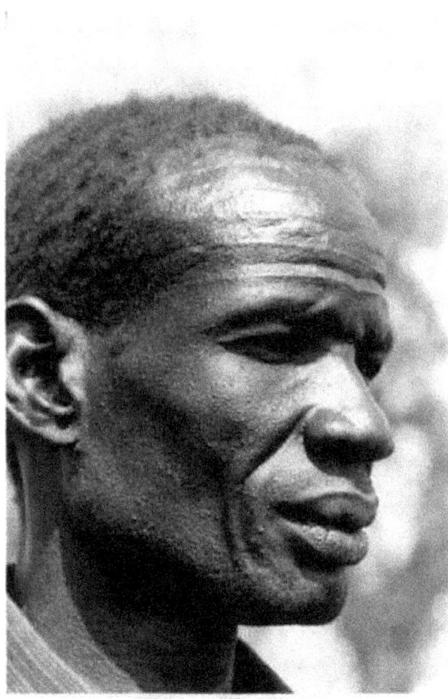

Photo 8. Nuer

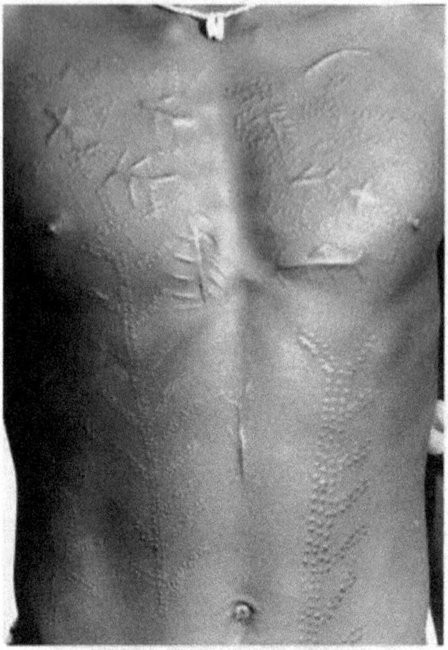

Photo 9. Scarifications

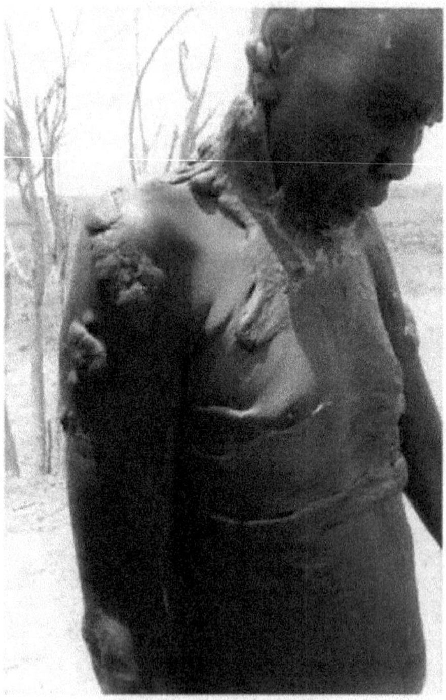

Photo 10. Kyloides

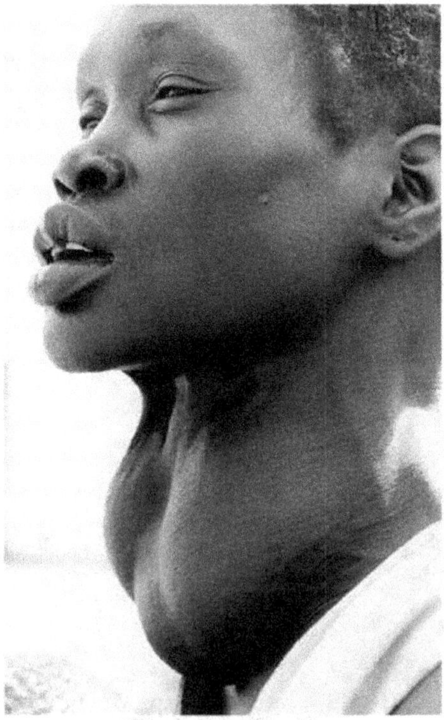

Photo 11. Ggoiter

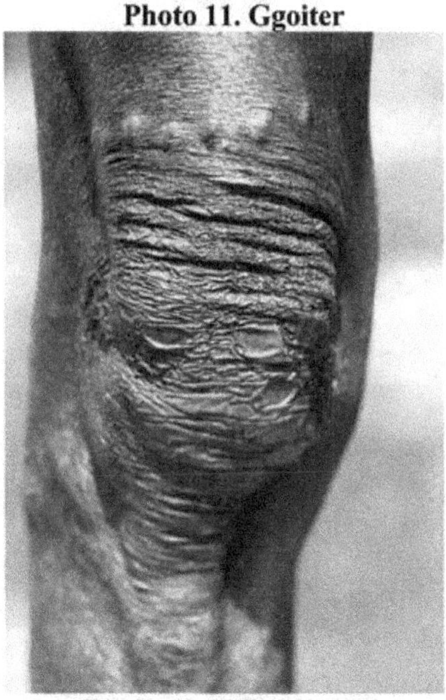

Photo 12. Hperkeratose

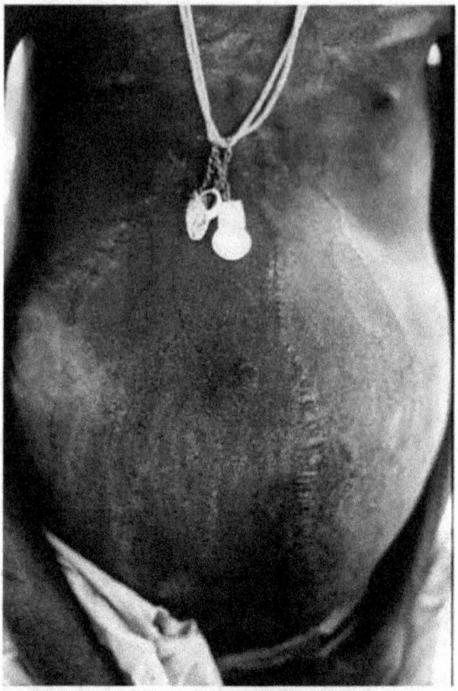

Photo 13. Spleno - hepatomegaly

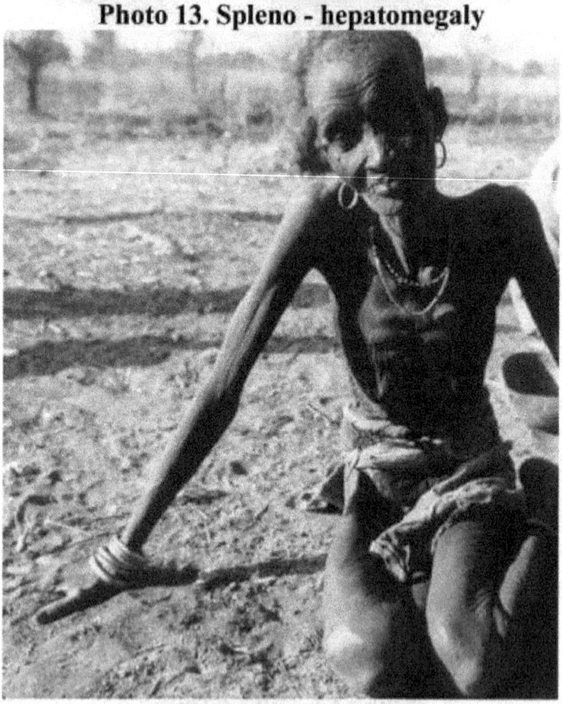

Photo 14. Cachexia

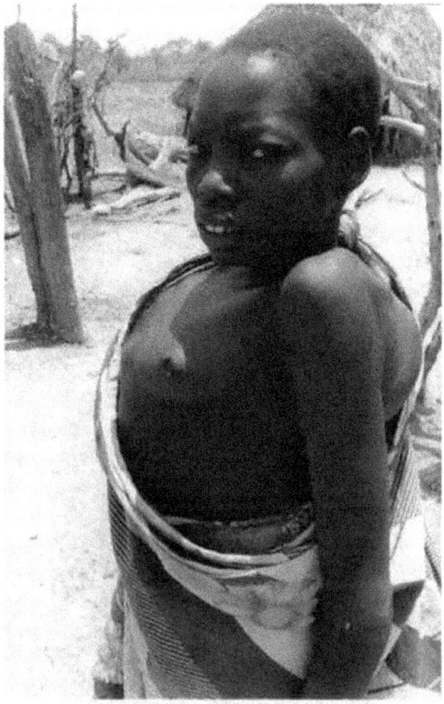

Photo 15. Hunchbacked

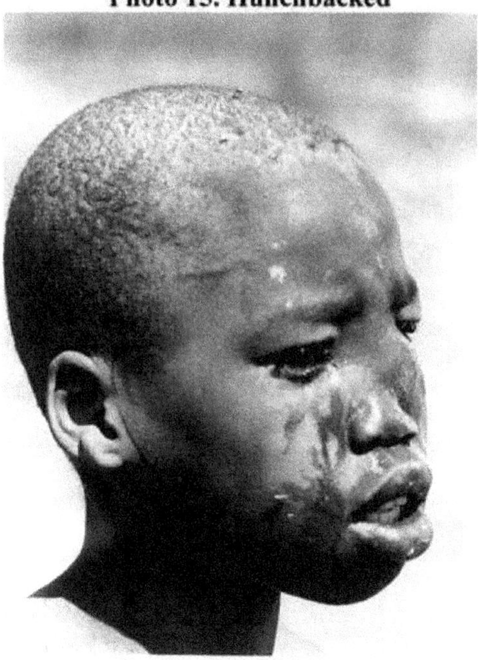

Photo 16. Fractures

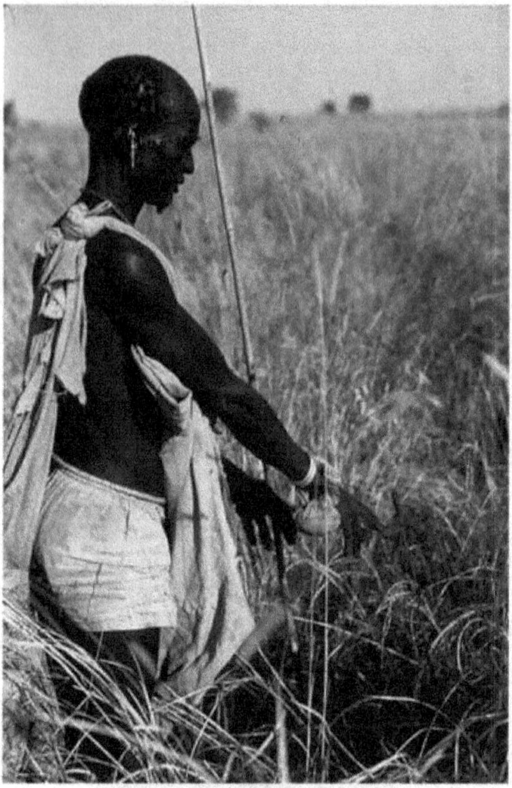

Photo 17. Witch doctor

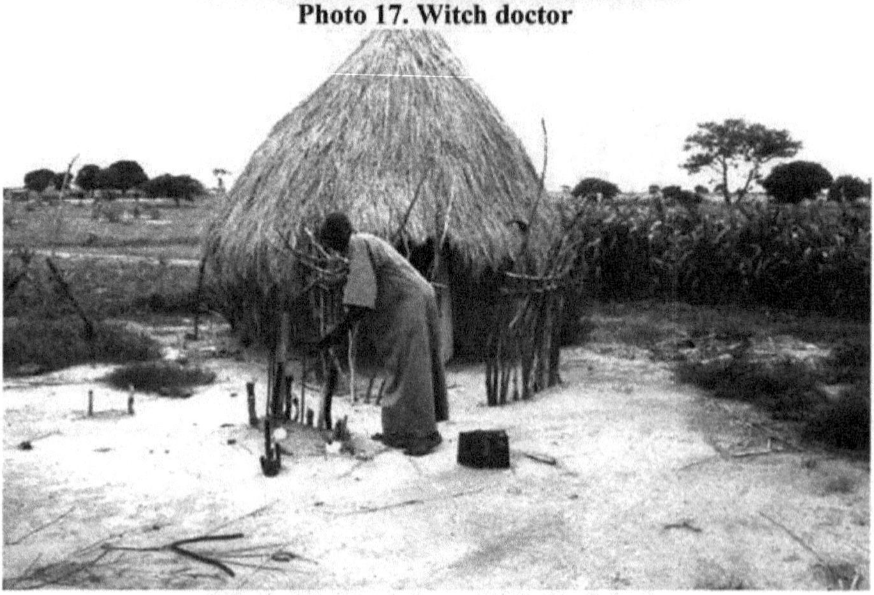

Photo 18. Magician outside the tukul

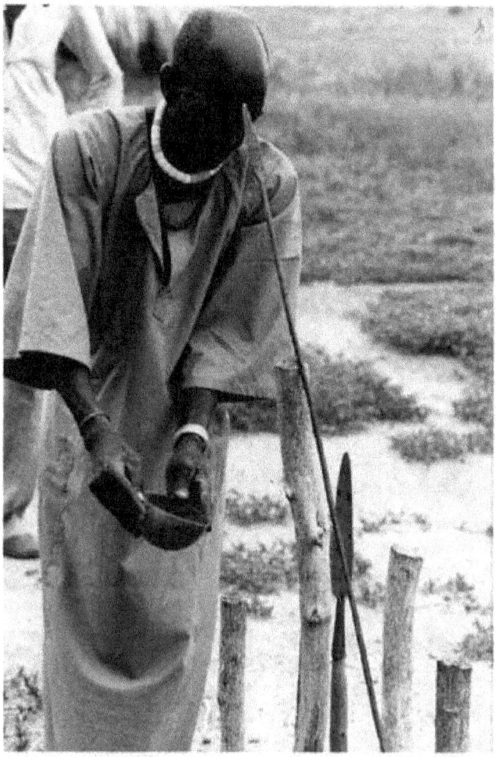

Photo 19. Magic ceremony – preparation

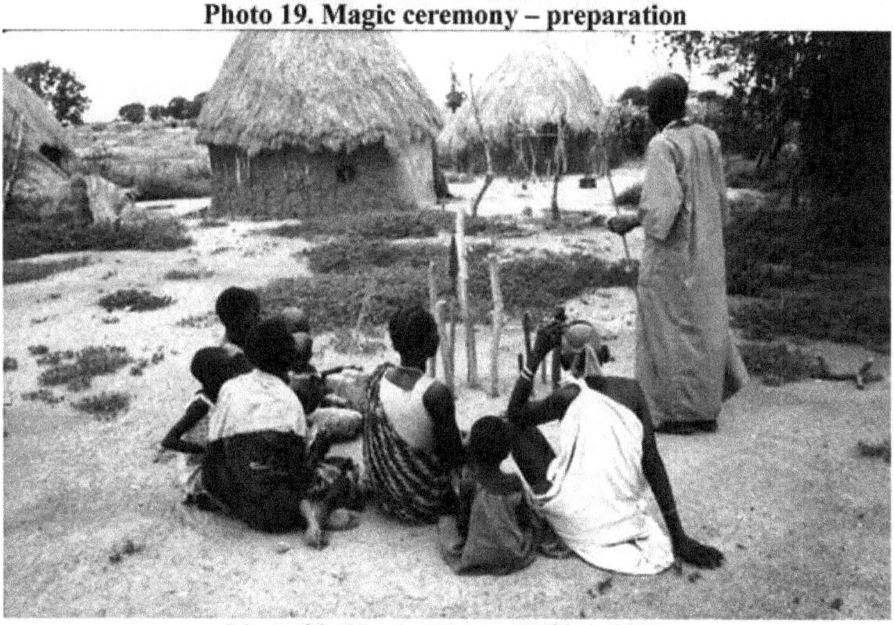

Photo 20. Magic ceremony for people

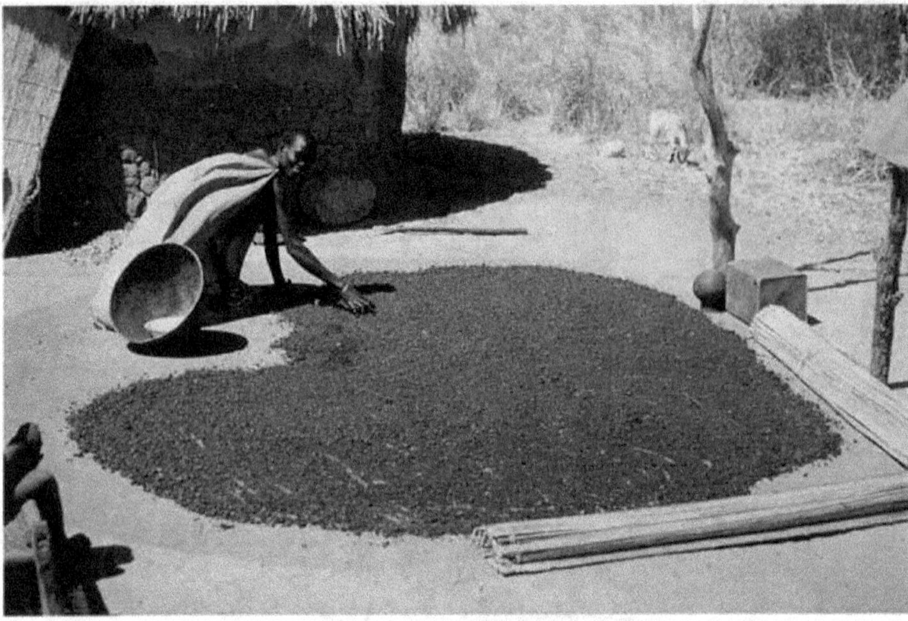

Photo 21. Sieving

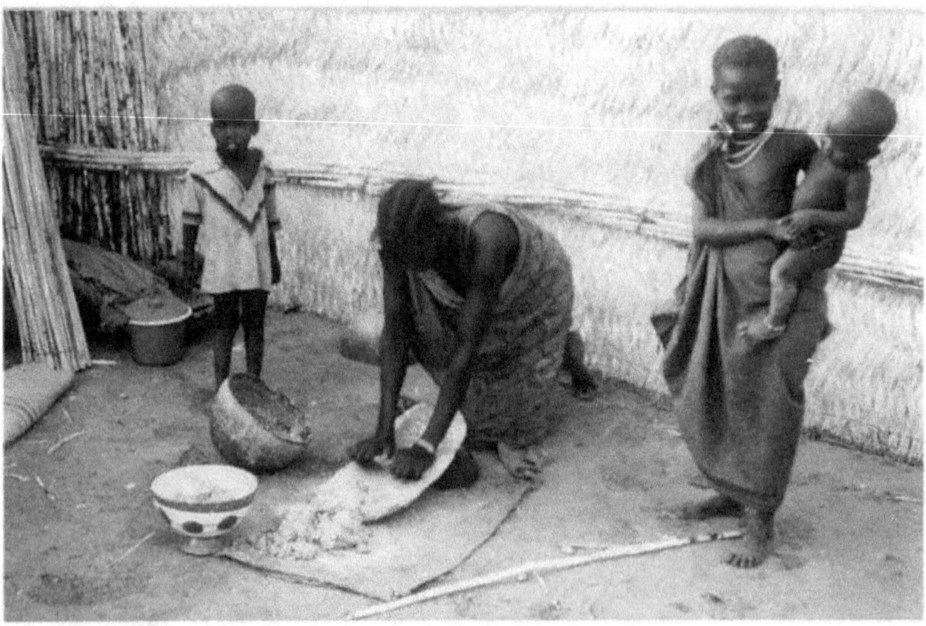

Photo 22. Grinding

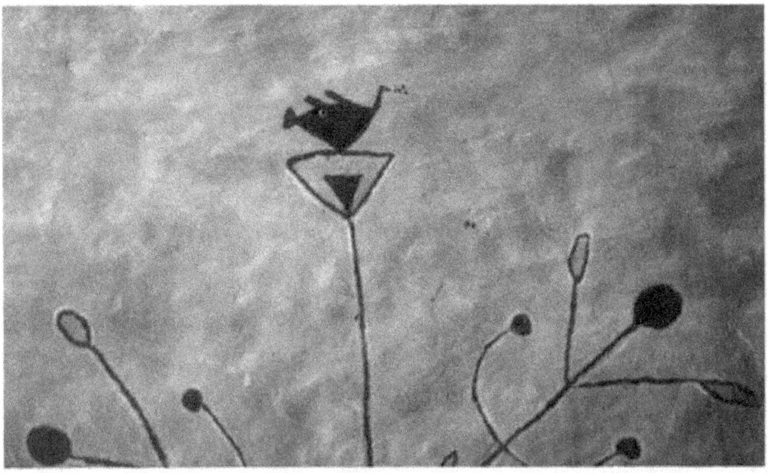

Photo 23. Wall drawings : flowers

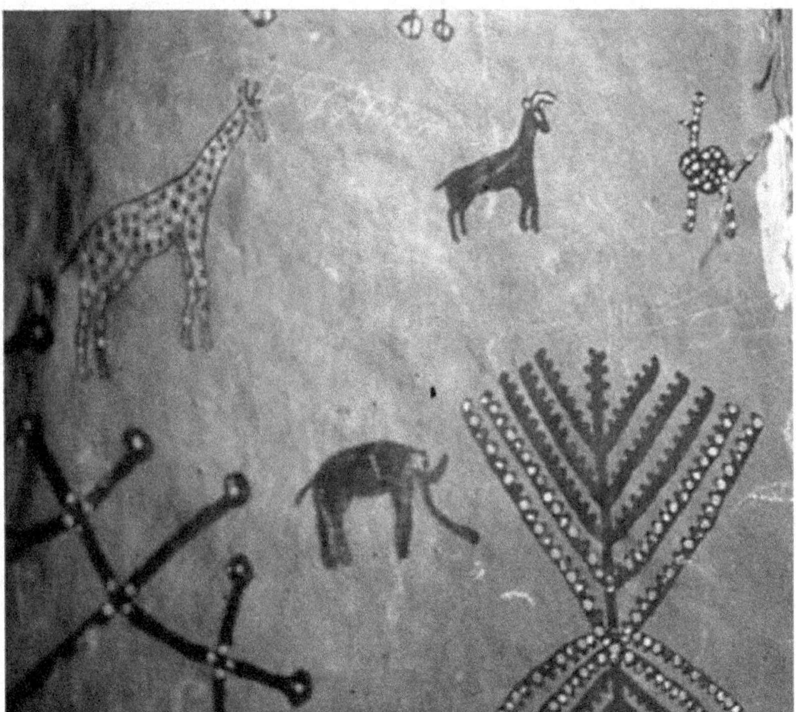

Photo 24. Wall drawings :animals

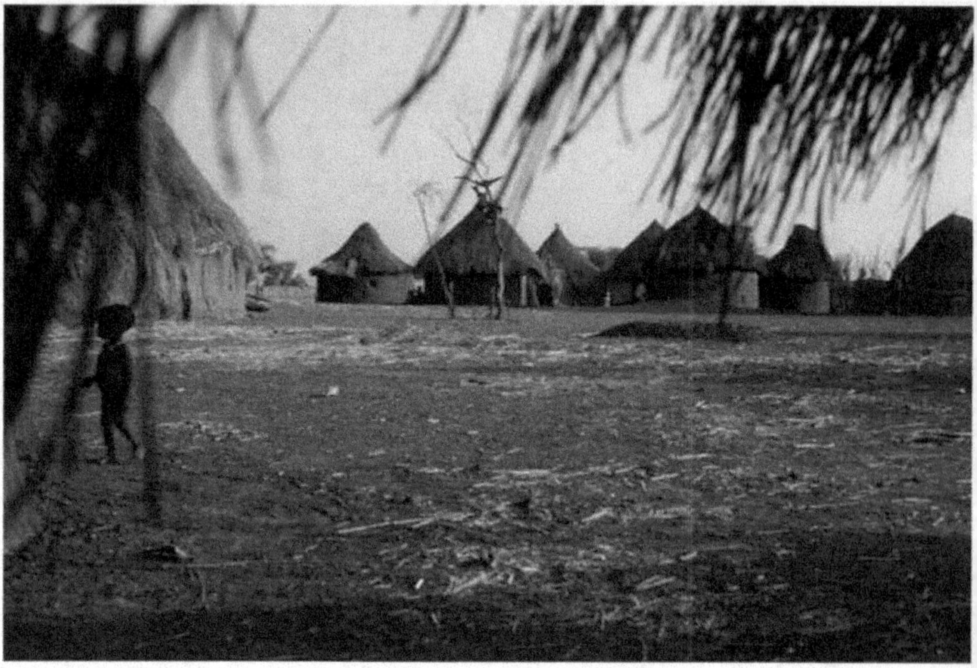

Photo 25. Village

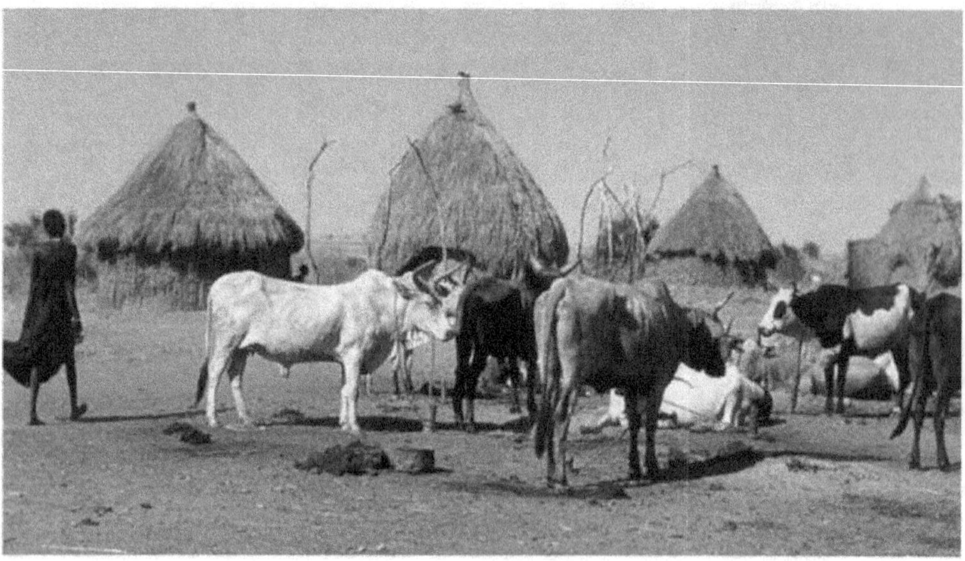

Photo 26. Cattle camp

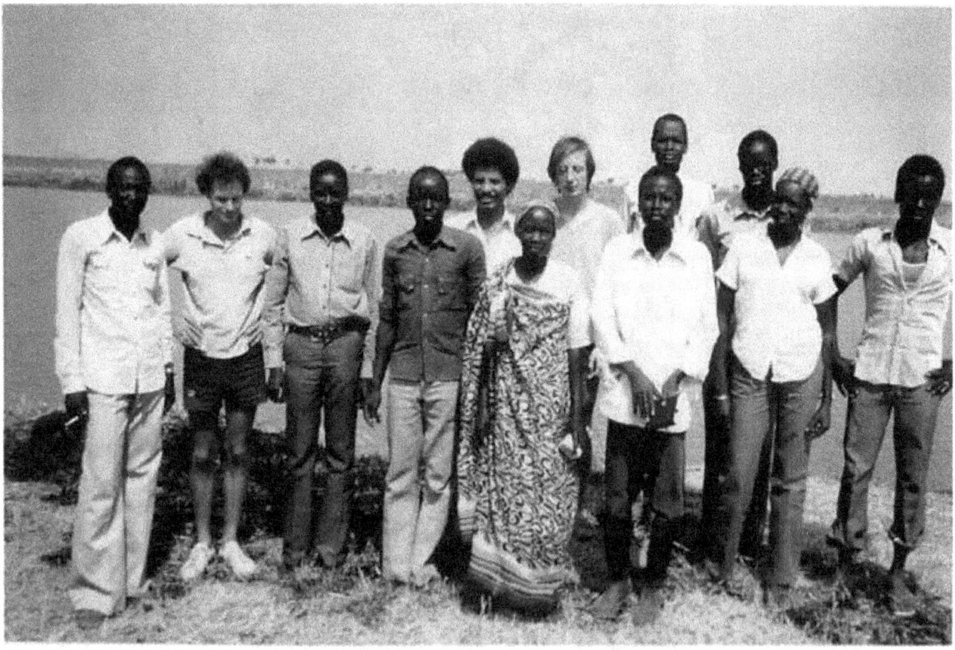

Photo 27. A.D.E. research team in Sobat

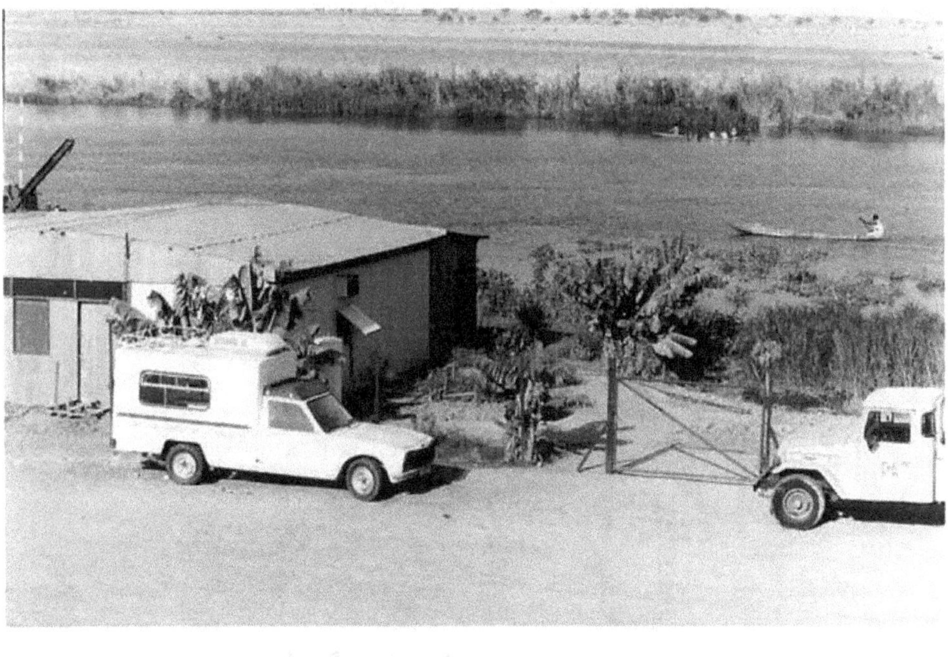

Photo 28. A.D.E. Research Center in Sobat

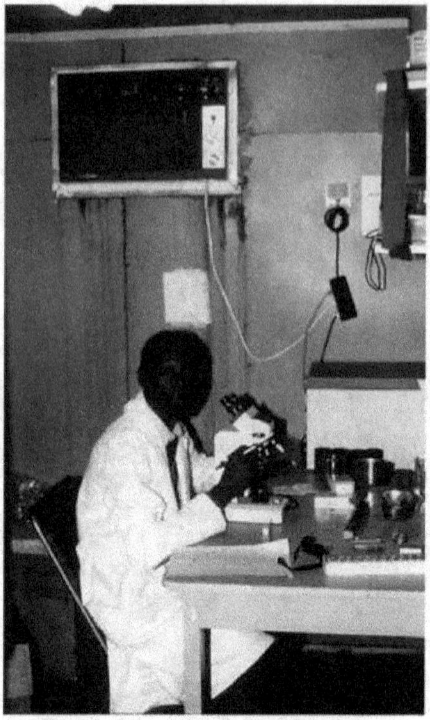

Photo 29. A.D.E. Laboratory

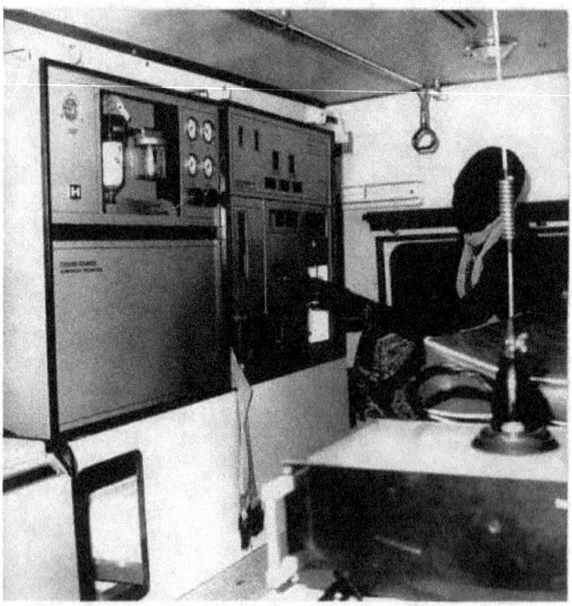

Photo 30. A.D.E. Laboratory – Kemo Mat

INDEX

L'HARMATTAN ITALIA
Via Degli Artisti 15; 10124 Torino
harmattan.italia@gmail.com

L'HARMATTAN HONGRIE
Könyvesbolt ; Kossuth L. u. 14-16
1053 Budapest

L'HARMATTAN KINSHASA
185, avenue Nyangwe
Commune de Lingwala
Kinshasa, R.D. Congo
(00243) 998697603 ou (00243) 999229662

L'HARMATTAN CONGO
67, av. E. P. Lumumba
Bât. – Congo Pharmacie (Bib. Nat.)
BP2874 Brazzaville
harmattan.congo@yahoo.fr

L'HARMATTAN GUINÉE
Almamya Rue KA 028, en face
du restaurant Le Cèdre
OKB agency BP 3470 Conakry
(00224) 657 20 85 08 / 664 28 91 96
harmattanguinee@yahoo.fr

L'HARMATTAN MALI
Rue 73, Porte 536, Niamakoro,
Cité Unicef, Bamako
Tél. 00 (223) 20205724 / +(223) 76378082
poudiougopaul@yahoo.fr
pp.harmattan@gmail.com

L'HARMATTAN CAMEROUN
TSINGA/FECAFOOT
BP 11486 Yaoundé
699198028/675441949
harmattancam@yahoo.com

L'HARMATTAN CÔTE D'IVOIRE
Résidence Karl / cité des arts
Abidjan-Cocody 03 BP 1588 Abidjan 03
(00225) 05 77 87 31
etien_nda@yahoo.fr

L'HARMATTAN BURKINA
Penou Achille Some
Ouagadougou
(+226) 70 26 88 27

L'HARMATTAN SÉNÉGAL
10 VDN en face Mermoz, après le pont de Fann
BP 45034 Dakar Fann
33 825 98 58 / 33 860 9858
senharmattan@gmail.com / senlibraire@gmail.com
www.harmattansenegal.com

www.ingramcontent.com/pod-product-compliance
Lightning Source LLC
LaVergne TN
LVHW080929071026
849535LV00013B/4147